Professional Practice in Engineering and Computing

Preparing for Future Careers

Professional Practice
in Engineering
and Computing
Preparing for Future Careers

Riadh Habash

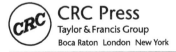

CRC Press
Taylor & Francis Group
Boca Raton London New York

CRC Press is an imprint of the
Taylor & Francis Group, an **informa** business

CRC Press
Taylor & Francis Group
6000 Broken Sound Parkway NW, Suite 300
Boca Raton, FL 33487-2742

First issued in paperback 2023

International Standard Book Number-13: 978-1-03-265390-7 (Paperback)
International Standard Book Number-13: 978-0-367-18036-2 (Hardback)
International Standard Book Number-13: 978-0-429-20273-5 (eBook)

DOI: 10.1201/9780429202735

Library of Congress Cataloging-in-Publication Data

Names: Habash, Riadh W. Y., author.
Title: Professional practice in engineering and computing : preparing for future careers / authored by Riadh Habash.
Description: Boca Raton : Taylor & Francis, 2019. | Includes bibliographical references.
Identifiers: LCCN 2018054588| ISBN 9780367180362 (hardback : alk. paper) | ISBN 9780429202735 (e-book)
Subjects: LCSH: Engineering--Vocational guidance. | Computer science--Vocational guidance.
Classification: LCC TA157 .H23 2019 | DDC 620.0023--dc23
LC record available at https://lccn.loc.gov/2018054588

Visit the Taylor & Francis Web site at
http://www.taylorandfrancis.com

and the CRC Press Web site at
http://www.crcpress.com

To my parents and family

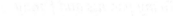

Perplexity is the beginning of knowledge.

Gibran Khalil Gibran

Contents

Part II   Communication skills and reflective practice

Part III   Practices of innovation, entrepreneurship, safety and sustainability in design

**Part IV   Contemporary issues in management, AI, and
career development**

Preface

The transition from the university learning context into the professional workplace environment and the integration of theoretical knowledge to real-world skills and experiences is an important component to begin students' professional careers. We are currently witnessing a fundamental shift in understanding the neuroscience of learning and key structural changes in the nature of society into which students will enter. This requires a need to support educators in enhancing their teaching practice and in the development of their own creative practices and entrepreneurial mindsets, so that they are best positioned to develop such mindsets in their students for the advancement of society.

The purpose of this book is to bring into focus some of the challenges and very specific qualities of graduates at the threshold of a professional career. Therefore, the engineering and computing professions expect the inclusion of professional-practice and engineering-management skills within a professional degree. Traditional topics like professionalism and ethics, law and property rights, risk and design safety, and leadership and communication skills are very well blended with contemporary topics such as innovation and entrepreneurship, design for sustainability, practice and project management, reflective practice, digital transformation and artificial intelligence (AI), and future career development to produce a highly correlated platform that meets the futuristic practice-driven engineering and computing professional goals. The benefit of the above combination is unique; readers will be cross-trained by drawing upon resources from a wide spectrum of traditional and contemporary world-class education.

The content of this book has been developed with an emphasis on clarity, with stress on the basic concepts as well as emerging ideas. To enhance the presentation of the material, every module of the book includes knowledge acquisition questions as well as sets of knowledge creation activities.

This educational textbook is suited for a professional practice course with an emphasis on engineering and computing technology. The development of the content revolves around the "futuristic knowledge platforms" of engineering, information and communication technology (ICT), and practice and project management. On the other hand, the book suits other courses, including sustainable design, innovation, and entrepreneurship, where professional thinking is now evident and in which there is increasingly visible activity worldwide.

Organization

This book is presented in four parts and twelve modules. Module 1 establishes the notion of "composite professional" that integrates technical expertise, business know-how, effective communication skills, and other talents to develop innovative and sustainable solutions to future society's challenges. Key topics that describe the evolvement of the broad fields of engineering and computing, practice management and project management overlaps, and students' preparation for professional practice have been extensively discussed.

Part I (Modules 2–4) deals with professionalism and ethics, the legal system, and leadership. Module 2 traces the roots of professionalism and the attributes of professional practice, including accreditation and licensing. The module discusses the historical perspectives of morals and ethics and their association with professional practice. It discusses the evolution of professional codes of ethics and organizations, with several corresponding examples. The module also provides knowledge about ethics, ethical theories, codes of ethics, and various categories of ethics including micro-, macro-, preventive, aspirational, technical, social, professional, and entrepreneurial ethics.

Module 3 introduces legal systems relevant to engineering and computing practice, including employment law; contract law; law of tort, including negligence, duty of care, and product liability; and intellectual property. A special emphasis is placed on intellectual property law, its building blocks including patent, copyright, trade secret, and trademark; and technology transfer including policy and process in the context of progress from initiation to commercialization.

An aptitude for leadership is significant to the individual professional development in this modern civilization. Module 4 deals with leadership practice, provides a historical perspective, and discusses several theories and qualities of leadership, including theories of management and motivation. It discusses the role of emotional intelligence, positive psychology, and systems thinking on leadership. It also presents authentic and innovative leadership practices, design thinking, and Lean leadership, and their impact on professional practice.

Part II (Modules 5 and 6) deals with communication skills and reflective practice. Module 5 provides the reader with a guide to communication skills in practice. Various arenas for professionally communicating, including speaking, listening, writing, presenting, and meeting, are extensively discussed. The focus is on the central concept of communicating ethically, actively, and reflectively. Achieving high levels of communication skills involves deep understanding of the notions of audience, range of audience, professionalism, teamwork, facial expression, body movements and posture, gestures, eye contact, personal space, and sensitivity.

Module 6 blends professional practice in reflection as a pedagogically and theoretically contentious concept that improves understanding of professional practice and action taken as a result of the reflective thinking. The three major reflection processes: reflection "in", "on", and "for" action and models of reflective practice, including common sense, the what, experiential learning, and iterative models, are initially discussed. In addition, conditions and situations that prompt engagement in the reflective process are examined. This module also presents the process of reflective listening, reading and writing, reflection on design, and tools of reflection on learning, including processes such as journaling, portfolios, and studios.

Part III (Modules 7–9) presents the practices of innovation, entrepreneurship, safety, and sustainability in design. Module 7 provides an extensive perspective of creativity and innovation and summarizes innovation milestones throughout history. This module also distinguishes invention from innovation, incremental from radical innovations, disruptive from sustaining innovation, and open from closed innovation. It presents the 16 habits of mind and six engineering habits of mind that aid in stimulating creativity and innovation in individuals. The module also introduces the practices of entrepreneurship and intrapreneurship. The emphasis is on how people think entrepreneurially and the role of entrepreneurship mindset. A great deal has been emphasized on the entrepreneurial process, including innovation, triggering, implementation, and growth. Importantly, the role of ethics in entrepreneurship practice has been discussed extensively.

Module 8 investigates the practice of safety in design. It discusses design methodology and process. The module explores the concepts of hazard, risk, risk assessment, risk management, and risk communication. It discusses also the approaches of system safety; functional safety; safety integrity; safety instrumented system; system safety analysis techniques, including failure modes and fault tree analysis; safety factor; and design margin. Presented also are ergonomics principles and types of standards and codes in engineering design.

Sustainability is a factor vital to successful and effective engineering. Module 9 introduces the concept of sustainable design and explains the application of sustainable methods to the engineering design process. It also covers important design tools, including triple bottom line, cradle-to-cradle approaches, and life cycle sustainability in product remanufacturing process

Part IV (Modules 10–12) presents the contemporary practices in management, AI, and career development. Module 10 presents the notion of project and practice management, including their scope and constraints. This instinct for management of people and organizations is a requisite for future successful professions. Extensively discussed are topics related to project risk management, project quality management, change management, management models including waterfall model, concurrent engineering, V-cycle development model, Lean and green project management, and Agile project management.

Module 11 discusses the substantial increase in the future applications of AI, historical evolution of AI, current enablers of AI, various focus technologies that enable AI, and industrial applications of AI. Also presented are the three pillars of AI, namely accountability, responsibility, transparency, safety, and privacy; moral, ethical, and philosophical impacts that AI will have on society; international ethical initiatives; legal implications of AI; intellectual property; and AI technologies.

Module 12 introduces professional and career development as activities that develop an individual's skills, knowledge, and expertise. It presents the future of work, workforce, and workplace that is influenced by the continuing march of technology, digital workplace paradigm, automation and AI, and the corresponding social, ethical, and legal impacts. The module also highlights types and categories of work and key skills and approaches for work readiness, basic attributes required by graduates before they join the workforce, and key elements of professionalism in the workplace.

Objectives and learning outcomes

The engineering and computing profession requires better kinds of learning by students. Accomplishing this requires new and better kinds of teaching and curricula, which in turn requires engineering faculty to think about teaching and learning in more scholarly ways. Professional practice is a broader topic for inclusion in engineering and computing curricula than is usually associated with engineering design. Practicing professionals require a working knowledge of numerous non-engineering disciplines and should interact with people of various backgrounds within a diversity of working contexts.

Both engineering and computing are not only applying scientific laws and solving technical problems. They are focused on caring about society, and as such, they bring workers into industry and business during these times of digital transformation and AI. Accordingly, all entry-level workers should become involved, at least laterally, with circumstances that call for some understanding of professional practice and project management, law and situations that call for ethical judgments, safe design and sustainability, entrepreneurial mindset, and career planning. This book will develop the following learning outcomes:

- Examine and reflect on topics related to the ethical and social impact of engineering and computing and the responsibilities that engineers and computing professionals have in shaping corresponding technologies and their applications
- Identify the values that are unique to the engineering and computing profession and promote a general compassion of what it means to be a member of the profession
- Explain how ethical considerations may play a role in the completion of engineering practice
- Enhance personal and professional communications skills and reflective practice
- Describe the important components, functions, and benefits of teamwork, partnering, client service, negotiation, and effective decision-making in professional practice
- Utilize appropriate methods and techniques to design and/or execute work-based or professionally focused project management projects, demonstrating capacity for independent and collaborative learning, addressing real-world industry issues
- Collaborate and work effectively in teams to demonstrate intellectual independence and autonomy and to solve problems that address industry issues and imperatives
- Critically analyze and apply predicted trends in project management, risk management, and decision-making techniques to engineering design tasks
- Examine and reflect on the profession, in local and/or global contexts, and question accepted interpretations and decision-making
- Explore contemporary issues in management, AI, and career development

Key pedagogical features

To help readers develop their understanding, several features have been built into this textbook, including:

- Each module opens with module objectives to inform the reader of the subject and scope of the topics to be covered.
- Each section begins with an opening quotation to stimulate interest in the content.
- The book in general introduces future professional practice concepts and ethical principles in the context of every subject under consideration.

- Many modules open with historical perspective that allows readers to think historically.
- All modules incorporate aspects of moral, ethics, and law, including the appropriate approaches and pedagogies.
- The book provides open-ended tasks for students and instructors at the end of each module. These tasks rely on two main approaches of pedagogical skill development, namely knowledge acquisition and knowledge creation. In general, the given tasks have no unique answers or solutions and can be adapted to every discipline easily.

Audience

This textbook is designed as a main resource for a two-semester undergraduate course in professional practice and professional career development in universities and colleges. Because of its comprehensive coverage and large number of topics, each part of the book can be used as a reference for a number of undergraduate courses.

How to teach the unteachable?

There is widespread acknowledgment among educators of a professional practice course. "Can the unteachable be taught?" is how the problem of teaching professional and managerial skills to engineering and computing students has sometimes been framed, thereby conveying the desperation that may exist. To effectively teach such diverse subjects under the platform of professional practice, a learner-centered environment pedagogy is needed, from among several other pedagogies, which calls for engaging students in the process of learning and knowledge creation. To accomplish this goal, all questions and tasks provided at the end of each module are transdisciplinary, open to debate, and mostly open-ended. Accordingly, the adopted pedagogy in this book calls instructors to develop course online libraries that may be shared with others and with the public. Such an approach gives the instructor the opportunity to treat the process of teaching as a design task and makes students more innovative in investigating problems, developing solutions, and creating new knowledge by using digital media. Instructors may benefit from the following technologies, among many more, in developing their classroom online libraries or blogs for multimedia presentations:

YouTube	Teachers can create YouTube channels to help students leverage videos they create to educate, engage, and inspire other students.
SlideShare	A web-based slide-hosting service. Users can upload files privately or publicly in various formats such as documents, PDF, slides, videos, and webinars.
VoiceThread	A free cloud application that allows professors to upload lessons and documents to discuss with students via microphone, webcam, text, phone, or audio.
Vidyo	A software-based video conferencing tool that can run on existing hardware.
Skype	An often free way to chat with students via phone or video call.
Blackboard	A web-based tool used by many instructors for online and hybrid courses. It provides discussion boards, calendars, and quizzes and tracks student progress.
Web	Instructors can develop their own online learning resources. You may see two such examples developed by the author: www.g9toengineering.com and www.greenengineers.ca.

Acknowledgments

I would like to thank my students and colleagues at the University of Ottawa, who have provided the reason and environment for writing this book. I am particularly grateful for the assistance given by Marina Habash, who largely contributed to the writing of Part IV of this book.

Author

Riadh Habash, PhD, is a continuing special appointment professor and professional engineer at the School of Electrical Engineering and Computer Science, University of Ottawa, Canada. He has been the recipient of many awards, including the National Wighton Fellowship Award, and has authored or co-authored over 80 professional articles, 5 books, and 5 book chapters. His most recent book is *Green Engineering: Innovation, Entrepreneurship, and Design* in 2017 (CRC Press), with the remaining previous books targeting specialty areas. Additional recent work includes several open educational resources that provide learning for inquiring minds by developing professionalism, entrepreneuria,l and employability attributes.

List of abbreviations

Module 1

AI	Artificial intelligence
AoA	Activity-on-Arrow
CPM	Critical path method
DSS	Decision support system
ENIAC	Electronic numerical integrator and computer
HR	Human resources
ICT	Information and communications technology
IT	Information technology
ITAA	Information Technology Association of America
LAN	Local area network
MIS	Management information systems
PC	Personal computer
PEP	Program evaluation procedure
PERT	Program evaluation and review technique
PM	Project Management
PMI	Project Management Institute
ST	Systems thinking
STEAM	Science, technology, engineering, arts, and math
UNESCO	United Nations Educational, Scientific and Cultural Organization

Module 2

ABET	Accreditation Board for Engineering and Technology
ACM	Association for Computing Machinery
ACS	Australian Computer Society
AICE	American Institute of Consulting Engineering
AIChE	American Institute of Chemical Engineers
AITP	Association of IT Professionals
ASAC	Applied Science Accreditation Commission

ASCE	American Society of Civil Engineers
ASME	American Society of Mechanical Engineers
CAC	Computing Accreditation Commission
CAP	Certified automation professional
CEAB	Canadian Engineering Accreditation Board
CEES	Center for Engineering Ethics and Society
CEQB	Canadian Engineering Qualifications Board
CET	Certified engineering technician
CSAB	Computing Sciences Accreditation Board
CSDP	Certified software development professional
EAC	Engineering Accreditation Commission
ETAC	Engineering Technology Accredited Commission
GDTP	Geometric dimensioning and tolerancing professional
IEA	International Engineering Alliance
IEEE	Institute of Electrical and Electronics Engineers
ISA	International Society of Automation
ISP	Information systems professionals
ITCP	Information technology certified professionals
NAE	National Academy of Engineering
NICET	National Institute for Certification in Engineering Technologies
NSPE	National Society of Professional Engineers
SANS	SysAdmin, Audit, Network, Security
WPI	Worcester Polytechnic Institute

Module 3

IP	Intellectual property
IPM	IP management
R&D	Research and development
TT	Technology transfer
WIPO	World Intellectual Property Organization

Module 4

APA	American Psychological Association
CoP	Community of practice
EQ	Emotional intelligence
IQ	Intelligence quotient
MIT	Massachusetts Institute of Technology
TMS	Toyota Management System
TPS	Toyota Production System

Module 5

IMRaD	Introduction, methods, results, and discussion
ISTE	International Society for Technology in Education
NvC	Non-verbal communication

Module 6

CR	Critical reflection
ERA	Experience, reflection, action
RP	Reflective practice

Module 7

EHoM	Engineering HoM
HoM	Habits of mind

Module 8

5M	Man, Machine, Medium, Mission, and Management
AFNOR	Association Française de Normalisation
AIDMO	Arabic Industrial Development and Mining Organization
ANSI	American National Standards Institute
ARSO	African Organization for Standardization
ASTM	American Society for Testing and Materials
BSI	British Standards Institute
CAE	Canadian Academy of Engineering
CCBFC	Canadian Commission on Building and Fire Codes
CENELEC	European Committee for Electrotechnical Standardization
CSA	Canadian Standards Association
DIN	Deutsches Institut für Normung
ETSI	European Telecommunications Standards Institute
FMEA	Failure mode and effects analysis
FS	Functional safety
FTA	Fault tree analysis
IEC	International Electrotechnical Commission
INCOSE	International Council on Systems Engineering
ISO	International Organization for Standardization
***it*SMF**	IT Service Management Forum
ITU	International Telecommunication Union
NSB	National Standards Bodies
OASIS	Organization for the Advancement of Structured Information Standards

PASC	Pacific Area Standards Congress
RA	Risk assessment
RC	Risk communication
RM	Risk management
SAE	Society of Automotive Engineers
SCC	Standards Council of Canada
SHEL	Software, Hardware, Environment, and Liveware
SI	Safety integrity
SIL	SI level
SIS	Safety instrumented system
SRS	Safety requirement specification
SrS	Safety-related system

Module 9

3Es	Economy, ecology, and equity
3Ps	People, planet, profit
3Rs	Reuse, remanufacturing, recycling
C2C	Cradle-to-cradle
CF	Carbon footprint
DfE	Design for environment
DfR	Design for recycling
DfS	Design for sustainability
GE	Green engineering
GHG	Greenhouse gas
ICE	Institution of Civil Engineers
LCA	Life cycle assessment
LCC	Life cycle costing
LCE	Life cycle engineering
LCIA	Life cycle impact assessment
LCSA	Life cycle sustainability assessment
LCT	Life cycle thinking
LEED	Leadership in Energy and Environmental Design
PLC	Product life cycle
SD	Sustainable development
SLCA	Social LCA
TBL	Triple bottom line
USGBC	U.S. Green Building Council
WF	Water footprint
WFEO	World Federation of Engineering Organizations

Module 10

ADKAR	Awareness– Desire–Knowledge Ability Reinforcement
APM	Agile project management
ASD	Adaptive software development
CE	Concurrent engineering
CM	Change management
DSDM	Dynamic systems development methodology
FDD	Feature driven development
JIT	Just-in-time
LPD	Lean product development
LSS	Lean six sigma
σ	Sigma
6σ	Six Sigma
DMAIC	Define, Measure, Analyze, Improve, Control
PDCA	Plan-Do-Check-Act
PPM	Project portfolio management
PQM	Project quality management
PRM	Project risk management
XP	Extreme programming

Module 11

AAAI	Association for the Advancement of AI
ASI	Artificial superintelligence
ASIC	Application-specific integrated circuit
EGE	European Group on Ethics
FPGA	Field-programmable gate array
GPU	Graphics processing unit
NLP	Natural language processing
SNARC	Stochastic neural analog reinforcement calculator

Module 12

IoT	Internet-of-Things
M2M	Machine-to-machine

module one

The composite professional

1.1   Knowledge and understanding

Having successfully completed this module, you should be able to demonstrate knowledge and understanding of:

- The impact of engineering, computing, and project management in developing the futuristic knowledge practice to facilitate innovative and sustainable solutions to society's greatest challenges
- Historical evolvement and development of engineering practice as one of the oldest professions which led to the rise of the Industrial Revolution
- Advances in computing technologies that generated a web of dynamic virtual networks that allow people worldwide to communicate and share information
- Management evolvement through the nineteenth and twentieth centuries in response to waves of innovation in business and society and its overall role on harmonizing planning, organizing, implementing, and controlling future work, workforce, and the workplace
- The notion of a "composite professional" who can integrate knowledge, competence, expertise, business know-how, communication skills, leadership, and entrepreneurial talents
- Instruction that prepares students for the route of professional and career development with emphasis on lateral thinking as well as on real-world problem-solving methodologies

1.2   Professional identity and practice

> *From Wi-Fi to space travel, engineers, project managers, and information technology professionals develop innovative and sustainable solutions to society's greatest problems.*

> **Futurist Michio Kaku**

Future development as perceived in the quotation above is not just about technology but is a synergy of broad knowledge platforms of engineering ingenuity, information technology (IT), and management (Figure 1.1). Ingenuity means the process of applying ideas to solve real-life problems

1

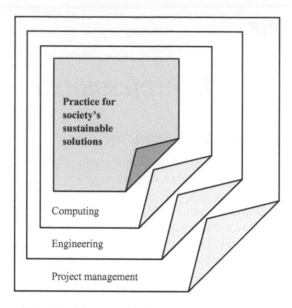

Figure 1.1 Futuristic knowledge platforms.

to meet new generational challenges. To increase synergy, there is a need to define and establish different educational and training platforms to help realization of the knowledge practice platforms.

The terms "professional", "professional identity", and "professionalism" are cited interchangeably in education. The American philosopher Mortimer J. Adler defined a professional as "a man or woman who does skilled work to achieve a useful social goal. In other words, the essential characteristic of a profession is the dedication of its members to the service they perform" (Manning and DeBakey 2003). Professional identity is part of a complex, multifaceted, continuous process of personal identity development. As part of this process, students simultaneously develop several identities, such as religious believer, partner, citizen, engineer, and others (Beam et al. 2009). Identities are the meaning that individuals hold for themselves, what it means to be who they are. These identities have bases in being members of groups (social identity), having certain roles (role identities), or being the unique biological entities that they are (personal identities) (Burke 2004). Professionalism will be discussed in detail in Module 2.

In the context of practice, knowledge represents a broad sense of theoretical and practical "knowledge" and "skills". Professional knowledge that accumulates through practice is organized and codified to facilitate importing concepts and ideas from other disciplines in the expansion of the knowledge base (Nilsson 2007).

Professionals learn and grow in various ways, and only part of their professional growth is intentionally enhanced by professional development interventions, programs, and activities. According to Cochran-Smith and Lytle (2001), knowledge in the process of practice development is classified into three types as shown in Figure 1.2. First, knowledge-for-practice, which represents formal knowledge for professionals to improve practice through education and lifelong training and learning. Second, knowledge-in-practice, which means knowledge embedded in the practice process. Third, knowledge-of-practice, which grows through reflection on the practice by using the process of inquiry.

Instead, competence is understood as a broader concept than knowledge but also an affective component, including attitudes, values, behaviors, and motives, as well as personal traits, such as self-efficacy and self-confidence, and socio-communicative skills (Nilsson 2007). Competence or "know-how" is the ability, not yet put into practice, to do something as a result of knowledge in the presence of experience and judgment. It is the strategy an individual would apply in practice if an opportunity exists. It is divided into a formal aspect (formal merits and credentials) and an actual aspect (an individual's capacity to appropriately manage a situation or complete a task).

$$Competence = knowledge + skills + ability + attitude$$

On the other hand, performance is based on competence but is adapted by system factors and other circumstances. It is the implementation of learned strategies. Professional performance may be influenced by knowledge, competence, or by other factors external to the individual, including the system within which one practices (for example, incentives, resources, expectations, or demands). In brief, performance is competence implemented, or applied in actual practice: "show-how".

The last leg of the journey is placing competence and performance into practice. This represents what professionals actually "do" during day-to-day practice. Having an impact on clients or society is often the result of more than just a single practitioner's performance. Figure 1.3 shows a modified version of George E. Miller's (1990) model. The different layers in Miller's model represent a developmental sequence of stages. All levels are needed and have their own important impact on professional practice.

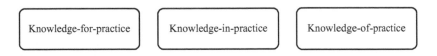

Figure 1.2 Knowledge in the process of practice development.

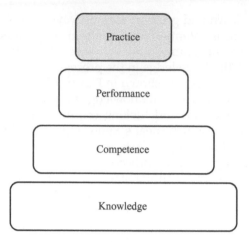

Figure 1.3 Developmental stages toward professional practice.

1.3   Engineering practice

> *Engineering is not only the study of 45 subjects but it is moral studies of intellectual life.*

> **Prakhar Srivastav**

Engineering is one of the oldest professions, along with medicine and law. However, it differs from the other professions in that doctors and lawyers generally provide their services to specific individuals or corporations. Engineering is a profoundly creative, social activity; it tends to design and build things under constraint, as well as providing services. An engineer's responsibility is more often to society than to specific people (Habash 2017).

1.3.1   Engineering defined

The word "engineer" has its root in the Latin word "ingeniator", which means ingenious, to devise, in the sense of construct, or craftsmanship. Several other words are related to ingeniator, including ingenuity (Johnston et al. 2000). The term "engineer" was used in the 1300s for a person who operated a military engine or machine such as a catapult or, later, cannon. The word "engine", in turn, is derived from the Latin "ingenium" for ingenuity or cleverness and invention. The terms "art" and "technical" are important because engineering arranges elements in a way that may or may not appeal to human senses and emotions, and relates also to the Greek "technikos", which involves art, craft, skill, and practical knowledge and language (UNESCO 2010).

While the objective of science is to understand nature, engineering's objective is to build useful things using science. Engineers must not only build things, they must also do so within budgetary, schedule, resource, regulatory, and operational constraints (Coallier 2007). Practically, engineering is problem identification, formulation, and solving. It is concerned with the transformation of knowledge to value, by establishing the knowledge in some physical and functional form. At its domain, engineering engages principles of science, mathematics, design, art, and business to practical ends. Engineering as a broad discipline, practice, and profession has a major role in the creation and implementation of materials, components, machines, structures, systems and processes, and organizations for well-defined purposes. It encompasses a range of specialized sub-disciplines that focus on developing a specific kind of product, service, or use a certain type of technology.

Engineering as a profession is an occupation based upon specialized education and training, as providers of professional advice, skills, and services (Habash 2017). It develops itself through the interaction of various professionals, engaged in a social context. It is, above all, an opinion leadership to build ideas from a benchmark set by the professional community (Ciampi 2010). Engineering yesterday, today, and tomorrow exhibit practical ingenuity (Johnston et al. 2000). It will remain identical with creativity: skill in planning, designing, building, and adapting.

1.3.2   History of engineering

> *If you only look to the past, you are blind in one eye. If you only look to the future, you are blind in both eyes.*

> **Russian saying**

History, like most subjects, represents a systematic way of thinking. A key insight necessary for deep learning of history is that history should be understood as an organized, integrated way of thinking (Elder et al. 2011). History lets people see how decisions made in the past affected societies and civilizations. A professional engineer must look in all directions, to the past to obtain the information from experienced engineers and to the future to use that information to improve performance and safety in the engineering process (Bond 2004).

Thinking historically introduces students and engineers to the wonders of the past and fosters the ability to make judgments about the present. To think historically is not straightforward but needs to be able to establish a sum of concepts, according to "Historical Thinking: www. historicalthinking.ca". This includes historical significance (events that resulted in great change over long periods of time for large numbers of people), use of primary source evidence (not source of information only);

continuity and change (history is not a list of events but is a complex mix of continuity and change); cause and consequence (how and why); historical perspectives (understanding the social, cultural, intellectual, and emotional settings that shaped people's lives and actions in the past); and the ethical dimension of historical interpretations (learn something from the past that helps to face the ethical issues of today) (Habash 2017).

Engineering has been around as a concept for a long time, because the history of human advancement has been one of technological development. In ancient times, many of the wonders of the world could be attributed to the skill and inventiveness of what were, essentially, civil engineers. After the rise of agriculture, powerful civilizations such as the Persians, Romans, and Mongols exploited and developed long-distance trade routes to expand their regional influence. The Roman aqueducts, Greek temples, the Great Wall of China, the Egyptian pyramids in the Nile Valley, and Sumer's wheels and carts present civilization with enduring models of the elegant art and science of problem-solving; that is, the power of engineering.

The history of engineering as a profession, where payment is made in cash or kind for services, began with tool and weapon making, indicating that engineering is one of the oldest professions. The professionalization of engineering is illustrated by Imhotep, who built the Step Pyramid at Saqqara in 3000 BC and was one of the few commoner mortals to be accorded divine status after his death. That continued with the development of craft and guild knowledge and the formalization of associated knowledge and education. Leonardo da Vinci, for example, had the official title of Ingegnere Generale, and his notebooks reveal an increasing engineering interest in how things worked (UNESCO 2010).

The modern professional identity of engineers began with the establishment of the École Polytechnique in France and the foundation of professional engineering societies in England. Engineers from the Victorian era in Britain, such as Isambard Kingdom Brunel and George Stephenson, enjoyed celebrity status. Brunel was responsible for bridges and dockyards, including the construction of the first major British railway, the Great Western Railway; a series of steamships, including the first propeller-driven transatlantic steamship; and important bridges and tunnels. Brunel's designs revolutionized public transport and modern engineering. George Stephenson was an English civil and mechanical engineer who built the first public railway line in the world to use steam locomotives. Electrical engineering can trace its origins to the experiments of Alessandro Volta in the 1800s, the experiments of Michael Faraday, Georg Ohm, and others, and the invention of the electric motor in 1872. Chemical engineering, as with mechanical, developed in the nineteenth century. Large-scale production of chemicals was needed, along with the demand for new materials and new industrial processes (EO 2016). Aeronautic engineering turned the ancient dream of flight into a travel convenience for people. Control engineering accelerated the pace of automation, while industrial engineering designed and managed mass production and distribution systems.

Germans in the sixteenth century, Dutch in the seventeenth century, and French in the eighteenth century have perhaps the best claims to be regarded as being at the forefront of engineering expertise, each with impressive achievements (Armytage 1976). However, engineering powered the Industrial Revolution that really took off in the UK in the eighteenth century, subsequently spreading to Europe, North America, and the world, replacing muscle by machine in a synergistic combination of knowledge, skills, and money.

1.3.3 Engineering and the Industrial Revolution

The Industrial Revolution and engineering are actually supporting each other. First due to engineering machines that came into the world and then industries. Regular advancement in engineering and technology actually boosted the growth of industries (Singh 2018).

The first Industrial Revolution took place from 1750 to 1850 in Western Europe. It was crucial for the inventions of spinning and weaving machines operated by water power. The second phase of the first Industrial Revolution, symbolized by the advent of electricity and mass production, was driven by many disciplines of engineering. The first phase of the second Industrial Revolution was based on steel, electricity, and heavy engineering from 1875. The second phase of the second Industrial Revolution was based on oil, automobile, and mass production, taking place between 1900 and 1950 and onward. The third Industrial Revolution started with the invention of the transistor, which largely accelerated the development of electronics. Electronics was and still is so significant to modern industry that electrical and electronics engineers today outnumber colleagues in any other engineering discipline. Since the early 1970s, the dominant business has been the age of information and communications technology (ICT), the second phase of the third Industrial Revolution.

The likely first phase of the fourth Industrial Revolution, based on sustainable "green" engineering and technology, is seen to have begun around 2000. Today, artificial intelligence (AI), if cared for, can level-up society into the fourth Industrial Revolution. With extensive automation and computational capability, this disruptive technology is blurring the lines between the digital, physical, and biological divides. Figure 1.4 outlines the predicted timelines of the Industrial Revolution.

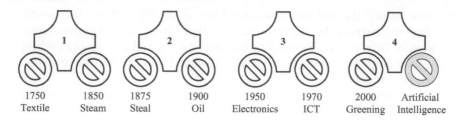

| 1750 | 1850 | 1875 | 1900 | 1950 | 1970 | 2000 | Artificial |
| Textile | Steam | Steal | Oil | Electronics | ICT | Greening | Intelligence |

Figure 1.4 Timeline of Industrial Revolution.

1.4   Computing practice

Today, computers are almost second nature to most of us.

James Dyson

Computing technology is ever-changing and ever-evolving in all aspects of calculation and the physical devices used to aid people in their attempts at automating the arithmetic process. Today, the world is witnessing major advances in arithmetic, from the beginning of counting through the most important developments in logarithms and the electronic computer.

1.4.1   IT and ICT defined

Computing technologies including IT and ICT are generating robust computing devices to make dynamic virtual networks that allow people worldwide to communicate and share information. IT is a general term that comprises the acquisition, processing, storage, and dissemination of information. It involves the use of computers, storage, networking, physical devices, infrastructure, and processes. The diversified and encouraging possibilities of IT have reduced distances between people, countries, and continents, and eventually have led to the emerging concepts "global society" and "global village".

The broadest definition of IT embraces not only the development of the technology employed in the manipulation of information but also human activities which employ that technology, such as knowledge management (Stoodley 2009). According to the Information Technology Association of America (ITAA), IT is "the study, design, development, implementation, support or management of computer-based information systems, particularly software applications and computer hardware". The United Nations Educational, Scientific and Cultural Organization (UNESCO) defines IT as "scientific technology and engineering disciplines and the management techniques used in information handling and processing their application, computers and their interaction with human and machines and associated social, economic and cultural matters".

ICT is broader than IT. It refers to all computer-based advanced technologies for contributing to innovative changes in business and daily life. The use of ICT is currently an integral part of modern society. Today, ICT is widely used by people within the workplace in exchanging information and data, as well as for a social interpersonal tool, particularly amongst younger generations. It has been evolving so rapidly and has developed into an expanded and massive knowledge area. Figure 1.5 shows the components of ICT and a typical flow of information through a medium of communication.

As the applications of ICTs continue to grow, it is significant to realize the importance of convergence and how convergence shapes the transmission of information and service delivery. This concept refers to "the coming together of IT (computer, consumer electronics, telecommunications) and gadgets (personal computer [PC], television, telephone), leading to a culmination of the digital revolution in which all types of information (voice, video, data) travel on the same network" (Coyle 2009).

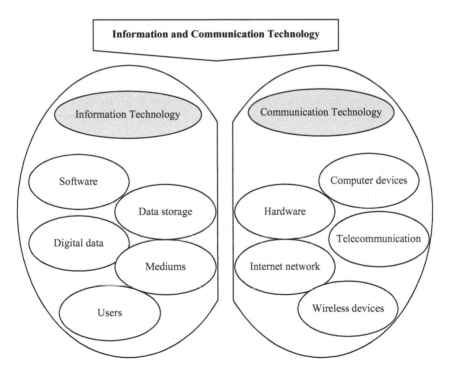

Figure 1.5 Components of ICT and flow of information through the medium of communication.

1.4.2 Evolution of computers

The origin of computers and IT goes back many centuries. The development of arithmetic led to the development of tools to establish the field of computing. Blaise Pascal (1623–1662), in France, was credited with building the first calculating machine. Pascal invented the Pascaline in 1642, a very popular mechanical computer capable of adding, subtracting, multiplying, and dividing two numbers. Initially called the arithmetic machine, it was presented to the public after 50 prototypes in 1645. In 1649, King Louis XIV of France granted a royal privilege to Pascal, similar to a patent.

The electromechanical age signaled the beginnings of telecommunications. This age can be outlined around the time between 1840 and 1940. Charles Babbage (1791–1871) worked on his "difference engine", a mechanical computer which could perform mathematical calculations. The world's first computer algorithm was written by Ada Lovelace (1815–1852) in the UK. In 1890, Herman Hollerith used punch cards to help classify information for the US Census Bureau. John Von Neumann (1903–1957) developed many concepts, including the "Von Neumann architecture". In the US, Alonzo Church (1903–1995) developed the key concepts of computability and computing, such as lambda calculus. In the UK, Alan Turing (1912–1954) introduced many core concepts of computer science, including "Turing machine", and "Turing test". Grace Brewster Murray Hopper (1906–1992), an American computer scientist and US Navy rear admiral, was a pioneer of computer programming who invented one of the first compiler-related tools. The first, most famous computer, called Electronic Numerical Integrator and Computer (ENIAC), was built in the 1940s, and the first hard-disk drive, weighing a ton and storing five megabytes, was built in 1956.

At the same time, the invention of the telegraph and telephone laid the groundwork for telecommunications and the development of the vacuum tube. This electronic device could be used to store information represented as binary patterns, on or off, one or zero. ENIAC was developed at the University of Pennsylvania in Philadelphia in 1946.

Until the 1970s, ICTs were still regarded as quite distinct. However, powerful technology changes in microelectronics, software, optics, and increasing integration of technologies have made this evolution a reality. Over the past 50 years, the evolution of ICTs can be divided into three eras, as shown in Figure 1.6. These include mainframe; PC plus local area network (LAN); and Internet computing.

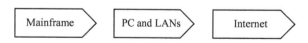

Figure 1.6 The three eras of ICT evolution.

The first large-scale automatic digital computer in the US was the Harvard Mark 1, created by IBM in 1944. In the 1960s, business computing revolved around the mainframe, which performed batch processing tasks. Users used to submit stacks of punched cards and wait for the printed results. Timeshared approaches gave more people access to mainframes in the 1970s, and minicomputers gave some people a less structured computer environment.

1.4.3   Data to information

The first microprocessor, which was invented by a young engineer, Marcian "Ted" Hoff, Jr. in 1971 at Intel, in California, changed the history of IT development. Hoff invented an integrated circuit with 2,300 transistors that was essentially equivalent to the central processing unit (CPU) of a computer, which paved the way for embedding intelligence in inanimate objects as well as the PC. The CPU on a chip became known as a microprocessor. Two memory chips were attached to the microprocessor: one to move data in and out of the CPU and another to provide the program to drive the CPU. This invention has proved to be one of the most significant technological innovations of the twentieth century.

The first PC, "Altair", was developed in 1975. Two years later, Radio Shack introduced the first PC with keyboard and display monitor. This was the first complete PC to be marketed to the general public.

The rapid advance of microcomputers and the demands for communications between microcomputers greatly stimulated the development of network computing and computer communication systems. LAN technology rapidly developed in the second half of the 1980s. Internetworking of LANs had been leading to the speedy development of wide area networks (WANs) technology during the 1980s and the early 1990s.

The project that initiated the groundwork of the Internet began in 1969. Known as the Advanced Research Projects Agency Network (ARPANET), it meant to build a computer network enabling researchers around various locations to exchange ideas. The initial plan of the ARPANET project was to connect four locations: the University of California, Los Angeles (UCLA), where the first "node" was located; the University of California, Santa Barbara; the Stanford Research Institute; and the University of Utah. There were nearly two dozen sites connected by 1971, including computers at the Massachusetts Institute of Technology (MIT) and Harvard University. Three years later, there were 62 and, by 1981, more than 200 sites.

The ARPANET itself was phased out in 1990 in favor of the more advanced National Science Foundation Network (NSFNET) backbone, a network established by the National Science Foundation of the US. As PCs became cheaper and easier to use in the late 1980s, anyone with a modem could get online. The NSFNET then served as the technical backbone of the Internet (a network of networks). It is a unique collection of networks throughout the world.

With the development of computer technologies, the focus of computer applications development was directed towards data and information management, which is used to support administration and management of an organization as well as its decision-making. During this period, numerous so-called management information systems (MIS) and Decision support systems (DSS) were developed worldwide. In this regard, the main content processed and managed by computers had shifted from data to information.

1.4.4　Information age to knowledge age

With the advent of computers, the Internet and computing explosion provided extraordinarily powerful tools. As such they have great potential both to benefit and to harm societies that embrace them. Today, the content processed and managed by computers has been shifted again, from information to knowledge.

The first decade of the twenty-first century started by the consolidation of the great achievements in computing technology: the appearance of the operating system Windows XP; the version from 2001 has brought important facilities regarding Internet, multimedia, and universal serial bus services (Vlada and Ţugui 2006).

Today, computing networks have terabytes of storage, and the world has more phones than people (Prentic 2012). Sustainability is converging with digitalized communication Internet and a digitalized automated transportation to create a super-Internet of Things (IoT). In the IoT era, sensors are embedded into every device and appliance, allowing them to communicate with each other and Internet users, providing up-to-the moment data on the managing, powering, and moving of economic activity in a smart digital world.

Technological advancement has transformed global society into a knowledge society. Today, more than ever, computing technologies are recognized as the means for sustainable human, social, and economic development. The IoT will fundamentally change how people go about their lives. It is anticipated that the number of objects connected to the Internet is set to exceed 20 billion by 2020. The scale of the IoT is set to have major economic, social, and environmental impacts; the intersection of which forms the future sustainable growth.

The digitization of information has had a profound impact on traditional media businesses, such as book publishing, the music industry, and television and cable networks. As information is increasingly described in digital form, businesses across many industries have refined their focus on how to exploit the Information Age.

The unprecedented availability of data and eventually of information is overwhelming, even for the smartest minds working in big data and cloud computing. That is why help is needed from machines, which have a much greater ability than humans to process large amounts of data points at the same time from multiple sources and multiple domains in real-time. Machine learning and more sophisticated deep learning or neural networks in general are living their most flourishing period in history (the renaissance of AI) and their application and use in a variety of industries is the proof that this is happening (Correani 2017).

Today, two central focus areas require work to do. One is about collecting data, and the second involves moving beyond the age of information into a space of knowledge. With the proper tools and guidance, society and industry may start turning the information into some sort of knowledge.

1.5   Two disciplines, one profession

> *My brother is an electrical engineer and went to computer science grad school at Stanford, and he'd tell me stories about the happy hours he'd organize.*
>
> **Alec Berg**

Two disciplines, engineering and computing, have paralleled and overlapped evolutions but followed a similar pattern. One of the most intriguing and influential developments in the history of engineering and computing has been the widespread adoption of the rhetoric and ideology of software engineering. When Presper Eckert first introduced the concept in 1965, it received little attention from industry pundits (Ensmenger 2001). Just several years later, however, the 1968 NATO Conference on Software Engineering firmly entrenched the language of software engineering in the vernacular of the computing community, thereby setting an agenda that influenced many of the technological, managerial, and professional developments in commercial computing for the next several decades.

Table 1.1 presents a review of the historical evolution of engineering, intertwining it with the history of computing. This retrospective represents a further step forward to understand the current state of both disciplines. It also defines a set of milestones that represent a convergence or divergence of engineering and computing development methodologies. These milestones do not appear at the same time, so lessons learned in one discipline can help in the development of the other.

Table 1.1 Historical milestones of engineering and computing

3500 BC	Sumer first used the wheel in making pottery.
3000 BC	Pyramids of Egypt.
1500 BC	Assyrian agricultural technology in the Empire capital Nineveh.
800 BC	The Romans built fortifications, sewers, roads, water distribution systems, and public buildings across the territories and cities they controlled.
600 BC	Walls of Babylon.
200 BC	Great Wall of China.
200 BC	A scientific approach to the physical sciences concerning civil engineering was implemented by Archimedes.
950 AD	Al-Biruni realized that measuring instruments were prone to error and bias, so proposed experiments needed replication many times before a commonsense average was possible.
1000 AD	Ibn Al-Haytham's work on optics revealed that controlled and systematic experimentation and measurement are essential to discovering new knowledge.
Mid-1600	Calculating machines.
Mid-1800s	Telephony.
Mid-1890s	Wireless telegraphy.
Beginning of the 1900s	Car industry; Building materials.
Beginning of the 1920s	Radio broadcast.
Beginning of 1930s	Telegraphy; Analog computers.
End of the 1930s	Airplane industry.
Beginning of the 1940s	Television broadcast; Electronic general computer; Atomic bomb.
End of the 1940s	Polaroid land camera; Gas turbine.
Beginning of the 1950s	Nuclear power plant.
Mid-1950s	Transistor; Color television.
End of the 1950s	Rockets, satellites, and space exploration; Microchip.
Beginning of the 1960s	Laser and satellite communications.
Mid-1960s	Computer operating system.
End of the 1960s	Beginning of Internet.

(Continued)

Table 1.1 (Continued) Historical milestones of engineering and computing

Beginning of the 1970s	Genetics and biotechnology.
Mid-1970s	Personal computer.
End of the 1970s	Apple II personal computer.
Beginning of the 1980s	Cellular communications.
Mid-1980s	Personal computers and Microsoft Windows.
End of the 1980s	Local and wide area networks.
Beginning of the 1990s	WWW and Netscape Web browser; 3D printing.
Mid-1990s	Evolution of Google.
End of the 1990s	Interactive television; Human genome.
Beginning of the 2000s	Wireless Internet; High-definition and 3D television; GPS; Hybrid car and renewable energy development; Text messaging; Wikipedia as user-generated content; Digital cameras; Nanotechnology.
Mid-2000s	iPhone; iPad; Digital music; Facebook; YouTube; LEED Green Building Rating System.
Beginning of the 2010s	Genetically engineered immune cells; Smart grid.
Mid-2010s	Cloud computing; Autonomous driving; Robotics; High-efficiency and less-expensive solar panels.
End of the 2010s	IoT; 5G technology; Humanized big data; Machine learning; 3D metal printing; Sensing city; Artificial intelligence for everybody; Seamless voice recognition; Dueling neural networks; Zero-carbon natural gas; Perfect online privacy; Genetic fortune-telling; Material's quantum leap; Augmented reality and virtual reality; Wearable technology; Physical-digital integration; Self-driving cars have attracted big corporations such as Google, Tesla, Mercedes, and more.

1.6   Project management (PM) and practice management overlaps

Management is, above all, a practice where art, science, and craft meet.

Henry Mintzberg
[from Simply Managing: What Managers Do and Can Do Better (2013)]

Management is important because it ensures that what is being delivered is right. It is important because it brings leadership, direction, and order to projects. With projects, the principal goal of professional practice is to acquire the right people and skills, measure progress, deliver results on time and to budget, to meet expectations, and importantly to adhere to standards, regulations, and codes of ethics.

1.6.1 PM and practice management defined

Practice management is all about how an engineer or computing professional should manage a firm. This requires an understanding of different types of business structures; laws, regulations, and ethics surrounding professional practice; financial issues and responsibilities; and other related aspects of a firm that must be in place before a client contract is signed. The main goal is to protect the public's health, safety, and welfare (Cohn 2016).

PM, on the other hand, is all about how to manage a project. A project is a planned temporary venture that consists of tasks to be executed over a fixed period and within a certain scope, budget, quality, timescale, deliverables, and limitations. The process focuses on establishing and delivering on contract requirements; project teams; client, fee, and schedule; risk management; effective communication skills; and quality control throughout the project. PM in this context have a complex set of components that have to be completed and assembled in a certain manner to create a functioning product or service.

The "divide line" between practice management and PM is the point at which a contract is signed and a project begins. PM covers the execution of all contracts, including owner-engineer agreements, engineer-consultant agreements, owner-consultant agreements, and others (Cohn 2016).

1.6.2 Evolution of PM

Historically, a vast number of projects of various magnitudes have been successfully undertaken across civilization. Starting with the Industrial Revolution, management science evolved through the nineteenth and twentieth centuries and various processes, tools, and techniques were developed to help identify and control business functions (Weaver 2007). WWII marked the beginning of the modern PM era; prior to then, projects were managed on an ad hoc basis using mostly informal techniques and tools.

The term PM was coined in the 1950s, where the basic principles of PM focus on the planning, scheduling, and execution of projects. This includes managing resources, maintaining schedules, and coordinating different activities and tasks. One key difference between the ancient marvels of PM and modern-day projects is the ancient marvels did not routinely involve schedule optimization.

In 1957, Kelley and Walker (1959) started developing the algorithms that became the "Activity-on-Arrow" (AoA) method of critical path scheduling after approval of funding for the project. The computer program they developed was trialed on plant shutdowns in 1957. Their 1959 paper discussed the critical path method (CPM) of scheduling. As computer-controlled options and complex algorithms were developed, project managers began to complete more work in less time with fewer errors than ever before (Collins 2015).

Dr. Martin Barnes (UK) first described the "iron triangle" of scope, time, and cost (the correct scope at the correct quality) in a course he developed in 1969 called "Time and Money in Contract Control". Whilst all three elements have always been important, the evolution of scope and cost control into relatively precise processes occurred with the Industrial Revolution in the eighteenth century. Whilst time control was important, and many projects were built in remarkably short times, scheduling lacked science and recognition until very much later.

In the early days, PM closely mirrored the classical school of management with a focus on scientific processes (scope, time, and cost). More recently, the emphasis has shifted towards the soft skills, more closely aligned with the human relations and human resources (HR) schools of management theory, including more focus on stakeholders, communications, and leadership.

These developments were closely followed by the development of the program evaluation and review technique (PERT) system. The US Air Force translated PERT into the program evaluation procedure (PEP), and a host of similar systems appeared over the next few years. Whilst CPM and PERT use the same basic approach, including the AoA network diagram, the PERT analyzed individual tasks by asserting a minimum amount of time for completion, while the CPM factored in a project's activities, how long the activities will take to complete, and the relationship between the activities and their end points.

1.6.3 Professional PM

Two major professional PM bodies, one from the US and the other European, were established in the 1960s. In the US, the first organization to propose the promotion and development of the PM, Project Management Institute (PMI), was founded in October 1969 at the Georgia Institute of Technology as a non-profit. PMI has grown into a multi-national, member-based organization in virtually every major country around the world, mainly thanks to PERT and CPM. According to the PMI, traditional PM is "the application of knowledge, skills, tools, and techniques to project activities to meet the requirements". This approach is widely regarded as stemming from the traditional waterfall model. This model is based on breaking down the work into stages that should be completed before moving to the next one. It will be discussed in Module 10.

The 1970s saw an unprecedented expansion in PM applications and in the development of PM as a distinctive discipline. The overall role of PM in this aspect is to harmonize the functions of planning, organizing, implementing, and controlling in order to meet the project objectives of cost, time, and quality in addition to scope as shown in Figure 1.7.

The addition of project scope management appears to be in recognition of the fact that a project's scope objectives need as precise a definition as time, cost, and quality (Stretton 2007). Thinking ahead of the project process reveals problems, which helps find proper solutions.

The advent of computing technology facilitated the "front-end" analysis. This increased focus on the front-end of projects helped redress the previous imbalance in effective PM of the project life cycle (Sievert 1991). As an extension of the above, there were increasing pressures to look at projects themselves in their broader contexts (Ireland 1991).

The growth of the Internet led to web-based PM applications being developed. The software used for PM began offering the option to connect and work jointly in an intranet or Internet network.

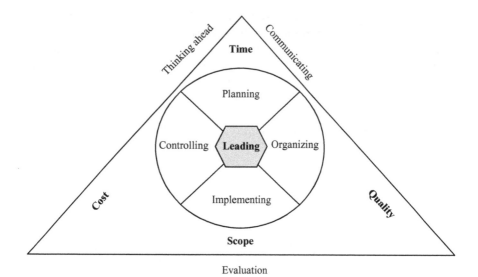

Figure 1.7 General functions of management.

1.7   The composite professional

> *The ideal engineer is a composite ... He is not a scientist, he is not a mathematician, he is not a sociologist or a writer; but he may use the knowledge and techniques of any or all of these disciplines in solving engineering problems.*

Nathan W. Dougherty

The future professional should be a composite of transdisciplinary competences. Such competences involve interacting dimensions of knowledge, skills, and attitudes. Knowledge primarily refers to the respective fields of knowledge that characterize each discipline. The specific knowledge that is gained through an educational program constitutes the foundation of the respective professional roles (Andersson and Andersson 2006). However, transdisciplinary competence requires an overall awareness of the knowledge fields represented by other closely related disciplines.

Nathan W. Dougherty, professor of civil engineering at the University of Tennessee, wrote these words in 1955: "Today's engineers require an interdisciplinary approach to solve current complex problems. The more they know about other fields, the more prepared they are to generate innovative ideas and solutions that are socially mindful and sustainable".

Currently, organizations are investing in hiring professionals who can integrate technical expertise, business know-how, and effective interpersonal communication skills. Those who can do this are prime candidates for positions in management. Successful engineering managers understand their role in taking an integrated view of management in order to rationalize operational activities, meet deliverables on time, and achieve goals.

Today, engineers are increasingly relying on computing technologies for the high-performance computers needed to run software programs and the networks that allow virtual operation and sharing data. There is a growing trend for ICTs to be used from conception to completion of any project process.

Professionals of the future, like professionals of yesterday, should maintain strong analytical skills. It is crucial to manage technological changes, be creative, take risks, manage stress, think conceptually, and recognize and respect people's diversity and individual differences. This leads to thinking of an engineer as a professional who combines in variable proportions the qualities of a scientist, a socialist, a designer, a manager and leader, and an entrepreneur. Figure 1.8 shows integrated traits of the future composite professional.

The composite professional will need not only awareness but an embedded ethical philosophy that stems from the foundation of their

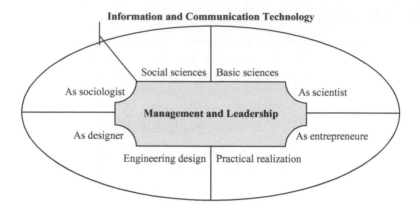

Figure 1.8 The composite professional.

engineering learning with understanding of and commitment to economy, society, and environment. This professional has a particular role to meet sustainability. The role should involve the enhancement of well-being, health, and safety, with the minimal use of natural resources and paying attention with regard to the environment and the sustainability of resources.

This new breed of engineers will be not only truly comprehensive problem solvers, but problem definers, leading transdisciplinary teams. This is an admirable aspiration, but significant reform of curricula will be required to prepare engineering graduates for their new responsibilities (Grasso and Martinelli 2007). Besides the above talents, one major quality is innovation and leadership, and one way to learn how to lead is to be creative. Professional engineers should also be inquisitive, analytical, and detail-oriented.

1.7.1   Professionalism in science

Professionalism is part of science. It encompasses knowledge ranging from basics to societal duties. Science provides objective information and raises moral issues. It offers valuable professional recognition among scientists across all disciplines and the wider community. Engineering principles means the professional application of the principles of mathematics, biology, chemistry, physics, or any related applied subject. When professionalism is integrated into basic science, engineers gain opportunities to develop competencies and understand interconnections between disciplines.

The dimension inspired by basic sciences views a professional as a scientist who applies the basics of natural and exact sciences, stresses the value of logic and rigor, and sees knowledge as produced through analysis and experimentation. The role of science in engineering education is not a static one. It must respond and evolve with the changes in both engineering and science, which are occurring continually.

Today, nearly every discipline has been converted into a science. The borderlines between the pure or epistemic sciences, on the one hand, and the action sciences or applied science, on the other hand, have become fuzzy. Thus, all disciplines have more or less theoretical, empirical, and practical issues as well. Any given science can act as an ancillary discipline to any other science. Whilst practical design seems to be only a matter of technology, the study of possibly alternative design is a task for the technological sciences (Kornwatchs 2016). The thinking in alternatives requires that the practical design has become also a scientific, not only a practical, task.

1.7.2   Professionalism in sociology

The sociologist dimension of a professional sees engineers not just as technologists but also as social experts in their abilities to recognize the social nature of the world they act upon. Engineers should try to establish relations with not only the machines and products they build but also with the operators and users of those machines and products. Therefore, it is very important to understand their problems, grievances, welfare, safety, and security from all points of view.

Technology alone cannot improve society. As social systems, communities have dynamic interactions among entities that occur in uncertain ways. Technologies co-evolve with societies; technological developments influence society, and vice versa. The questions about who makes decisions about the development and direction of new technologies have seldom been asked and even less often answered. The successful development and adoption of new technologies, however, requires a model which includes social elements (Habash 2017).

1.7.3   Professionalism in design

Design is one of the oldest endeavors among intellectual and technological pursuits. It is a field of innovation; at its core is the creation of something new and unique. Design as problem-setting views design as a systemic activity needing the discovery and possible negotiation of unstated goals, implications, and criteria before a problem can be formulated and, subsequently, solved (Simon 1973).

The designer dimension sees engineering as the art of design. As discussed before, engineering exists and operates at the interface between science and society. It values systems thinking (ST) much more than the analytical thinking that characterizes traditional science. Professionally, managers, engineers, architects, scientists, etc. all act designerly in the context of industry while they conceive and plan out in the mind and devise for a specific function or end (Habash 2017).

Academically, design is in humanities (literature, history, philosophy, etc.), in sciences (natural, mathematical, behavioral, physical, economical, etc.), in engineering (electrical, civil, chemical, human, etc.), and in arts in the means of personal expression and research context (Kocabiyik 2004).

1.7.4   Professionalism in entrepreneurship

Engineers and computing professionals should have all the skills necessary to be successful entrepreneurs. The technical skills and innovation required of future engineers are vital to convert innovative ideas into reality for common use. An entrepreneurially minded engineer places product benefits before design features and leverages technology to fill unmet customer needs. The purpose of entrepreneurial mindset is to design value-added products and processes that create demand through innovation, resulting in positive revenue and regenerative profits for the enterprise producing the product (Kriewall and Mekemson 2010).

The entrepreneurial professional should have the ability to transform information into knowledge. Such an engineer can do anything possible; can understand basics to quickly assess what needs to be done; and can acquire the tools needed and use these tools proficiently. This engineer should work with anybody, anywhere and have the communication skills, team skills, and understanding of global and current issues necessary to work effectively with other people (Habash 2017).

1.8   Preparing students for professional practice

> *I never teach my pupils, I only attempt to provide the conditions in which they can learn.*
>
> **Albert Einstein**

Student preparation for future professional practice is a major aim of the education system. Such education should integrate highly specialized knowledge with skills of contextual factors that impact the contemporary engineering and computing practice.

1.8.1   Route to professional practice

A key objective of any engineering education program is to provide graduates with the tools necessary to begin the professional practice journey. It contributes to the application of systematic synthesis and design processes and to the conduct and management of projects. Also, it introduces ethical conduct and professional accountability, effective communication skills in professional and lay domains.

The typical route to professional practice is shown in Figure 1.9. Professional education in the broadest sense provides specialized knowledge needed to pursue a particular craft, trade, vocation, or profession. In engineering and computing, professional education provides knowledge of an advanced type or learning customarily acquired by a prolonged course of specialized intellectual instruction and study (Bachelor or Master level). It is typically delivered by lecture, individual assignments, and team projects. Many instructors are not properly prepared to teach professional practice or imbed its components into other subjects due to various reasons, including lack of experience in professional practice in their discipline; focus on their research and teaching on a narrow subfield of the discipline; lack of motivation to engage in collaboration (such as team teaching); and lack of preparation in teaching techniques that best serve preparing students for professional practice (Hilburn 2013). Faculty need a better understanding of professional practice through gaining more professional experience; engaging with industry through guest lecturers, helping industry to solve problems, establishing industrial advisory boards; and embracing active learning.

Skills development takes many forms. Historically, one of the most common forms of skills development was apprenticeship. Today, most professional programs include skills development in the form of lab sessions, team projects, design competitions, special summer off-campus programs, or cooperative education (Ford and Gibbs 1996).

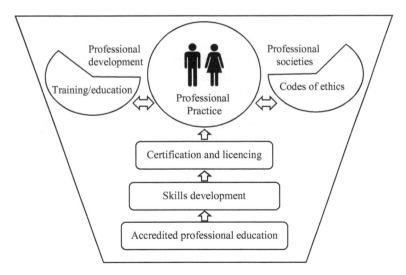

Figure 1.9 The route to professionalism.

The interactions among the components of a profession are substantially more complex than might be suggested in Figure 1.9. For example, the requirements for professional licensing may have a significant effect on the content of initial professional education. A professional society may manage the certification process or may develop the code of ethics. Certification guidelines can influence the content of professional development. More details about these components are given in Module 2.

1.8.2 Lateral thinking versus vertical thinking

Concerns regarding education have been raised with a list of components which are lacking in curriculum (Bordogna et al. 1993). In order to become competent engineers, students have to acquire academic and engineering knowledge, knowledge of the social role of the engineering profession, as well as knowledge of the professional practice as a community of practice (CoP) (Dehing 2012). Therefore, curriculum must provide both breadth and depth across the range of engineering and computing topics entailed by the title and objectives of the program. The problem is more of failing to teach an adequate breadth of skills than in imparting additional knowledge. The curriculum must prepare graduates to analyze, design, verify, validate, implement, apply, and maintain engineering systems; to appropriately apply mathematics and relevant topics in engineering and computing as well as supporting disciplines to complex systems; to work in one or more significant application domains; and to manage the development of engineering systems.

Although education has made much progress in the past 20 years, there are still serious problems in meeting these challenges. By using a survey of 4,000 alumni of engineering programs, Passow (2012) identified the four highest-rated competencies: ability to function on a team; engineering problem-solving skills; ability to analyze and interpret data; written and oral communication skills.

Comparing the two dimensions in Figure 1.10 indicates that the problem is more of failing to teach an adequate breadth of skills than in imparting additional knowledge. It is clear that vertical thinking is a rigid way of thinking. It is about sticking to one approach from the beginning and excluding any other approach. Lateral thinking is flexible. It is about thinking on a problem from different angles and generating new approaches. It is a common concept that it is virtually identical with creative thinking. Lateral thinking is concerned with the generation of new ideas. It is quite different from vertical thinking, which is the conventional way of thinking. In vertical thinking, learning moves forward by selective sequential steps, each of which must be validated. However, lateral thinking is not a substitute for vertical thinking; both are complementary.

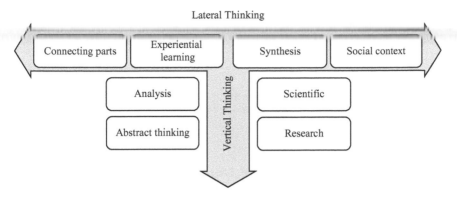

Figure 1.10 Lateral thinking versus vertical thinking.

Because the lacking components broaden the engineer's perspective, the new knowledge involved tends to fall outside the boundaries of the subject discipline and the field of engineering. The lacking components are consistent with the definition of professional practice. Also, they are consistent with the premise that the practice of engineering involves significant interaction with subjects that fall outside those traditionally associated with engineering.

1.8.3 *Methodologies for professional practice instruction*

The current concepts-oriented curriculum is well suited for preparing research graduates but not the practice-oriented graduate on which their competitive advantage progressively depends (Denning 1992). Tackling such complex challenges requires a capacity to understand how relationships and interactions between parts of a system result in dynamic behavior of the whole systems. This requires an education that focuses on ST of the whole rather than parts; on real life topics rather than disjointed subjects.

Such education works when learners are enthusiastically involved in activities or experiences. It is participative, either making or doing, which takes diverse forms. Students would learn through doing and reflect on those activities by applying knowledge to practical experience in order to develop skills or new ways of thinking. Crucial success requirements of this experiential education include space and resources, actual whole problems of no right answer, and a structure developed by the teacher who leads from alongside students in new and creative ways. Cultivating the results of such education demands that the learning environment should be transformed to support growth. Since reflection is such an important element of a successful experiential education, it is essential that students

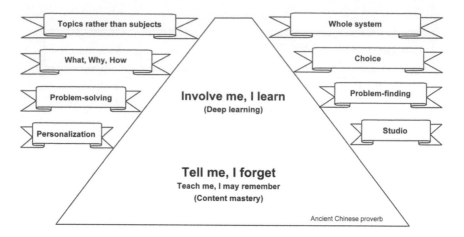

Figure 1.11 Integration of methodologies for professional practice.

realize exactly what reflection is and how to utilize the process to develop their learning (Habash 2018). Figure 1.11 shows the integration of instruction methodologies for professional practice.

It is important to understand the role of engineering and computing within our society. Graduates are the members of society that will be engaged in systematic development of technology and application of that technology to the benefit of society. In the present globalized world, the impact of these professions is growing in importance, and society is becoming more aware of their role. Education institutions should assume the responsibility that their expertise affords graduates the proper knowledge and skills to demonstrate awareness of social responsibility while practicing their professions.

Conventional instruction with lectures geared to structured problem-solving and controlled laboratory settings do not provide learning of the kind expressed in Figure 1.10. Other approaches of instruction should be used to meet the needs of professional practice education. These may include project-based and case research methods of learning. Both methods provide the context for a sense of real-world problem-solving. The experience of developing and using the above methodologies provides an excellent opportunity for instructors to begin exploring their impact in the classroom.

In addition, there is a wide range of design models that aims to embed learning within real-world contexts, including laboratories, workshops, and studio work. The main focus of these methods of instruction is the analysis/solution process, which can be individualistic or group-oriented. Thus, this instructional approach can deal with issues outside the bounds of any one discipline and can help develop the skills of professional practice. Such instruction is one method of teaching topics that are fundamental to practice. This provides the student with a sense of real-world problem-solving and a context for learning skills as well as knowledge.

1.9   Knowledge acquisition

Attempting to answer the following questions involves acquisition of knowledge from this book and other books, documents, and the Internet.

- Differentiate between knowledge, competence, performance, and practice in the design of professional activities.
- Define engineering, the types of questions engineers usually ask, and the tools they use to answer those questions.
- What does thinking historically mean for professionals? What can they learn from the past?
- How is ICT affecting the efficiency of projects and/or project organizations? What are the impacts of its use?
- How does one become a professional?
- What distinguishes engineers from other professionals?
- What distinguishes computing professionals from other professionals?
- What is the difference between practice management and PM?
- How quickly are changes in work, the workforce, and the workplace happening?
- What are the main traits of future composite professionals?
- What key trait would you recommend entrepreneurs invest their time in?
- What is the difference between lateral thinking and vertical thinking?

1.10   Knowledge creation

Collaborate with peers on learning, or you may work with others outside the class to narrow down the objectives of each activity. You may access online resources and analyze data and information to create new ideas and balanced solutions. High-level digital tools may be used to develop multimedia presentations, simulations or animations, videos and visual displays, digital portfolios, reflective practice (online publishing and blogging), or well-researched and up-to-date reports.

1.10.1   Alternative paradigm professional development

The rise of the constructive approach to learning, coupled with analysis of traditional engineering and computing professional development efforts, will lead to an alternative paradigm of professional development. For this task, develop alternative paradigms against typical paradigms in the following table.

Typical paradigm	Alternative paradigm
The goal is to have professionals who are competent in rigid and prescribed classroom routines	
Professionals are trained to follow patterns	
Positivist base	
Expert-driven	
Passive learning	

1.10.2 Campaign for future engineering

More than 50 years ago, Dean William L. Everitt wrote a visionary essay (Everitt 1962) about "Educating Engineers in the Future". His future was 2012. His essay asserted that "educating engineers means fostering innovative minds, the ability to create and navigate a world that, at any given time, we are only beginning to imagine" (Chartoff 2014). In this task, propose a vision for a "futuristic composite engineer" based on realizing the future, in particular 2020. The vision may be reflected in the form of a logo, poster, video, simulation, animation, or any sort of digital media.

1.10.3 Inspiring pre-university students about engineering and computing

The world is living in an innovation revolution characterized by exponential development and accelerating change, particularly in the fields of science, technology, engineering, arts, and math (STEAM). It is an exciting time for the new generation to be thinking about a career in this domain. For this task, develop a colorful poster to inspire pre-university students to consider careers in engineering and/or computing.

1.10.4 Computing as a change agent

Computing is a very rapidly changing field. It is an example of a technology that is a powerful change agent. This swift pace of change is a major challenge to existing educational systems. Computing in education may pose challenges of how to deal with prospective changes in curriculum content, instructional tools and processes, and assessment in a manner that leads to students receiving a better education. By reflecting on the above, develop an e-Poster or a video that views computing as a challenging mind tool. Provide specific example(s) that have significant impact on learning.

1.10.5   Computing, IT, and ICT

To the layperson, computer science, computer engineering, software engineering, IT, and ICT may seem like the same thing. This task is to investigate the above programs and to produce an e-Poster or pamphlet that can benefit high school students when applying to one or more of the programs.

References

Andersson, N., and P. H. Andersson. 2006. Interdisciplinary skills in architectural and engineering education programs: The pedagogical challenge. Technical University of Denmark. http://orbit.dtu.dk/files/2447002/Interdisciplinar y%20skills.pdf.

Armytage, W. H. G. 1976. *A Social History of Engineering*. Fourth Edition. London, UK: Faber and Faber.

Beam, T., O. Pierrakos, J. Constantz, A. Johri, and R. Anderson. 2009. Preliminary findings on freshmen engineering students' professional identity: Implications for recruitment and retention. Annual Conference and Exposition, Austin, Texas. https://peer.asee.org/5112.

Bond, J. 2004. The professional engineer and his enhanced duty of care. https://www.icheme.org/communities/subject_groups/safety%20and%20 loss%20prevention/resources/hazards%20archive/~/media/Documents/ Subject%20Groups/Safety_Loss_Prevention/Hazards%20Archive/XVIII/ XVIII-Paper-57.pdf.

Bordogna, J., E. Fromm, and W. W. Ernst. 1993. Engineering education: Innovation through integration. *Journal of Engineering Education* 82(1): 3–8.

Burke, P. 2004. Identities and social structure: The 2003 Cooley-Mead award address. *Social Psychology Quarterly* 67(1): 5–15.

Chartoff, R. 2014. Engineering education: Past, present and future. Academy for Excellence in Engineering Education. http://ae3.engineering.illinois.edu /2014/08/29/engineering-education-illinois-past-present-and-future/.

Coallier, F. 2007. Standards, agility, and engineering. *IEEE Computer* 40(9): 100–102.

Cochran-Smith, M., and S. L. Lytle. 2001. Beyond certainty: Taking an inquiry stance on practice. In Lieberman, A., and L. Miller (eds.). *Teachers Caught in the Action: Professional Development that Matters*. New York, NY: Teachers College Press.

Cohn, M. 2016. Understanding the ARE 5.0 divisions: Practice management vs. project management. https://www.ncarb.org/blog/understanding-are- 50-divisions-practice-management-vs-project-management.

Collins, F. 2015. A brief history of project management. https://www.ims-web. com/blog/a-brief-history-of-project-management.

Correani, A. 2017. Is information age equal to knowledge age? https://www.lin kedin.com/pulse/information-age-equal-knowledge-alessia-correani-phd.

Coyle, D. M. 2009. *Computers Are Your Future*. Tenth Edition. Upper Saddle River, NJ: Pearson.

Dehing, A. J. M. 2012. Preparing students for workplace learning in higher engineering education. Eindhoven, Netherlands: Technische Universiteit Eindhoven. https://pure.tue.nl/ws/files/3440648/733802.pdf.

Denning, P. J. 1992. Educating a new engineer. *Communications of the ACM* 16(12): 83–97.

Elder, L., M. Gorzycki, and R. Paul. 2011. *Student Guide to Historical Thinking.* Tomales, CA: Foundation for Critical Thinking.

Ensmenger, N. L. 2001. The 'question of professionalism' in the computer fields. *IEEE Annals of the History of Computing* 23(4): 56–74.

Everitt, W. L. 1962. Engineering education-circa 2012 A.D. *Communication and Electronics* May 50(5): 571–572.

Ford, G., and N. E. Gibbs. 1996. A mature profession of software engineering. CMU/SEI-96-TR-004, Software Engineering Institute, Carnegie Mellon University, Pittsburgh, PA. https://resources.sei.cmu.edu/asset_files/Tec hnicalReport/1996_005_001_16460.pdf.

Grasso, D., and D. Martinelli. 2007. Holistic engineering. *The Chronical Review* 53(28): B8.

Habash, R. 2017. *Green Engineering: Innovation, Entrepreneurship, and Design.* Boca Raton, FL: CRC Taylor and Francis.

Habash, R. 2018. Unleashing knowledge creation and sharing in a reflective open education. Proceedings of the 2018 Canadian Engineering Education Association (CEEA-ACEG 18) Conference, Vancouver, BC.

Hilburn, T. B. 2013. Preparing students for professional practice. http://conferen ces.computer.org/cseet/2013/slides/CS2013CSEETKeynote.-Hilburn.pdf.

Ireland, L. R. 1991. *Quality Management for Projects and Programs.* Upper Darby, PA: Project Management Institute.

Johnston, S., J. P. Gostelow, and W. J. King. 2000. *Engineering and Society.* New York, NY: Prentice Hall. https://www.criticalthinking.org/store/get_file.php?inv entories_id=453&inventories_files_id=358.

Kelley, E. J., and M. R. Walker. 1959. Critical path planning and scheduling. https://www.computer.org/csdl/proceedings/afips/1959/5055/00/5055 0160.pdf.

Kocabiyik, E. 2004. Engineering concepts in industrial product design with a case study of bicycle design. Master of Industrial Design, Izmir Institute of Technology, İzmir, Turkey.

Kornwatchs, K. 2016. Design technoscience: What's up with responsibility? Proceeding of the Design 14th International Design Conference, Cavtat, Dubrovnik, Croatia, May 16–19.

Kriewall, T. J., and K. Mekemson. 2010. Instilling the entrepreneurial mindset into engineering understanding. *The Journal of Engineering Entrepreneurship* 1(1): 5–19.

Manning, P. R., and L. DeBakey. 2003. *Preserving the Passion in the 21st Century.* 2nd edition. New York, NY: Springer.

Miller, G. E. 1990. The assessment of clinical skills/competence/performance. *Academic Medicine* 65(9): S63–S67.

Mintzberg, H. 2013. *Simply Managing: What Managers Do-and Can Do Better.* San Francisco, CA: Berrett-Koehler Publishers.

Nilsson, S. 2007. From higher education to professional practice: A comparative study of physicians' and engineers' learning and competence use. Linköping Studies in Behavioural Science. Linköping, Sweden: Department of Behavioural Sciences and Learning, Linköping University. https://pd fs.semanticscholar.org/80e4/2b95e1f3ee7c9e511108c5df14c7440bee4d.pdf.

Passow, H. J. 2012. Which ABET competencies do engineering graduates find most important in their work? *Journal of Engineering Education* 101(1): 95–118.

Prentic, J. 2012. Technological revolutions through the ages: Lessons for leading the cleantech revolution. Business 485: Business Leadership and the Liberal Arts.

Sievert, R. W. Jr. 1991. A review of value engineering as an effective system for planning building projects. *Project Management Journal* XXII(1): 31–38.

Simon, H. A. 1973. The structure of ill-structured problems. *Artificial Intelligence* 4(3–4): 181–201.

Singh, A. K. 2018. What is the relation between industrial revolution and engineering? https://www.quora.com/What-is-the-relation-between-Industrial-Revolution-and-Engineering.

Stoodley, I. 2009. IT professionals' experience of ethics and its implications for IT education. PhD Thesis, Queensland: Faculty of Science and Technology University of Technology, Brisbane, Australia.

Stretton, A. 2007. A short history of modern project management. *PM World Today* IX(X): 1–18.

UNESCO. 2010. Engineering: Issues, challenges, and opportunities for development. United Nations Educational Report, Scientific and Cultural Organization, Paris, France, UNESCO Publishing.

Vlada, M., and A. Ţugui. 2006. Information society technologies - The four waves of information technologies. The 1st International Conference on Virtual Learning (ICVL), Bucharest, Romania, pp. 69–82.

Weaver, P. 2007. The origins of modern project management. Fourth Annual PMI College of Scheduling Conference, Vancouver, Canada, April 15–18. https://mosaicprojects.com.au/PDF_Papers/P050_Origins_of_Modern_PM.pdf.

WSP. 2018. The emerging workforce. http://www.wal-staf.com/blog/the-emerging-workforce.

part one

Professional, ethical, legal, and leadership practices

part one

Professionalism and ethical practice

2.1 Knowledge and understanding

Having successfully completed this module, you should be able to demonstrate knowledge and understanding of:

- Various concepts of professionalism in practice
- Characteristics and attributes of professional practice
- Professional attributes, knowledge, and skills in practice
- Professionals, including profession maturation, professional nature, and future professionals
- Professional programs accreditation, stakeholders who benefit from it, and ways professional programs gain accreditation
- Licensing according to professional standards and several examples of certification programs
- Morals and ethics, ethical theories, and approaches
- Evolution of professional codes of ethics and related organizations with several corresponding examples
- Categories of ethics including technical, social, professional, and entrepreneurial
- Common ethical issues in engineering and computing professions
- Distinction between ethics, including microethics, macroethics, preventive ethics, and aspirational ethics

2.2 Professionalism

> *Professionalism: It's not the job you do; it's how you do the job.*

Anonymous

Professionalism, in the sense perceived in the quotation above, is more than doing a job; it is a key cluster of social and ethical responsibility, commitment, knowledge and skills, and judgment in the sociologies of work, occupations, professions, and organizations (Figure 2.1). Hurd (1967)

35

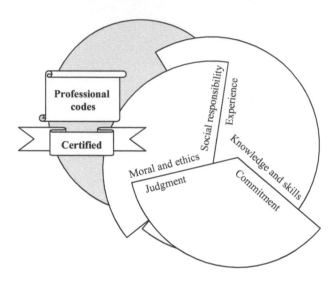

Figure 2.1 Main characteristics of professionalism.

suggests that professionalism should be perceived as a scale or continuum process, rather than as a cluster of characteristics. The main idea behind this module is that this process of wide range is relevant to engineering and computing.

Professionalism is perceived as a force for stability and freedom against the threat of encroaching industrial and governmental bureaucracies (Carr-Saunders and Wilson 1933). The early American sociological theorists of professions developed similar interpretations, and again the key concept was the occupational value of professionalism based on trust, competence, a strong occupational identity, and cooperation (Evetts 2012).

The concepts of professions and professionalism are somewhat indistinct and vague, and this can be attributed to the fact that they are used in everyday language at the same time as researchers are trying to fill them with a formal content. Goode (1957) has argued that a profession is a community characterized by the members' sense of identity that binds them together, and usually membership is a permanent status.

Professionalism is the conduct and standards which guide the work of professionals. It describes the qualities, skills, competence, and behaviors they are expected to bring to the workplace. Traditionally, professionalism has been seen in terms of fulfilling a list of requirements, including membership of a professional body (which includes agreeing to a code of ethics), attainment of a specified training level, pursuit of ongoing professional development, and licensing from the government (Sizer 1996). With respect to ethical responsibility, a proper standard of professionalism is the quality of professionals' relationships with others (Stoodley 2009).

Professionalism reflects the professional competence of a professional and not only the individual's behavior

Professionalism is a multidimensional term that encompasses many subcomponents, including the pillars of excellence, humanism, account-ability, and altruism resting on a base of ethical and legal understanding, communication skills, and competence (Ludwig 2013). Professionalism requires professionals to be worthy of trust, to put clients first, to maintain confidentiality, and not to use their knowledge for deceptive purposes. In return for professionalism in client relations, some professionals are rewarded with authority, privileged rewards, and high status (Evetts 2012).

Finally, professionalism in the workplace means taking responsibility for work; pride in the quality of work; acting ethically to clients, colleagues, management, community, and the environment; understanding risks and inhibiting failures; and persistent improvement of the profession and technology.

2.3   Approaches to professional practice

> *Practice does not make perfect. Only perfect practice makes perfect.*
>
> **Vince Lombardi**

The original meaning of "professional" is derived from the Middle English "profes", an adjective meaning having professed one's vows, which itself is derived from Medieval Latin "professus", which meant to profess and confess (Balthazard 2015). The idea was that professionals were those who professed their specialized knowledge and skill to others, vowed to perform their profession to the highest standard, and acquired special rights and responsibilities.

2.3.1   Characteristics of practice

Practice involves "practical reasoning", using knowledge in the face of uncertainty, understanding that action is always a kind of exploration of what might possibly be done, and understanding that the historical consequences of practice in a particular case will only become apparent in the future and then only if people reflect critically on what was done (Green 2009).

The concept of professional practice refers to the work that professionals actually do and the context within which the work is done. It is based on the competence of the professionals, which is associated with the knowledge base of the professional practice. From a traditional perspective, professional practice is regarded as referring to applied science, technology, and policy; applications of knowledge grounded in theories, technologies, and techniques developed through science; or as instrumental problem-solving (Nilsson 2007). It is a social activity, involving teams working in concert towards a common goal. It reflects the commitment to relationships with society and strong ethical values; utilization of specialized knowledge, critical inquiry, and evidence-informed decision-making; continuous development of self and others; and accountability and responsibility for insightful competent practice (AHS 2016).

True professionals possess a number of important characteristics that can apply to virtually any type of discipline. All practices are enacted based on certain theories, public or private. What is important in this section is to help students understand the practice as a composite of "saying: talk", "doing: action", and "relating: relationship", which helps to constitute practices as being of a particular type. Also, these practices do not exist in and of themselves, but are always and everywhere influenced by existing provisions which affect how practices play out – and which are themselves concurrently influenced by these practices. In terms of sayings, different professional practices involve particular ways of thinking and learning about what the practice is and its means.

In terms of doing, different practices involve different activities and work for professional practitioners and different kinds of activities and consequences for others involved in and affected by the practice. Professionals must obey a strict code of ethics. Even if the organization does not have a written code, displaying ethical behavior is mandatory at all times.

In terms of relationships, different kinds of professional practices similarly involve different kinds and complexes of relationships between practitioners and those involved in and affected by their practices (Schatzki 2002). Responding to people and duties promptly and following through on actions in a timely manner is also important, as this demonstrates reliability.

In regard to the workplace, professional practice may be identified as any practice situation in the workplace, good or poor. A good workplace practice involves staying positive, being responsible, taking initiative, and thinking critically to be able to solve problems. Poor workplace practice involves prohibited practices, incompetent attitudes, abusing agreements, and making choices for one's own personal advantage.

The vital question to ask in such cases is whether practices as they are represented or enshrined in laws, regulations, rules, policies, or social technologies (like funding and accounting systems) are sustainable (Green 2009). In general, practices are not sustainable if they do not meet criteria necessary for their continuation in one or more of several dimensions: personal, social, political, environmental, and economic.

2.3.2   Professional attributes, knowledge, and skills in practice

A profession remains what it was thought to be a few centuries ago, namely, an occupation the practice of which requires more than an ordinary amount of knowledge, acquired by persistent and systematic study and authoritatively certified (Henninger 1991). With regard to practice, it might be useful to think in terms of three distinct but interrelated categories, namely, "activity", "experience", and "context". These are of course relatively familiar and even commonsense terms that may be kept in mind. Rather than thinking of them in linear or sequential terms, it is perhaps more appropriate and generative to conceive of them and their interrelations as layering and unfolding (Green 2009). Activity is to be regarded as a primary category of action or operation. Professional experience is often understood as a replacement for practicum, which refers to engagement in pre-service practice of the profession before being immersed in the real world. Finally, practice is always contextualized; it cannot be thought of outside of a situation within which activity or experience exists or happens. Beyond the above, practice also constitutes relationships between people that take place in a material context of action (work or labor) in the physical world Kemmis and McTaggart 2000).

The so-called élite professions, such as engineering, medicine, education, nursing, and law, share that common set of principles. These include providing valuable services in the pursuit of important human and social ends; possessing fundamental knowledge and skills; developing the capacity to engage in complex forms of practice; making judgments under conditions of uncertainty; learning from past experiences; and creating and participating in a responsible professional community (Shulman 1998). Accordingly, professionals enjoy a level of self-control in their work and a standard of good work that they apply to it, which other occupations do not regularly enjoy. Being a professional involves the recognition of responsibility to the public. Such professions require involvement in an intellectual effort that requires advanced formal education, sophisticated skills, judgment, and exercise of responsibility that benefits society.

A profession requires high standards of learning, a focus on individual responsibility, resilience under pressure, a sense of fairness, honesty, attention to details in perspectives, and practical experience and judgment in the application of needed skills (Erdogmus 2011). It demands the acquisition and creation of a body of specialized knowledge, problem-solving skills, and good judgment for the service of society. These three domains are aimed at forming professionals who are intellectually trained, practically adept, and ethically responsible for their work.

Most professions have developed clear notions of what it means to do a competent job by having their own professional organizations and journals, formal training programs, examination and review procedures, codes of practice, and so on. It is therefore clear to most professionals, as well as to the public, what criteria determine whether one is a member of a professional community, holds to its regulations, and is considered a competent professional (Ulrich 2011). To teach and learn these domains in a setting is a challenge. Ideally, the educational processes in a university setting integrate these domains, and thereby education serves as an apprenticeship to the profession (Sheppard et al. 2006).

2.4   The push toward professionalism

Breakthrough innovation occurs when we bring down boundaries and encourage disciplines to learn from each.

Gyan Nagpal
[from Talent Economics: The Fine Line Between Winning and Losing the Global War for Talent (2013)]

As technology advances and spins off into specialized disciplines, so do the careers, professions, and educational programs that reinforce them. As these programs and disciplines gradually narrow their fields of focus, it may be useful to realize how they perform into the wider technology background by breaking them down into several underlying curricula. And while there is shared background between them, knowing where these disciplines both overlap and wander is a good place to begin.

2.4.1   Computing profession maturation

The debate about professionalism in the computer field originated in the programmer labor shortages of the early 1950s. The supply of programmers had been a problem for the commercial computing industry from the beginning. As the market for commercial computers changed and expanded in the early 1960s, the demand for computer specialists increased accordingly (Ensmenger 2001). The professionalization of programming and other computer specialties was appealing to practitioners because professionalism offered increased social status, greater autonomy, improved opportunities for advancement, and better pay (Wilensky 1964). In 1962, the Data Processing Management Association (DPMA), inclined toward business programmers, announced its ambitious "Six Measures of Professionalism Program", which included provisions for certification standards, continuing education, public service, and the development of a professional code of ethics. In 1966, the Association for Computing Machinery (ACM), inclined toward academically oriented computer scientists, announced a professional development program that included skill upgrade seminars offered at the national computer conferences, a traveling course series, and self-study materials. Both efforts appear to have been responses to a larger groundswell of support for increased professionalism in the computer fields (DPMA 1962; Oettinger 1966). As the programming community broke down into competing factions, theoretical versus practical, certified versus uncertified, ACM versus DPMA, its members lost the influence necessary to push through any particular professionalization agenda. In the decades following the 1960s, the question of professionalism has remained one of the dominant themes in the computing industry.

Today, computing contributes significantly to almost every domain, including engineering, business, and government. Professionals in the computing sector are primarily concerned with the information that computer systems can provide to aid an enterprise in defining and achieving its goals. Compared with many disciplines, computing is relatively young and is constantly developing, with new types of roles emerging as technologies evolve. These new roles respond to the increased variety of tasks computers can perform, and both of these phenomena enable more opportunities for the undesirable consequences of computing misuse (Leicester 2016). Therefore, the progress in computing can leave an ethical vacuum. To deal with ethical issues facing computing specialists as technology began to grow and diversify, codes of ethics began to emerge in the 1960s through professional associations of technology workers, which had recently come into existence. Today, there are many professional bodies around the world to promote good practice, diligence, and ethical behavior in computing and technology-related professions.

Many computing specialists have duties, backgrounds, and training that qualify them to be classified as professionals, including specialists such as mobile application developers, software engineers, systems analysts, and network administrators. One could argue, however, that not every role requires "knowledge of an advanced type in a field of science or learning customarily acquired by a prolonged course of specialized intellectual instruction and study", to quote again from the labor code. From a legal perspective, a cluster of computing specialists might not be recognized as professionals because they are not licensed by the government (Reynolds 2015). Computing specialists typically are involved in many different relationships, including those with users, suppliers, and other professionals; and economy, society, and environment at large, as illustrated in Figure 2.2.

While skills and technologies related to computing have changed in the past few years, the profession itself has not been recognized in official statistics as an industry sector in its own rights. Many of the concerns relating to low levels of professionalism in the past might still be valid today. Given the role of computing as an enabler of emerging and future

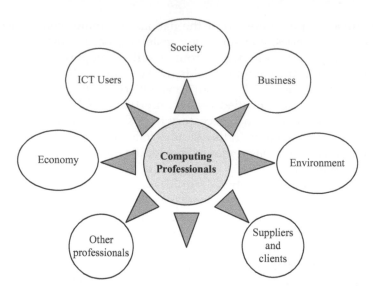

Figure 2.2 Domains of computing professionals and specialists.

technologies, including AI, this has important implications for competitiveness. Moreover, the increasingly prevalent nature of computing means that society at large is at more risk from low levels of professionalism. The risks posed to society dictate that actions be taken to develop the profession.

Creating a recognition system for computing professionals, for example, certification, should be a priority due to the impact of computer specialists in a global profession, the widening gap between skills and the supply of qualified practitioners, the lack of regulation of the computing skills market, and the lack of agility in responding to skills gaps (Aynsley 2018). Today, no universal code of ethics for computing professionals clearly exits. Also, no single, formal organization has emerged as leaders. However, several most prominent organizations exist to contribute to the field of computing and have developed their code of ethics, including ACM, founded in 1947; Institute of Electrical and Electronics Engineers (IEEE, founded in 1946); Computer Society (IEEE-CS); Association of IT Professionals (AITP, founded in 1951); and SysAdmin, Audit, Network, Security (SANS Institute, founded in 1989).

2.4.2   *Professional nature*

Engineering that puts scientific and other knowledge to practical use has been regarded as a profession in Europe and North America since the nineteenth century. The real professional will then incorporate ethics into the daily decision-making situations. It is clear that engineering meets all of the definitions of a profession.

A profession depends on belief of two kinds for efficient activity of work, the personal belief of the client or employer in the technical competence of the professional, and the belief of the public at large in the integrity and ethical conduct of the professions as a whole. Therefore, the nature of profession varies to a large extent among various practices. For example, physicians and lawyers have direct, individual interactions with their clients, but engineers and computing professionals usually are employed within organizations and firms. The majority of these professionals work for either industry or government, and only a small percentage are in direct contact with the public as consultants or university educators. Therefore, the service feature of engineering and computing is less noticeable to the public than that of medicine and law. The particularities of the profession as compared with other professions are reflected in the domain of ethics. Because engineering and computing lack the homogeneous character of such professions, it is common to find that there is no widely accepted code of ethics. Most professional societies have implemented their own codes.

Yet again, engineers and computing specialists who are employees by either business or government face different ethical problems than self-employed professionals. These arise from the conflict between the professional's desire to gain a maximum profit for the employer and the desire to adhere to a standard of ethics that places the public welfare ahead of corporate profit (Perry 1981).

2.4.3 The future professional

Looking ahead a decade or so, professionals including engineers and those in computing will need attributes similar to those that sufficed in the past; however, those attributes will need to be expanded and refined due to inevitable change. More specifically, the future's successful and relevant professionals will need the following attributes (NSPE 2013): to be analytical and practical; thorough and detail-oriented in design; creative and innovative; communicative; knowledgeable about the application of sciences and math; thoroughly knowledgeable in a selected field and conversant in related technical fields; knowledgeable about and skillful in business and management; able to provide leadership with ability to make change in strategies, tactics, policies, and procedures; professional and positive in attitude; aware of societal and historical considerations in the global context; aware of and compliant with relevant laws, regulations, standards, and codes; licensed as a professional engineer and knowledgeable about ethics and applicable codes of professional conduct; and dedicated to lifelong learning

On the other hand, the National Academy of Engineering (NAE 2004) presents guiding principles for the "The Engineer of 2020" as follows:

- The pace of technological innovation will continue to be accelerating.
- The world will be intensely globally interconnected.
- The presence of technology in everyday lives will be seamless, transparent, and more significant than ever.
- The population of individuals who are involved with or affected by technology (for example, designers, manufacturers, distributors, and government users) will be increasingly diverse and multidisciplinary.
- Social, cultural, political, and economic forces will continue to shape and affect the success of technological innovation.

2.5   *Professional programs accreditation*

> *Intelligence plus character; that is the goal of true education.*

> **Dr. Martin Luther King, Jr.**

Accreditation is the public recognition accorded to a professional program that meets recognized professional qualifications and educational standards through initial and periodic evaluation.

2.5.1   *Why accreditation?*

Accreditation is a review process to assure the quality of educational programs and determine if these programs meet defined standards. Once achieved, accreditation is not permanent; it is renewed periodically to ensure that the quality of the educational program is maintained. Accreditation concerns itself with both quality assurance and program enhancement. It applies to programs and is to be distinguished from certification or licensure, which applies to individuals. These accreditation standards embrace the philosophy that program graduates should have acquired general and special knowledge, general to avoid the constraints of too narrow, and special to provide a basis for critical professional evaluations (CCAPP 2018).

Professional accreditation is conducted by professional bodies and/ or accreditation agencies on behalf of the professions. Its principal aim is to maintain the standards of professional training with the ultimate goal of providing the community with the confidence of a professional practice that meets competency standards, ethical standards, and ensures public safety (PKPA 2017). In the US, for example, academic accreditation is voluntary, decentralized, and carried out by many non-governmental, non-profit organizations.

All professional accreditations are reviewed regularly by their professional body to ensure that the content of educational programs, teaching resources, and research outputs are of high quality to meet competency expectations and to support future professionals in their disciplines of expertise.

2.5.2   Who benefits from accreditation?

In general, professional accreditation is valued by all stakeholders. Most accreditors and education providers stress the value of accreditation as a stimulus to self and peer review, a benchmarking process and an opportunity for continuing quality assurance and improvement (PKPA 2017). Students benefit from accreditation by providing a measure of educational quality, and in many professions, students are required to complete an accredited program of study in order to be eligible for certification or state licensure for practice. On the other hand, employers benefit from accreditation by assuring prospective employers that graduates come from a program or school where the content and quality satisfy established standards.

Accreditation provides educators and institutions with validation of higher education programs, as well as the opportunity for academic administrators, faculty, and practitioners to build consensus on expected learning outcomes and graduate competencies. Regulators and lawmakers benefit from accreditation by providing assurance that higher education programs are evaluated against nationally accepted standards and that graduates are competent for entry into the workplace or for advanced practice (ASPA 2013).

2.5.3   How does a professional program gain accreditation?

Any specialized or professional study program seeking accreditation goes through a thorough review process. It begins with self-evaluation and comprises a comprehensive, on-site review and an ongoing process of continual improvement. An important factor in the accreditation process is peer review by experts in the fields of study. A team selected by the accrediting agency visits the institution or program to determine if the applicant meets established standards. Usually, evaluators are volunteers who are a merge of practitioners and academics with professional knowledge in the specialized area under evaluation.

While specific guidelines vary by agency, most accreditors review the following areas: teaching and research; professional or specialized program curriculum; ethics and integrity; evaluation and assessment of outcomes; faculty qualifications; financial resources; library, information, and learning resources; mission and planning; organization and administration, physical, laboratory, and training facilities; and student support services.

2.5.4 Accreditation bodies

In many countries, educational accreditation for higher education professional programs is conducted by a government organization, such as a ministry of education. However, in the US, the quality assurance process is independent of government and is performed by private agencies. The accreditation boards accredit undergraduate engineering programs. These programs provide the academic requirements for licensure. The Accreditation Board for Engineering and Technology (ABET), founded in 1932, is a not-for-profit body which accredits associate, bachelor's, and master's degree programs in the applied sciences, computing, engineering, and engineering technology. Programs in computer science can be accredited by the Computing Sciences Accreditation Board (CSAB).

Programs applying for ABET accreditation are evaluated by one of the body's four commissions based upon their academic discipline: Applied Science Accreditation Commission (ASAC); Computing Accreditation Commission (CAC); Engineering Accreditation Commission (EAC); and Engineering Technology Accredited Commission (ETAC) (Manley 2017). In addition to the US, ABET provides accreditation services to programs in 30 countries across the world, with the exclusion of Canada.

The general ABET criteria is under the following headings: students, program educational objectives, student outcomes, continuous improvement, curriculum, faculty, facilities, and institutional support. Concerning students, EAC and CAC student outcomes are listed in Table 2.1.

In 1965, Engineers Canada established the Canadian Engineering Accreditation Board (CEAB), a board of specialists tasked with accrediting Canadian undergraduate engineering programs that meet or exceed educational standards acceptable for professional engineering registration in Canada (CAA 2016). Programs eligible for CEAB accreditation must be in Canada, delivered at the undergraduate level, and include the word "engineering" in their title. While the CEAB does not accredit international programs, it has established equivalency terms with engineering programs in 18 countries across the world (Manley 2017). The ABET and CEAB share a similar accreditation process that includes internal evaluation, on-campus evaluation, external review reports, and notification of decision.

In Europe, the European Network for Accreditation of Engineering Education (ENAEE) authorizes accreditation and quality assurance

Table 2.1 ABET student outcomes (Carroll 2015)

EAC	CAC
An understanding of professional and ethical responsibility	An understanding of professional, ethical, legal, security, and social responsibilities
An ability to communicate effectively	An ability to communicate effectively with a range of audiences
An understanding of the impact of engineering solutions in a global, economic, environmental, and societal context	An ability to analyze the local and global impact of computing on individuals, organizations, and society
A recognition of the need for, and an ability to engage in, lifelong learning	A recognition of the need for and an ability to engage in continuing professional development
A knowledge of contemporary issues	A knowledge of contemporary issues

agencies to award the EUR-ACE label to accredited engineering degree programs.

In Australia, professional accreditation of entry to practice engineering programs is the responsibility of Engineers Australia and is normally carried out every five years.

The USA, UK, Hong Kong, New Zealand, Canada, South Africa, China, Chinese Taipei, India, Ireland, Japan, Korea, Malaysia, Russia, Singapore, Sri Lanka, and Turkey are co-signatories to international agreements which provide greater international mobility through mutual recognition of accredited programs.

The Washington Accord, the Sydney Accord, and the Dublin Accord recognize the substantial equivalence of accreditation systems and accredited programs across international boundaries at the professional engineer, engineering technologist, and engineering associate levels, respectively. The link to the International Engineering Alliance (IEA) can be found at: www.ieagreements.org.

2.6   Licensing and certification

> *Liberty is the right to do what I like; license, the right to do what you like.*
>
> **Bertrand Russell**

Licensing and certification processes often co-exist in a single jurisdiction and complement one another. They are often confused, because they are both intended as mechanisms to assure the competence of professionals. These two processes may be distinguished somewhat in this sense:

licensing is a mandatory process administered by a governmental authority, while certification is a voluntary process administered by a profession
(Ford and Gibbs 1996). The term registration is also sometimes used for
similar mechanisms.

2.6.1   Licensing for practice

The objective of licensing is the protection of the public. Engineering is a
licensed profession. Licensure is the highest restrictive form of credential-
ing and implies the granting of a license by a governmental or delegated
(for example, regulatory) body to practice a profession. The primary purpose of licensure is to protect the health, safety, and welfare of the public
by restricting practice of the profession to individuals who possess the
knowledge, skills, and abilities required to do so safely and competently.

Licensure is a regulatory process which permits an individual to
engage in an occupation if it is determined that an applicant has attained
the necessary degree of competency required. It forbids anyone from
practicing the profession who is not licensed, regardless of whether or
not the individual has been certified by an organization. Only licensed
engineers can practice engineering in most of the world. Although many
engineers work in an industrial setting where a license is not required to
do engineering work inside a company, engineers involved in services
directly for the public require licensing.

For licensing, one typically has to meet eligibility requirements and
pass an examination that covers a comprehensive range of knowledge
and skills, usually at the entry level. Education and experience prepare
a graduate for technical engineering work. The license legally allows an
engineer to take personal responsibility for the engineering work performed for public and private clients. A licensed engineer may achieve
an enhanced status in the eyes of the public, which equates the holder
with professionals licensed in other fields, such as physicians, lawyers,
and accountants. Private practicing, like engineering consulting or a firm,
is only possible with licensing. Many agencies require that certain responsible engineering positions, particularly those considered higher level, be
filled only by licensed engineers. Engineering educators who provide
fundamental knowledge to those who study engineering and serve as role
models should go through licensure.

Licensure also aids engineers and the profession in the important area
of ethics. While technical societies have codes of ethics for guidance, none
of these codes have legal standing in the practice of engineering. On the
other hand, licensing boards have standards of ethical conduct that are
legally binding. The identification and implementation of these standards
gives greater definition to the profession and considerably enhances the
image of licensed engineers.

2.6.2   Professional certification

Professional certification is a designation earned by a person to ensure qualification to perform a work or task. It is a license that provides the authority to independently practice and take legal responsibility for work done by way of a seal or stamp on the relevant produced documents, including design, drawings, specifications, reports, and calculations.

Certification is an earned credential awarded through an evaluation process. It indicates the command of advanced or specialized knowledge and expertise. Therefore, it provides an individual's capability as measured against a highest standard of competence, a symbol of achievement, and an assurance of quality, while ensuring a key point of accountability.

Certification is voluntary, involves no legal requirement, and does not grant permission to practice. It is usually managed by a professional society. It attests to certain qualifications and demonstrates specialty expertise beyond a minimum competence. Some certifications must be renewed regularly or may be valid for a certain period of time. They may also be withdrawn by the issuing organization. It would serve to enhance the importance, reputation, and standing of professionals in society.

Today, engineering and computing are universally recognized as a learned profession characterized by competency and the sustained activity of knowledge and experience. Figure 2.3 outlines three major requirements for professional certification. The first requirement is formal education consisting of a bachelor's degree in engineering or computing plus a master's degree in a recognized field of study, with exceptions in certain cases (for example, 10–15 years of working experience). The second requirement is cumulative working experience (several years or a certain number of working hours) in the desired field with strong references (current or former supervisors or coworkers). Knowledge as a third requirement means passing certification examination.

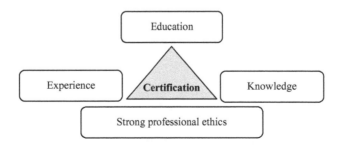

Figure 2.3 Professional certification requirements.

Table 2.2 Several examples of certification programs

Certifying body	Certificate
The National Institute for Certification in Engineering Technologies (NICET)	Certified Engineering Technician (CET). Certification in graduated levels for a range of engineering technologies.
International Society of Automation (ISA)	Certified Automation Professional (CAP). Generally requires an engineering degree.
Institute of Electrical and Electronics Engineers (IEEE)	Certified Software Development Professional (CSDP). Typically requires an engineering degree.
American Society of Mechanical Engineers (ASME)	Geometric Dimensioning and Tolerancing Professional (GDTP). This certification does not require an engineering degree or license to qualify.
Canadian Engineering Qualifications Board (CEQB)	Develops guidelines which seek to bring about uniform requirements for registration across Canada (licensing is a provincial responsibility).
Information Systems Professionals (ISP)	Canada's legally recognized designation for IT professionals.
Information Technology Certified Professionals (ITCP)	This certification is intended for senior IT specialists and academics who have demonstrated an ability to apply their organizational experience to tough problems and achieve ambitious goals.

Certification mostly implies to an earned certificate awarded by a private sector, non-profit, professional association, or independent board to those members who, through an assessment process, demonstrate competence of knowledge and skills required by the certifying organization. Certification supports licensure because certification requires licensure. A few examples of certification programs are listed in Table 2.2.

2.7   Morals and ethics

> *In civilized life, law floats in a sea of ethics.*

Earl Warren

Generally, the terms *"morals"* and *"ethics"* are used interchangeably, although a few different settings (academic, community, legal, or field) will sometimes make a difference (Grannan 2018). Both morals and ethics have to do with differentiating the difference between good and bad or right and wrong.

2.7.1   Combination of morals, ethics, and law

Morals refer to social conventions about right and wrong that are widely shared so that they become the basis for an established consensus. However, individual views of what behavior is moral may vary by age, cultural group, ethnic background, religion, life experiences, education, and gender (Stoodley 2009).

Ethics comes from the Greek word "ethos" and is defined as the study of standards and codes of behavior expected of an individual by a group. It is that part of science and philosophy dealing with moral conduct, duty, and judgment (Velasquez et al. 1987). Ethics is a major characteristic of professionalism. It is about developing the ability of practitioners to see the ethical dimensions of problems, to reflect on issues, to take difficult decisions, and to be able to justify these decisions and act with integrity (NYA 2004). Ethics is the collection of value concepts and principles into a code that can be lived. These values center what is considered basically good (Levine 1993). Ethics include attitude, communication skills, behavior toward colleagues, honesty, and responsibility. What distinguishes a positive ethic apart from a negative ethic is the focus on confidence and encouraging interactions with colleagues. All ethics are based on the concept of free choice and the responsibility of the individual.

Law is a system of rules that tells what one can and cannot do. Laws are enforced by a set of institutions such as the police, courts, and law-making bodies. The legal system is a set of acts that conform to the law. Moral acts conform to what an individual believes to be the right thing to do. Laws can proclaim an act as legal, although many people may consider the act immoral (Stoodley 2009).

This combination of morals, ethics, and law makes the study of the principles of conduct that oversee the behavior of an individual or a profession. It provides a framework of the rules of behavior that are moral, fair, and proper for a true professional. Ethical conduct is behavior anticipated by society and is above and beyond the minimum standards of the law. Therefore, morals, ethics, and law, while different, are not independent.

2.7.2   Evolution of morals and ethics

Ethical ideas were continually refined during the course of history. Many great thinkers have turned their attention to ethics and morals and have tried to provide insight into these issues through their writings (Fleddermann 2012).

In Western history, much of what is known about formal moral reasoning generally began with the ancient Greeks, especially with the philosophers Socrates (470–399 BC), Plato (427–347 BC), and Aristotle (384–322 BC). Socrates argued that there was only one true moral code, and it was simple: "No person should ever willingly do evil". Socrates never wrote down any of his philosophy. But his student, Plato (427–347 BC), made Socrates the hero of almost all of his many philosophical dialogues. Plato was the first professional philosopher in the West. He established a school of philosophy called the Academy, where the word academic comes from. He published a great number of books both for general readers and his own students and formed arguments on virtually every subject in philosophy (Reynolds 2015). Aristotle, on the other hand, focused on the moral character of the individual, which prepares them for ethical challenges.

Chinese ethical philosophy begins with the writings of Kongzi, known in the West by his Latinized name, Confucius, who lived from 551 to 479 BC in what is now the southern portion of Shandong province in China. Confucius' written works reflect a practical rather than a theoretical approach to moral problems, unlike Western philosophy after Plato that emphasizes more theoretical thinking. This way of thinking is often called "pre-theoretical". Confucian ethics emphasizes the role of ideal character traits. As such, it has much in common with the Western concept of virtue ethics (Fleddermann 2012).

The philosophical traditions of the Indian subcontinent are the oldest surviving written philosophical systems in human civilization. Discussing Indian philosophy and Indian ethics is made very difficult by the diversity and richness of the various cultures that make up the modern nation of India, each with its own literature and philosophical background. Indian philosophical and ethical thinking have their origins in the ancient texts known as the Vedas, further developed through the Upanishads, Jainism, Buddhism, and also expressed in the Bhagavad-Gita. These ancient traditions continue to inform current philosophical thinking in India, though more contemporary thinkers such as Tagore, Gandhi, and Nehru have adapted these traditions to the modern world (Sharma and Daugert 1965).

It was seen from the time of Ancient Greece up to the present day that there were two principal schools of ethics. Some moralists maintained that ethical conceptions are inspired in humans from above, and they accordingly connected ethics with religion. Other thinkers saw the source of morality in humans and endeavored to free ethics from the consent of religion and to create a realistic morality.

Beginning in the 1500s, modern history saw an emerging change in the understanding of ethics, one related to a revolution in science and technology. Immanuel Kant (1724–1804) connected duty to ethics. His ethics relies on the notion that "morality is grounded in reason, not in tradition, intuition, conscience, emotion, or attitudes such as sympathy". Kant recognizes two general categories of duties. A perfect duty is one everyone must always observe, such as duty not to harm another person, and imperfect duties, such as acting with kindness.

John Stuart Mill (1806–1873), an English philosopher of the early modern period, stressed that actions are ethical if they promote happiness. Throughout his life, he tried to persuade the British public for the need of a scientific method to understanding social, political, and economic change. He believed that there is no such thing as inborn ideas, no such thing as moral principles.

The work of Darwin (1809–1882) was not only limited to biology. Already in 1837, when he had just written a rough outline of his theory of the origin of species, he entered in his notebook this significant remark: "My theory will lead to a new philosophy". And so it did in reality. By introducing the idea of evolution into the study of organic life, he opened a new era in philosophy, and his later sketch of the development of the moral sense turned a new page in ethics (Kropotkin 1922).

2.8 Ethical theories and approaches

> *The platform of an Ethical Society is itself the altar; the address must be the fire that burns thereon.*

Felix Adler

For centuries, philosophers have come up with various theoretical approaches about good and bad or right and wrong within a society and for providing guidelines about how to live and act ethically. They have demonstrated a nurturing interest in applying moral theories to real-world problems.

2.8.1 Philosophical branches of ethics

Ethics can be divided into three branches that have been developed and explained throughout the history of philosophy. To summarize, ethics is distinguished in the following three branches: metaethics, normative, and applied, as shown in Table 2.3.

2.8.2 Ethical tools for problem-solving

Ethics as a discipline explores how the world should be understood and how people ought to act. There are many schools of thought within the study of ethics, which differ not only in the answers that they offer but in the ways they formulate basic questions of how to understand the world and to respond to the ethical challenges it presents. Most (though not all) work in ethics, both academically and in the wider world, has a normative purpose: that is, it argues how people ought to act (Burton et al. 2017).

Most approaches to understanding the world through ethics adopt one of the three major critical orientations: deontological ethics, utilitarianism

Table 2.3 Three branches of ethics

Branch	Outline
Metaethics	This theory addresses the origin and definition of people's ethical principles. Metaethics deals with whether morality exists. Universal truths, God's will, the meaning of ethical terms, and how reason plays a role in ethical decisions are all a part of metaethics.
Normative	Morals refer to generally accepted standards of right and wrong in society, often learned during childhood, but ethics are learned at the time of conflict of the problems. Normative ethics assumes an assenting answer to the existence question, deals with the rational structure of moral principles, and at its maximum level, determines what the ultimate principle of morality is.
Applied	Applied ethics involves the application of normative ethical theories to particular cases. It deals with difficult moral questions and controversial moral issues that people actually face in their lives in various areas, including for instance social and political ethics, computer ethics, medical ethics, bioethics, environmental ethics, business ethics, and it also relates to different forms of professional ethics. The basic goal of applied ethics is to establish a desirable principle of conduct in specific areas to which it relates. Given their situational nature, they are often distinct from one another.

(sometimes called consequentialism), and virtue ethics (Burton et al. 2017). Table 2.4 outlines the above three moral and ethical tools.

In order to develop workable ethical problem-solving techniques, it is necessary first to look at several theories of ethics in order to have a framework for decision-making. Ethical problem-solving is not as cut and dried as problem-solving in engineering classes. In most engineering classes, there is generally just one theory to consider when tackling a problem. In studying engineering ethics, there are several theories that will be considered. The relatively large number of theories does not indicate a weakness in theoretical understanding of ethics or a "fuzziness" of ethical thinking. It somewhat reflects the complexity of ethical problems and the diversity of approaches to ethical problem-solving that have been developed over the centuries. Having multiple theories to apply essentially enhances the problem-solving process, allowing problems to be looked at from various perspectives, since each theory emphasizes different aspects of a problem (Fleddermann 2012).

Ethical decision-making is not easy. However, the chances for successfully resolving an ethical conflict can be greatly increased by following a

Table 2.4 Basic moral and ethical tools

Approach and question	Summary
Deontology *What is my duty?*	Deontology understands ethics to be about following the moral law. It was developed by Immanuel Kant in the late 18th century but has ancient roots in both Divine Command traditions (such as ancient Israelite religion, the source of the Ten Commandments and the basis of Judaism, Christianity, and Islam) and in other legal codes.
Utilitarianism or Consequentialism *What is the greatest possible good for the greatest number?*	Utilitarian ethics was developed by Jeremy Bentham and John Stuart Mill in the late eighteenth to mid-nineteenth century. In computer science, and broadly in the social sciences, we use "utility" as a proxy for individual goodness and the sum of individual utilities as a measure of social welfare, often without reflecting on the possibility of thinking about social good in other ways.
Virtue or Teleological *Who should I be?*	Virtue ethics is focused on ends or goals. Grounded in Aristotle and outlined most clearly in the Nicomachean ethics, virtue ethics is organized around developing habits and dispositions that help a person achieve his or her goals, and, by extension, to help them flourish as an individual.

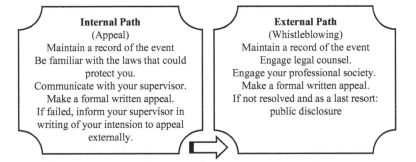

Figure 2.4 Path of resolving ethical problems.

systematic procedure. Figure 2.4 presents one set of guidelines that will help ensure meeting one's professional responsibilities. Except under the uncommon situations of imminent danger to the public, it is important that all inner procedures should be investigated before seeking options outside of the organization.

2.9   Codes of ethics and professional conduct

*If you do not know the laws of right conduct, you cannot
form your character.*

Swami Sivananda

It is not possible to separate professionalism from ethics nor consider professional ethics different from general ethics. The fear of this possibility often contributes to the formation of professional codes as guides of principles designed to help professionals conduct business decently and with integrity. It results when a discipline organizes itself into a profession. The resulting code is vital to guide professionals, to judge their conduct, and to recognize their profession.

2.9.1   Integrity and professional ethics

Professional integrity and honesty are crucial for personal credibility and professional success. Integrity is one of the central values that employers pursue in those that they employ. It is the trait of a person who demonstrates sound moral and ethical principles in the workplace. On the other hand, honesty is an optimal example of integrity in the workplace. It fosters communication between employers and employees. Acting with honor and openness are also basic ideologies in a person with integrity.

Confidentiality is a major example of integrity in the workplace. It is also a legal necessity. Employers have a duty to keep certain information private. Breach of privacy could lead to fines, penalties, and possible lawsuits. Confidentiality implants trust and encourages honest consideration of the privacy of others. Another related principle of integrity is credibility, which allows employers and their employees to build good relations based on mutual respect and trust. A key element of credibility involves transparency and certainty.

Employers and employees can display integrity in the workplace through "leading by example". When individuals lead by example, they set the basis for proper workplace behavior. Leading by example improves personal awareness, sensitivity to others, and accountability, which are all necessary for ethical behavior and integrity (Scott 2018).

Integrity requires strong moral principles, good character, honor, and honesty. It is an individual choice to hold one's self to consistent standards. In professional relationships, integrity is a much sought-after trait, while in ethics, integrity is considered as the honesty and truthfulness or accuracy of one's actions. Professional integrity and ethical behavior are crucial for personal credibility and professional success within any organization. Therefore, professional integrity means that the individual will operate in a professional and ethical manner within the workforce, regardless of whatever situation the individual is faced with.

2.9.2   Incorporating ethics into practice

A code is seen as one of the hallmarks of a profession, because people who form the profession are often in positions of power and those whom they serve are dependent upon the competence and integrity of the professionals. A code of ethics frequently includes a set of formal, written statements about the purpose of an organization, its values, and the principles that should guide its employees' actions. An effective code of ethics helps ensure that employees abide by the law, follow necessary regulations, and behave in an ethical manner (Reynolds 2015). Codes of ethics are a key component of the membership of professional organizations (Leicester 2016).

A code of ethics defines the overall aims of the profession, the ideals to which organizations aspire, so that they provide a sense of direction. It generally emerges when an occupation organizes itself into a profession. A code lays down the minimum standards of conduct that are considered suitable. It expresses the rights, duties, and obligations of the members of the profession. Largely, a code of ethics provides a context for ethical judgment for a profession. However, no code can be entirely complete and cover all possible ethical situations that a professional may encounter. Codes may serve somewhat as an initial point for ethical decision-making. Importantly, a code of ethics may designate to the public that the profession is genuinely concerned about responsible and professional conduct.

Mostly, a code of ethics provides broad standards that make a framework for ethical judgment for a profession. No code can be totally comprehensive and cover all possible ethical situations that a professional is likely to encounter. Rather, codes serve as a starting point for ethical decision-making. A code can also express the commitment to ethical conduct shared by members of a profession (Harris et al. 1995). In general, codes of ethics include what the organization aspires to become and rules and principles by which members of the organization are expected to act.

When ethics is applied to a profession, it defines a code of standards governing fair and responsible conduct with other members of a profession and the general public. In association with engineering and computing, ethics concerns the relationship of technology, society, and the people who use them. Most recently, the concept of engineering and computing ethics has extended philosophical consideration well beyond human behavior to explore the ethical properties of information objects (Floridi 2008). In general, ethical standards include legal requirements, codes of ethics, and moral and personal values. Many codes also contain obligations to continue education for members who practice the profession.

2.9.3   Codes and organizations

Most codes of ethics created by professional organizations have two kinds of harmonizing standards: the first outlines what the organization aspires to become (code of ethics), and the second typically lists rules and principles by which members of the organization are expected to abide in order to avoid possible disciplinary action (code of professional conduct) (Reynolds 2015). Both codes are an aspirational system of principles or guidelines that set satisfactory behaviors for a profession. They are useful to define accepted and acceptable behaviors and to promote high standards of professional practice. Their task is not to derive obligations but to spell out what the public anticipates from the profession. They express the rights, duties, and obligations of members of the profession. Professionally, the code of ethics is a comprehensive guide to professional conduct. Many codes also include a commitment to continuing education for those who practice the profession. Every profession has its professional ethics; for example, engineers, lawyers, and physicians typically adhere to a code of ethics. No computing professional organization has emerged as preeminent, so there is no universal code of ethics for computing specialists. It is important to note that a code of ethics is not a legal document, so a professional cannot be arrested for violating its provisions.

2.9.4   Evolution of codes

Professional engineering societies in the US began to be structured in the late nineteenth century, with new societies created as new engineering fields developed. Codes of ethics for engineers were established along with their corresponding professional societies. As these societies matured, many of them created codes of ethics to guide practicing engineers. The first engineering organization in the US, the Boston Society of Civil Engineers, was founded in 1848. The American Society of Civil Engineers (ASCE) was founded four years later. In 1906, the American Institute of Electrical Engineers (AIEE) voted to embody in a code the ideas expressed in an address by its president, Schuyler Wheeler. After much debate and many revisions, the AIEE board of directors adopted a code in 1912. The AIEE code was adopted by the ASME in 1914. Meanwhile, the American Institute of Consulting Engineering (AICE), the American Institute of Chemical Engineers (AIChE), and ASCE each adopted their own code. By 1915, every major engineering organization in the US had a code of ethics.

In the mid-20th century there was a proliferation of important codes of ethics that still guide engineering professional behavior and research activities. The first reference to the National Society of Professional Engineers (NSPE) code of ethics is found in the May 1935 issue of *The*

American engineer in the form of a suggestion for membership consideration. In 1946, the NSPE board of directors approved the canons of ethics for engineers (NSPE 2018).

2.10   Examples of professional codes

> *Ethics is in origin the art of recommending to others the*
> *sacrifices required for cooperation with oneself.*
>
> **Bertrand Russell**
> *[from Russell on Ethics: Selections from the*
> *Writings of Bertrand Russell (1999)]*

2.10.1   NSPE

In July 2007, the NSPE approved its professional obligations as follows: Engineers shall at all times strive to serve the public interest (NSPE 2018), as outlined. Engineers in the fulfillment of their professional duties shall:

- Hold paramount the safety, health, and welfare of the public
- Perform services only in areas of their competence
- Issue public statements only in an objective and truthful manner
- Act for each employer or client as faithful agents or trustees
- Avoid deceptive acts
- Conduct themselves honorably, responsibly, ethically, and lawfully so as to enhance the honor, reputation, and usefulness of the profession

2.10.2   IEEE

Today, the IEEE code of ethics, as part of the IEEE policies, begins with the phrase: "to accept responsibility in making engineering decisions consistent with the safety, health and welfare of the public, and to disclose promptly factors that might endanger the public or the environment". This clearly outlines that the safety of the public and environment is of utmost importance to the IEEE. Clearly, this code is very general, aiming to provide ethical rules for all electrical and electronic engineers. The IEEE code for conduct, approved and issued in June 2014, is given in IEEE (2014). This code has ten attributes of ethical commitment:

- To accept responsibility in making decisions consistent with the safety, health, and welfare of the public, and to disclose promptly factors that might endanger the public or the environment
- To avoid real or perceived conflicts of interest whenever possible, and to disclose them to affected parties when they do exist

- To be honest and realistic in stating claims or estimates based on available data
- To reject bribery in all its forms
- To improve the understanding of technology, its appropriate application, and potential consequences
- To maintain and improve our technical competence and to undertake technological tasks for others only if qualified by training or experience, or after full disclosure of pertinent limitations
- To seek, accept, and offer honest criticism of technical work, to acknowledge and correct errors, and to credit properly the contributions of others
- To treat fairly all persons regardless of such factors as race, religion, gender, disability, age, or national origin
- To avoid injuring others, their property, reputation, or employment by false or malicious action
- To assist colleagues and coworkers in their professional development and to support them in following this code of ethics

2.10.3   Engineers Canada

Engineers Canada's code of ethics sets out broad principles related to ethics and professionalism, while a complementary code of conduct provides more detailed guidance based on the application of the code to business practices. Violations of both the code of ethics and the code of conduct are clearly defined as professional misconduct. The code of ethics applies to all registrants, including limited license/permit holders and engineers-in-training. The code of ethics states that registrants:

- Shall conduct themselves with integrity and in an honorable and ethical manner
- Shall uphold the values of truth, honesty, and trustworthiness and safeguard human life and welfare and the environment
- Hold paramount the safety, health, and welfare of the public and the protection of the environment, and promote health and safety within the workplace
- Offer services, advise on or undertake engineering assignments only in areas of their competence, and practice in a careful and diligent manner and in compliance with applicable legislation
- Act as faithful agents of their clients or employers, maintain confidentiality, and avoid conflicts of interest but, where such conflicts arise, fully disclose the circumstances without delay to the employer or client
- Keep themselves informed in order to maintain their competence and advance their knowledge in the field within which they practice

- Conduct themselves with integrity, equity, fairness, courtesy, and good faith towards clients, colleagues, and others, give credit where it is due; and accept, as well as give, honest and fair professional criticism
- Present clearly to employers and clients the possible consequences if engineering decisions or judgments are overruled or disregarded
- Report to their association or other appropriate agencies any illegal or unethical engineering decisions or practices by engineers or others
- Be aware of and ensure that clients and employers are made aware of societal and environmental consequences of actions or projects and endeavor to interpret engineering issues to the public in an objective and truthful manner
- Treat equitably and promote the equitable and dignified treatment of people in accordance with human rights legislation
- Uphold and enhance the honor and dignity of the profession

2.10.4 *Worcester Polytechnic Institute (WPI) code for robotics*

As stated in WPI (2010), this code was written to address the current state of robotics engineering and cannot be expected to account for all possible future developments in such a rapidly developing field:

- Consider and respect people's physical well-being and rights
- Not knowingly misinform, and if misinformation is spread, do my best to correct it
- Respect and follow local, national, and international laws whenever applicable
- Recognize and disclose any conflicts of interest
- Accept and offer constructive criticism
- Help and assist colleagues in their professional development and in following this code

2.10.5 *Australian Computer Society (ACS)*

This ACS code of professional conduct identifies six core ethical values and the associated requirements for professional conduct. The ACS requires its members to abide by these values and act with responsibility and integrity in all of their professional dealings (ACS 2014).

- **The primacy of the public interest:** Place the interests of the public above those of personal, business, or sectional interests.
- **The enhancement of quality of life:** Strive to enhance the quality of life of those affected by your work.

- **Honesty:** Be honest in your representation of skills, knowledge, services, and products.
- **Competence:** Work competently and diligently for your stakeholders.
- **Professional development:** Enhance one's own professional development and that of staff.
- **Professionalism:** Enhance the integrity of the ACS and the respect of its members for each other.

2.11   Applied ethics

To have a sense of education and ethics is important.

Soleil Moon Frye

This section deals with applied ethics and systems of moral principles that relate to the practice of engineering and computing. It involves responsibilities and rights that ought to be recognized by those engaged in these practices.

2.11.1   Categories of engineering ethics

McLean (1993), an engineer, uses three categories in discussing engineering ethics. These include professional ethics, dealing with interactions among managers, engineers, and employers; technical ethics, covering technical decisions by engineers; and social ethics, concerning sociopolitical decisions about technology. Figure 2.5 shows the above three categories of ethics.

Professional ethics implies the ethics that a person must hold with respect to their interactions and business dealings in their professional life.

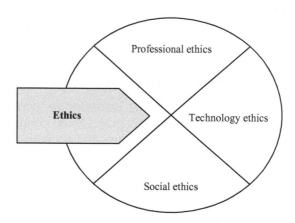

Figure 2.5 Categories of ethics related to engineering.

They provide guidance for interaction between professionals such that they can serve both each other and the whole society in the best way, without the fear of other professionals undercutting them with less ethical actions (Beabout and Wennenmann 1993). Such codes are available in most professions and are different from moral codes, which are used in the education and religion of an entire larger society. Ethical codes are more specialized than moral codes, more internally consistent, and typically simple to be applied by an ordinary practitioner of the profession, without the need for extensive interpretation (Rowan and Sinaich 2002).

Technology ethics is a transdisciplinary area that draws on theories and techniques from several knowledge domains such as engineering, computing, science, and social sciences to provide insights on ethical dimensions of technological systems and practices for advancing a technological society. It views technology and ethics as socially embedded enterprises and aims to discover the ethical use of technology, protecting against the misuse of technology and devising common principles to guide new advances in technological development and application to benefit society (Luppicini 2010).

Social ethics deals with human needs. It comprises demanding, careful reflection on the means that moral ideas and practices are exemplified in collective contexts. It deals with human needs and aspirations. It involves a code of conduct created by a society in order to ensure a smooth functioning of the said society.

Engineering has an enormous role to help provide benefits to society, and the idea of social responsibility is very common in engineering ethics. It helps to provide basic needs such as water, food, housing, and energy, and does that in a way that is crucial for the industrial sector to function. One of the most powerful gifts of engineering is how it improves lives. But, in the wrong hands, it can be just the opposite. The work of engineers is critical to many aspects of the economic and social progress of humanity. Contributing in this way requires not only technical competence but also imagination, persistence, and integrity (Murray 2009). At work, engineers and scientists regularly make decisions that have ethical significance or moral relevance at varying scales and aspects of life.

2.11.2   Common ethical issues for computing

Computing is a relatively new discipline and is in a continuous state of innovation. This discipline's infancy and the state of change place computing professionals in a susceptible position ethically, with little discipline-specific precedent or accumulated wisdom on which to base ethical practice (Stoodley 2009). National and cultural differences may make it difficult to determine what is and is not ethical, especially when it comes to computing. People of different nationalities and cultures have different perspectives; difficulties arise when one nationality's or culture's ethical behavior violates the ethics of another nationality or culture.

Computing ethics involves the nature and grounds of moral judgment, standards, and rules of conduct in using computing for decision-making. Computing users encounter more ethical challenges in the age of computing because using computing to do something that is not illegal does not imply it is ethical. Some of main ones are debated below.

There are ways in which computing has brought benefits to society. There are also ways in which computing has been misused, leading to serious ethical issues. The professional's roles of designer, manager, and user of computing bring with them a responsibility to help foster the ethical use of computers (Fleddermann 2012). Today, computing is facing some serious ethical challenges, and it is up to the experts and users to be ready for these challenges. As more emerging computing pops up on the market, most of the experts and users do not know how to go about the challenges brought about by these technologies. At the same time, computing is facing major challenges, which are lack of privacy, security, identity theft, stalking, copyright infringement, and various computer crimes. Criminals have been eagerly utilizing the many loopholes technology offers (Ramey 2012).

Making ethical judgments is not simply like expressing opinions, subjective conclusions that cannot be reasonably debated. Engineers and computing professionals, as well as other professionals, have a similar ethical responsibility to not cause harm or unreasonable risk of harm not only to individuals affected by their work but also to public welfare or the public interest (McGinn 2018). They must always work to serve the interest of the client and the public to the best of their ability, taking into consideration that no conflict of interest shall exist.

2.11.3   *Online resource on ethics*

Ethical problems are more open-ended, like design problems and are not as susceptible to formulaic answers as are problems assigned in typical engineering classes. They rarely have a correct answer that will be arrived at by everyone in the class (Fleddermann 2012).

An online resource on ethics for engineering and science maintained by the Center for Engineering Ethics and Society (CEES) at the NAE is available at: www.onlineethics.org. It provides engineers, scientists, faculty, and students with resources for understanding and addressing ethically significant issues that arise in scientific and engineering practice and from the developments of science and engineering; and serves those who promote learning and advance understanding of responsible research and practice in engineering and science.

2.12 Distinction between ethics

> More often there's a compromise between ethics and expediency.

Peter Singer

The distinction between ethics is useful for mapping the role of professionals on its negative and positive faces in making decisions consistent with safety, health, and welfare of the public.

2.12.1 Microethics and macroethics

Engineering ethics entails three frames of reference: individual, professional, and social. Microethics considers individual and internal relations of the profession, including health and safety, and bribes and gifts. On the other hand, macroethics applies to the collective social responsibility of the profession and to societal decisions about technology, including sustainable development and product liability (Herkert 2005). Social ethics deals with human needs and aspirations. Engineering has an enormous role to help provide benefits to society, and the idea of social responsibility is very common in professional ethics.

Vanderburg (1995) draws a distinction between microlevel analysis of individual technologies or practitioners and macrolevel analysis of technology as a whole. Also, Ladd (1980), an ethicist, argues that professional ethics can be delineated as microethics or macroethics depending on whether the focus is on relationships between individuals and their clients, colleagues, and employers or on the collective social responsibility of the profession.

Many engineers and ethicists are critical of the traditional preoccupation of engineering ethics with specific moral dilemmas confronting individuals and call for greater attention to macroethical issues related to the societal implications of technology as a complement to the traditional microethical approach that focuses on individual cases. One response to this critique would be to broaden discussions of engineering ethics so as to include the ethical implications of public policy issues relevant to engineering, such as risk and product liability, sustainable development, globalization, healthcare, and IT (Herkert 2000). Research and teaching related to engineering ethics have for the most part focused on microanalysis of individual ethical dilemmas in areas like health and safety issues in engineering design, conflict of interest, representation of test data, whistle-blowing, quality control, trade secrets, and gift giving, with little attention being paid to macroethics in engineering, and still fewer attempts to integrate both microethical and macroethical approaches to engineering ethics (Herket 2005).

2.12.2 *Preventive to aspirational ethics*

Ethics can be divided into a negative part, which focuses on preventing disasters and professional misconduct, and a positive part, which is oriented toward producing a better life for mankind through technology.

Preventive ethics describes activities performed by an individual or group on behalf of an organization to identify, prioritize, and address systemic ethics quality gaps. The overall goal of preventive ethics is to measurably improve ethics quality by identifying, prioritizing, and addressing ethics quality gaps on a systems level. Thus, the central focus of preventive ethics is to reduce unjustifiable variation in ethical practices, thereby improving overall ethics quality within an organization. To be effective, the preventive ethics function requires adequate integration, leadership support, expertise, staff time, and resources (Cook et al. 2015). Critical success factors also include access, accountability, organizational learning, and evaluation.

A look at engineering codes of ethics will show not only that they are primarily sets of rules but also that these rules are for the most part negative in character. The rules are often in the form of prohibitions, or statements that probably should be understood primarily as prohibitions. This negative character of the codes is probably entirely appropriate, and it is easy to think of several reasons for this negative orientation (Harris et al. 1995). One of the limitations of negative ethics is the relative absence of the motivational dimension. Engineers do not choose engineering as a career in order to prevent disasters and avoid professional misconduct. A related term for aspirational ethics is macroethics, the effort to collectively make the best possible engineering decisions on critical issues that have global impact, such as sustainable development, stem cell research, and climate change (Crawford 2012).

To be sure, many engineering students desire the financial rewards and social aspiration that an engineering career promises, and this is legitimate. This positive aspect of the profession is recognized to some extent in codes of ethics. The first fundamental canon of the NSPE code of ethics, for example, requires engineers to promote the "welfare" of the public, as well as to prevent violations of safety and health. Virtually all of the major engineering codes begin with similar statements. Therefore, there is a need to re-focus from preventive to aspirational ethics (Harris et al. 1995). This would be a shift away from preventive ethics, which concerns itself with the prevention of professional misconduct and harm to the public from technology.

2.13 *Knowledge acquisition*

Attempting to answer the following questions involves acquisition of knowledge from this book and other books, documents, and the Internet.

- What is a profession? Who is a professional?
- What is a professional practice?
- What is expected from a professional?
- What does good professional practice in the workplace consist of? Provide three examples.
- What does poor professional practice in the workplace consist of? Provide three examples.
- Why did software engineering emerge as such a compelling model for professional development?
- Why is professional accreditation important?
- What must one do to maintain professional certification?
- What is specialty certification and why is needed?
- How does certification relate to licensure?
- For what reason can a certificate of authorization be canceled?
- Why does the software engineering model appeal to employers?
- What is ethics about? Are there universal ethical principles?
- What is the meaning of "duty" or "right" or "morally good"?
- Explain the difference between values, morality, and professional ethics.
- Explain the difference between moral and legal responsibility.
- What are the three major ethical theories?
- What ethics can professionals learn from the past?
- How does ethics differ from law?
- What is a conflict of interest?
- Is integrity the main principle in professional behavior? If yes, why?
- Is there a need to enforce the membership of professional associations in order to ensure people adhere to an ethical code in order to practice?
- Can a code of ethics be unwritten?
- What is the meaning of ethical responsibility?
- What do code and standards cover?
- What do professional ethics include?
- What is applied ethics? When and why did applied ethics appear?
- What is the purpose of professional code?
- What are the factors that influence social ethics?
- How do computing professionals experience ethics these days?
- Why should engineers and computing specialists study ethics?
- What are the critical success factors for preventive ethics?
- What trends have increased the risk of using computing in an unethical manner?
- How do codes of ethics, professional organizations, certification, and licensing affect the ethical behavior of computing professionals?
- What are some of the key ethical issues associated with the use of social networking Web sites?

- Discuss how and when engineers and computing specialists are not the guardians of their profession?
- What are traits of professional character that make a good engineer?
- What is whistle-blowing, and what ethical issues are associated with it?
- Conduct an Internet search for landmark cases in engineering and computing ethics. Summarize two important cases.
- Is a professional required to keep up-to-date with technical developments in the professional's specific field of interest?
- What are the greatest ethical challenges engineers and computing specialists currently face in their workplaces?
- Explain by example how the development and use of technology poses ethical challenges.
- What are the consequences to an organization that uses persons without professional qualifications in positions which are generally considered to require professional engineering expertise?
- Can an organization, holding a Certificate of Authorization, still provide services to the public if the professional engineer named on the certificate is fired or resigns?

2.14   Knowledge creation

Collaborate with peers on learning or you may work with others outside the class to narrow down the objectives of each activity. You may access class and online resources and analyze data and information to create new ideas and balanced solutions. High-level digital tools may be used to develop multimedia presentations, simulations or animations, videos and visual displays, digital portfolios, reflective practice (online publishing and blogging), or well-researched and up-to-date reports.

2.14.1   Case for discussion

An electrical engineer works for a consulting company that designs small substations for wind energy farms. The supervisor asked the engineer to replicate a set of drawings and changed the name of the client, stating that a new client has a wind farm with identical specifications to the last project the engineer worked on, so the same design will work. When the engineer asked how to bill the time, the answer was to enter the same number of hours that were billed for the initial design work. What do you think about this process? Analyze and report this ethical scenario in a one-page written report.

2.14.2 Preventive ethics and aspirational ethics

The OEC (www.onlineethics.org) seeks submission of high-quality ethics education resources in science and engineering for inclusion in its collection. Interdisciplinary materials are particularly welcome, as are resources that promote active learning at the undergraduate or graduate level. For this task, students may visit the online resource, and in particular the "Resources" section, where they will come across hundreds of case studies, essays, codes and policies, and multimedia activities. Students may work in teams to develop a video that distinguishes preventive ethics from aspirational ethics using real-life examples and cases related to engineering and/or computing. Although the distinction between these two categories is not always sharp, it is believed that such a distinction is useful. For submission, see the "Submit Materials" page.

2.14.3 Piece of art on macroethics

Promoting the welfare of the public may be done in various ways, ranging from designing a sustainable energy efficient system in the course of an engineer's ordinary employment to using one's vacation time to develop a water purification system in an underdeveloped country. For this activity, use an example of a project based on macroethics that involves a spectrum of engineering activities and reflect issues related to positive aspects of ethics in a digital poster or video.

2.14.4 Embedded ethics content on future technologies

To create an environment where expertise from various discipline can be exchanged, discussed, debated, and shared about ethics of AI. In this task, collaborate with peers or work with others outside the class to develop the ethical content for a typical computing course. The content component could be a lab session where students can gain access to information about future technologies. This method provides an opportunity to help students understand the ethical and social implications of their work. It empowers students to build models that shape the direction of innovation to be more reflective on the social implications of their work. For this task, propose approaches to address the issue in general and your view in particular. Ethical perspectives employed in content range from traditional ethics (which considers whether actions are required, recommended, or forbidden) to issues of individual (microethical) and collective (macroethical) responsibility. The focus throughout the task may focus on responsibilities rather than outcomes. This ethical development may include allocations of cost and benefits, risks and rewards, social and environmental justice, and professional and organizational ethics.

2.14.5   Online discussion forum

As a supplementary course support, an online discussion forum may be established by a group of students in which an ethical subject that will be discussed in the class should be published in advance. Several examples from everyday life can be proposed, in particular from engineering and computing, such as AI and elements drawn from science fiction literature. The purpose is to demonstrate the importance of moral imagination and to connect the philosophical reflection with the real world. This aims to show that ethical thinking does not involve theoretical principles only but stems from real-life and professional circumstances.

References

ACS. 2014. ACS code of professional conduct professional standards board Australian computer society. https://www.acs.org.au/content/dam/acs/rules-and-regulations/Code-of-Professional-Conduct_v2.1.pdf.

AHS. 2016. Professional practice in action: A guide to professional practice at Alberta health services. https://www.albertahealthservices.ca/assets/about/msd/ahs-msd-com-ppa-guid-professional-practice-guide.pdf.

ASPA. 2013. The authoritative voice of specialized and professional accreditation. Association of Specialized and Professional Accreditors. http://www.aspa-usa.org/wp-content/uploads/2015/02/ASPA_WhoWeAre_June11-edited.pdf.

Aynsley, B. 2018. Common understandings of the challenges facing the ICT profession: An Australian case study. https://www.itu.int/en/ITU-D/Regional-Presence/Europe/Documents/Brenda-ACS%20Slides-2.pdf.

Balthazard, C. 2015. What does it mean to be a professional? Human Resources Professionals Association. https://www.hrpa.ca/Documents/Designations/Job-Ready-Program/What-it-means-to-be-a-professional.pdf.

Beabout, G. R., and D. J. Wennenmann. 1993. *Applied Professional Ethics*. Milburn, NJ: University Press of America.

Burton, E., J. Goldsmith, S. Koenig, B. Kuipers, N. Mattei, and T. Walsh. 2017. Ethical considerations in artificial intelligence courses. White Paper. https://arxiv.org/pdf/1701.07769.pdf.

CAA. 2016. Engineering instruction and accreditation. Consultation on Advances in Accreditation. https://engineerscanada.ca/sites/default/files/ec-consultation-document.pdf.

Carroll, B. 2015. A professional practices course in computer science and engineering. 122nd ASEE Annual Conference and Exposition, Seattle, June 17. file:///C:/Users/Dr%20Habash/Downloads/A_Professional_Practices_Course_for_CSE__Final_04032015.pdf.

Carr-Saunders, A. M., and P. A. Wilson. 1933. *The Professions*. Oxford, UK: Clarendon Press.

CCAPP. 2018. Accreditation standards for Canadian first professional degree in pharmacy programs. The Canadian Council for Accreditation of Pharmacy Programs. http://ccapp-accredit.ca/wp-content/uploads/2016/01/Accredit ation-Standards-for-Canadian-First-Professional-Degree-in-Pharmacy-Pro grams.pdf.

Cook, R. S., M. B. Foglia, M. K. Landon, and M. M. Bottrell. 2015. *Preventive Ethics: Addressing Ethics Quality Gaps on a Systems Level.* Second Edition. National Center for Ethics in Health Care. Washington, DC: U.S. Department of Veterans Affairs. https://www.ethics.va.gov/docs/integratedethics/pe _primer_2_edition_042015.pdf.

Crawford, M. 2012. Engineers must embrace aspirational ethics. https://ww w.asme.org/engineering-topics/articles/engineering-ethics/engineers-mu st-embrace-aspirational-ethics.

DPMA. 1962. Report, Six Measures of Professionalism, Charles Babbage Institute. Archives, CBI 88, Box 21, Fld. 40., University of Minnesota, Minneapolis.

Ensmenger, N. L. 2001. The "question of professionalism" in the computer fields. *IEEE Annals of the History of Computing* 23(4): 56–74.

Erdogmus, H. 2011. The seven traits of superprofessionals. *IEEE Software* 26(4): 4–6.

Evetts, J. 2012. Professionalism: Value and ideology. University of Nottingham, UK. http://www.sagepub.net/isa/resources/pdf/Professionalism.pdf.

Fleddermann, C. B. 2012. *Engineering Ethics.* Fourth Edition. Upper Saddle River, NJ: Prentice Hall.

Floridi, L. 2008. Information ethics: Its nature and scope. In van den Hoven, J., and J. Weckert (eds.). *Moral Philosophy and Information Technology.* Cambridge, UK: Cambridge University Press.

Ford, G., and N. E. Gibbs. 1996. A mature profession of software engineering. CMU/SEI-96-TR-004, Software Engineering Institute, Carnegie Mellon University, Pittsburgh, PA. https://resources.sei.cmu.edu/asset_files/Tec hnicalReport/1996_005_001_16460.pdf.

Goode, W. J. 1957. Community within a community: The professions. *American Sociological Review* 22(2): 194–200.

Grannan, C. 2018. What's the difference between morality and ethics? https:// www.britannica.com/story/whats-the-difference-between-morality-and-ethics.

Green, B. (ed.). 2009. *Understanding and Researching Professional Practice.* Rotterdam, the Netherlands: Sense Publications.

Harris, C. E., M. S. Pritchard Jr., and M. J. Rabins. 1995. *Engineering Ethics.* Belmont, CA: Wadsworth Publishing Company.

Henninger, E. H. 1991. Ethics and professionalism in higher education. IEEE Frontiers in Education Conference, pp. 156–159. https://ieeexplore.ieee.org/ stamp/stamp.jsp?tp=&arnumber=187460.

Herkert, J. R. 2000. *Engineering Ethics and Public Policy.* Hoboken, NJ: Wiley-IEEE Press.

Herkert, J. R. 2005. Ways of thinking about and teaching ethical problem solving: Microethics and macroethics in engineering. *Science and Engineering Ethics* 11(3): 373–385.

Hurd, H. G. 1967. Who is a professional? *Journal of Cooperative Extension* 85: 77–84.

IEEE. 2014. IEEE code of ethics. https://www.ieee.org/about/corporate/governance/ p7–8.html.

Kemmis, S., and R. McTaggart. 2000. Participatory action research. In Denzin, N., and Y. Lincoln (eds.). *Handbook of Qualitative Research*. Second Edition. Beverly Hills, CA: Sage.

Kropotkin, P. 1922. Ethics: Origin and development. White Paper, New York. https://theanarchistlibrary.org/library/petr-kropotkin-ethics-origin-a nddevelopment.pdf.

Ladd, J. 1980. The quest for a code of professional ethics: An intellectual and moral confusion. In Chalk, R., M. Frankel, and S. Chafer (eds.). *AAAS Professional Ethics Project: Professional Ethics Activities in the Scientific and Engineering Societies*. Washington, DC: AAAS, pp. 154–159.

Leicester, N. 2016. Ethics in the IT profession: Does a code of ethics have an effect on professional behavior. Victoria University of Wellington. https://researc harchive.vuw.ac.nz/xmlui/bitstream/handle/10063/5127/project.pdf? sequence=1.

Levine, M. 1993. Professionalism: The need for a workable code of ethics. https:// ieeexplore.ieee.org/stamp/stamp.jsp?tp=&arnumber=282285.

Ludwig, S. 2013. Domain of competence: Professionalism. https://www.acgme.or g/Portals/0/PDFs/Milestones/ProfessionalismPediatrics.pdf.

Luppicini, R. 2010. *Technoethics and the Evolving Knowledge Society: Ethical Issues in Technological Design, Research, Development, and Innovation*. Hershy, PA: IGI Global.

Manley, D. 2017. ABET versus CEAB accreditation. https://crowdmark.com/blog/ abet-vs-ceab-accreditation/.

McGrinn, R. 2018. *The Ethical Engineer: Contemporary Concepts and Cases*. Princeton, NJ: Princeton University Press.

McLean, G. F. 1993. Integrating ethics with design. *IEEE Technology and Society* 12(3): 18–30.

Murray, T. 2009. An introduction to principles of ethics and morality for scientists and engineers. IDEESE: International Dimensions of Ethics Education in Science and Engineering, University of Massachusetts Amherst, Amherst, MA. http://www.umass.edu/sts/ethics.

NAE. 2004. *The Engineer of 2020: Visions of Engineering in the New Centuries*. Washington, DC: National Academies Press.

Nilsson, S. 2007. From higher education to professional practice: A comparative study of physicians' and engineers' learning and competence use. Linköping studies in Behavioural Science No. 120, Linköping University, Department of Behavioural Sciences and learning, Linköping. https://pdfs.semanticscho lar.org/80e4/2b95e1f3ee7c9e511108c5df14c7440bee4d.pdf.

NSPE. 2013. Professional engineering body of knowledge. Licensure and Qualifications for Practice Committee of the National Society of Professional Engineers. https://www.nspe.org/sites/default/files/resources/nspe-body -of-knowledge.pdf.

NSPE. 2018. History of the code of ethics for engineers. https://www.nspe.org/ resources/ethics/code-ethics/history-code-ethics-engineers.

NYA. 2004. Ethical conduct in youth work: A statement of values and principles from the National Youth Agency. http://www.nya.org.uk/wp-content/up loads/2014/06/Ethical_conduct_in_Youth-Work.pdf.

Oettinger, A. 1966. ACM sponsors professional development program (President's letter to ACM membership). *Communication ACM* 9(10): 712–713.

Perry, T. S. 1981. Knowing how to blow the whistle. *IEEE Spectrum*, 18(9): : 56–61.

PKPA. 2017. Professional accreditation: Mapping the territory. PhillipsKPA Pty Ltd. https://docs.education.gov.au/system/files/doc/other/professional _accreditation_mapping_final_report.pdf.

Ramey, K. 2012. Five ethical challenges of information technology. https://www. useoftechnology.com/5-ethical-challenges-information-technology.

Reynolds, G. W. 2015. *Ethics in Information Technology*. Fifth Edition. Boston, MA: Cengage Learning.

Rowan, J. R., and S. Sinaich Jr. 2002. *Ethics for the Professions*. Boston, MA: Cengage Learning.

Schatzki, T. 2002. *The Site of the Social: A Philosophical Account of the Constitution of Social Life and Change*. University Park, PA: University of Pennsylvania Press.

Scott, S. 2018. Examples of integrity in the workplace. https://smallbusiness.chr on.com/examples-integrity-workplace-10906.html.

Sharma, I. C., and S. Daugert. 1965. *Ethical Philosophies of India*. London, UK: George Allen and Unwin Ltd.

Sheppard, S., A. Colby, K. Macatangay, and W. Sullivan. 2006. What is engineering practice? *International Journal of Engineering Education* 22(3): 429–438.

Shulman, L. S. 1998. Theory, practice, and the education of professionals. *The Elementary School Journal* 98(5): 511–526.

Sizer, R. 1996. A brief history of professionalism and its relevance to IFIP. In Berleur, J., and K. Brunnstein (eds.). *Ethics of Computing: Codes, Spaces for Discussion and Law*. London, UK: Chapman and Hall.

Stoodley, I. 2009. IT professionals' experience of ethics and its implications for IT education. PhD Thesis, Faculty of Science and Technology, Queensland University of Technology, Brisbane, Australia.

Ulrich, W. 2011. What is good performance practice? http://wulrich.com/downlo ads/bimonthly_march2011.pdf.

Vanderburg, W. 1995. Preventive engineering: Strategy for dealing with negative social and environmental implications of technology. *Journal of Professional Issues in Engineering Education and Practice* 121: 155–160.

Velasquez, M., C. Andre, S. J. Shanks, and M. Meyer. 1987. What is ethics? *Journal of Issues in Ethics* 1(1): 44–67.

Wilensky, H. 1964. The professionalization of everyone? *American Journal of Sociology* 70(2): 137–158.

WPI. 2010. Code of ethics for robotics engineers. http://ethics.iit.edu/ecodes/ node/4391.

Legal systems in practice

3.1 Knowledge and understanding

Having successfully completed this module, you should be able to demonstrate knowledge and understanding of:

- Legal systems relevant to engineering and computing, including employment law, contract law, tort, and intellectual property
- The nature and scope in which the employment relationship is regulated by both voluntary and legal measures
- Legal rights and duties important to engineers and computing workers in their professions
- Types and forms of contract negotiation and agreement practices
- Discharge and breach of contract
- Areas of potential exposure to liability in negligence
- Law of tort, its categories, professional negligence, duty of care, standard of care, product liability, and strict liability
- Intellectual property law, management, and building blocks, including patent, copyright, trade secret, and trademark
- Technology transfer practice, including policy and process in the context of progress from initiation to commercialization

3.2 Legal system

At the end of the day you are your own lawmaker.

Bangambiki Habyarimana
[from Book of Wisdom (2017)]

The legal system, in the sense perceived in the quotation above, is not just about a set of laws as shown in Figure 3.1, but goes beyond that to embrace morality, professionalism, codes of ethics, discipline, and rules of law.

The main difference between laws and ethics is that laws carry the authority of a governing body and ethics do not. The purpose of the legal system is to protect each member of society. The legal system is divided into criminal law and civil law. The law is a formalized code of conduct describing what society feels is the proper way to behave. Laws reflect

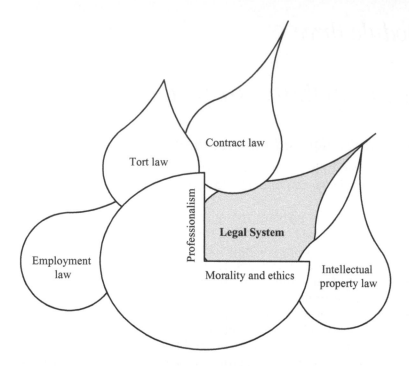

Figure 3.1 Legal system in the context of engineering and computing.

what society's values are. As society evolves, its attitude towards behavior changes, and the laws change as well.

Civil law covers a body of laws that govern a country or state and deal with the relationships and encounters between organizational entities, private affairs, and citizens. Civil law cases are concerned with the law of property, law of contracts, law of torts, and employment law. In this brief module, the latter four categories are discussed. It deals with behaviors that form an injury to an individual or other private party, such as a corporation. Examples are libel and slander, breach of contract, negligence resulting in injury or death, and property damage. In civil law, cases are initiated and suits are filed by a private party (the plaintiff). Cases are usually decided by a judge, though significant cases may involve juries; punishments mostly consist of a monetary award.

Criminal law deals with crimes against society such as murder, arson, bribery, perjury, etc. It addresses activities and conduct harmful to society and is actively enforced by the state. Law can also be categorized as private or public. Private law includes family law, commercial law, and labor law and regulates the relationship between individuals and organizations.

Public law regulates the structure and administration of government agencies and their relationships with citizens, employees, and other governments. Public law includes criminal, administrative, and constitutional law.

3.3   Why legal system for engineers?

If you're a lawyer, you talk about great law cases. If you're an engineer, you talk about giant monuments or innovations.

Rae Drew

Why should engineering and computing students learn about law? While they may be reluctant to dedicate some time to a subject like law, there are certain laws that professionals should be familiar with in order to solve or avoid problems during their careers.

3.3.1   Thinking like a lawyer

The label of "thinking like a lawyer" involves critical reasoning that is typically abstract and backward-looking, confronting uncertainties and questions that seldom have right answers. Thinking like a lawyer demands a severe commitment to logic and the sacrifice of one's own bias. On the other hand, "thinking like an engineer" is quantitative and includes being adept at seeing interrelations, adaptive, and comfortable with trial and error (Ottino 2016).

Law is basically different from engineering, since it is completely a human paradigm. People write laws, interpret laws, and enforce laws. Usually, a lawyer usually thinks about duties for action and recognizing the danger of not being properly qualified to do something. A lawyer is likely to look to rules on how to act in certain situations considering the policies that guide the workplace and the consequences of breaching these policies. Finally, the lawyer puts a premium on being convincing (as opposed to being right). The engineer, on the other hand, puts being right well ahead of being convincing (Buckland 2012). Is it any wonder then that both lawyers and engineers cannot believe the other and do not understand the real world? In a way, both are right.

Obviously, some key similarities bridge the gap. However, the two professions have essentially different principles and different ways of seeing the world. A dynamic partnership between law and engineering is needed. This will establish a constant dialogue to think of questions about the practice of law to new technology and the adjustment within law due to technological change. How does one bridge the real gap of having engineers and lawyers appreciate and work with one another, perhaps even learn how to better think like the other? What are the creative educational opportunities to approach that?

3.3.2   *Law basics for a future career*

Bridging the above contrast is reason enough for the student to learn about legal systems relevant to engineering and computing. One's motivation should be that it is professionally useful to be familiar with various aspects of law. Also the topic is interesting, especially in gaining additional legal knowledge. In general, at some time in their career, professionals have to deal with the law, such as contractual relationships, tort law, and intellectual property (IP) law. They have to deal with other parties such as vendors, contractors, consultants, and insurance companies either on behalf of the firm they work for or for their own firm. It is therefore worthwhile to learn the law and to be familiar with legal terminology in order to follow regulations, protect work, avoid lawsuits, know the boundaries of liability, and comply with government rules.

Contracts may potentially play a big part in a professional's career. They like safety systems when it comes to design. Reading a contract is similar to reading a computer program where it is necessary to read for every word, every statement, and pay attention to everything. Also, professionals may need to understand the various laws regulating employment and the workplace. Usually, laws cover everything from hiring practices to workers' compensation. Health and safety laws can be especially important in the field. There are also laws stopping discrimination in the workplace, laws regulating medical leave, and laws defending workers' rights.

For technical specialists working in a research and development (R&D) environment, a working knowledge of legal aspects of IP rights and patents would be essential. Then, for such specialists who move into management, they should additionally know about the legal aspects of licensing agreements and joint venture agreements. For entrepreneurs who want to initiate their own firms, all of the above are significant.

Recognition of the value of business aspects of technology in society is becoming very important in today's world. In terms of a career path for young practicing engineers and computing professionals, learning law relevant to their work not only provides students with an opportunity to take a peek into another world and try their hand at another discipline, it provides them with knowledge of the legal framework in a specialized environment. Such knowledge is effective whether they remain in the profession or not (Ng 1997). Should the engineers decide to become lawyers, their technological perspectives will be useful in understanding law grounded in an engineering or computing context.

Legal system familiarity is useful to become a patent specialist who operates as a liaison between a company and the patent lawyers. Patent specialists identify innovations within the company. They work closely with engineers and scientists to facilitate the drafting and internal review of invention disclosures and the approval and implementation of application filing projects. They may also administer inventor incentive programs for the company.

Another related career worth considering is licensing, which is the vehicle that allows companies to share technology with each other to the advantage of all parties. Licensing professionals have expertise in business and technology and are instrumental in monetizing a company's IP assets. They define licensing opportunities, valuate IP assets, develop strategic alliances, and administer license agreements. After developing expertise in their field, licensing professionals may become certified licensing professionals (Williams 2013).

3.4 Employment law

> When employees are happy, they are your very best ambassadors.

James Sinegal

Employment or labor law is defined as the negotiated relationships between employers and employees. In general, the employment relationship is regulated by both voluntary and legal measures. Voluntary measures comprise agreements and other decisions that derive from collective bargaining, arbitration, conciliation, mediation, and grievance and discipline handling. Legal measures are treaties and directives, statute law, the common law of contract and of tort, case law, statutory codes of practice, and some international standards (Willey 2012).

3.4.1 Employment obligations

Most employment relationships are not governed by a written employment agreement. Furthermore, in many instances where there are documents between an employee and employer, the document does not include all of the terms of the employment relationship. Where there is no written contract, or where the written contract is not complete, the common law will imply terms into the relationship and impose duties onto both the employer and the employee.

Under the common law for example, the duties an employer owes to an employee include (LEG 2004):

- An employer must not dismiss an employee without cause or reasonable notice of termination, which must be clear and unequivocal.
- In carrying out any dismissal, the employer must not act in bad faith.
- An employer must not force an employee to take a demotion without notice or cause.

Under the common law, the duties an employee owes to an employer include:

- To attend to work
- To carry out the lawful orders of an employer
- To perform duties in a competent manner
- To serve the employer honestly and faithfully
- Not to engage in a "conflict of interest"

In addition to the above, employees owe increased duties of confidentiality and have a fiduciary obligation to act at all times in the best interests of their employer. This is a common law duty that draws its name from the duty of loyalty. The employee's fiduciary duty is to act primarily for the benefit of their employer in matters related to the employment. Among the employee's specific fiduciary duties are the duty to account for profits or render benefits of the undertaking to the employer, the duty not to act as, or on account of, an adverse party without the employer's consent, the duty not to compete on their own account or for others in matters relating to the subject matter of the employment, and the duty to deal fairly with their employer in all transactions between them.

An employee is subject to a duty not to compete with the employer concerning the subject matter of the employment. This duty exists even though the employee does not use the employers' facilities or time. In the case of an engineer employed to conduct research and/or development for a firm or an institution, these fiduciary duties obligate the employee to offer all benefits of the work conducted for the employer to the employer. Further, the engineer is bound not to conduct similar R&D for any competitor or potential competitor without the authorization from their employer. In general, the engineer is obligated not to act in opposition to the interests of the firm. For example, some firms are currently in the business of selling and leasing the technologies developed in their labs. Therefore, an engineer hired by a firm to conduct research in certain fields cannot compete with the firm by creating an own company.

On the other hand, faculty members are clearly agents of their institutions. This is because, by accepting employment, a faculty member agrees to act on behalf of their institution in conducting its business (Walter and Richards 1995). Further, a university professor cannot be employed as a consultant by any private firm that competes with the university for funding or income from the sale of technologies.

3.4.2 Examples of employment laws

Considering North America, Canadian employees enjoy stronger protections and rights than their American counterparts in terms of severance, overtime eligibility, privacy within the workplace, and disabilities

(Monkhouse 2018). In the US, an employer may be able to terminate its employee "at-will". In Canada, unless there is a legal justification for the employee's termination (or the employee has a written employment agreement specifying a termination package), the employer is obligated to provide reasonable notice or pay in lieu of notice (McCarthy 2012).

In Canada, the power to make laws is divided between the federal and provincial governments. In the area of employment law, the federal government only has jurisdiction over specific works and undertakings within exclusive federal constitutional jurisdiction (McMillan 2011). The Québec Civil Code defines an employment contract as such: "a contract by which a person, the employee, undertakes for a limited period to do work for remuneration, according to the instructions and under the direction or control of another person, the employer" (Dupuis 2010).

European employment laws differ significantly from US employment laws. One of the biggest conceptual differences is the unique US employment at-will doctrine, which does not exist in European employment law (Bruce 2013).

3.5   Contract and agreement practice

A valid contract requires voluntary offer, acceptance, and consideration.

Robert Higgs

This section describes how a professional's agreement with the client should reflect the goals and expectations of both parties and determine the conditions under which services will be provided.

3.5.1   What is a contract?

A contract is an exchange of promises, verbal or written, between two or more parties, to do or refrain from doing an act enforceable in a court of law. Several elements must be met in order for a court to consider a contract legally enforceable. The three most important contractual elements are offer, acceptance, and consideration, and they all must exist whether the contract is written or oral.

Contract = Offer + Acceptance + Consideration

In order for a contract to be binding, there must first be an offer. The offer must be specifically made by one person (the offeror) who leads another person to expect that the offeror wishes to create an agreement with no serious misunderstanding. An acceptance of the offer is necessary to make a contract legally binding. Both the offer and the acceptance must be voluntary acts. A contract is not valid by law unless it contains an agreement to exchange promises with consideration. Some types of agreements are unenforceable as a matter of public policy. Consideration can take the form of money or something else, but it must be something of value. In order to be enforceable, persons contracting must not be under a legal disability, such as being minors or being adults who are mentally disabled, and the purpose of a contract cannot be illegal or against public policy.

3.5.2   Types of contracts

There are many types of contracts, but the main ones are: express, implied, unilateral, and bilateral. Also, a contract may be either "written" or "verbal". As stated, contracts may take many forms. Examples of contracts are purchase contracts, leases, a contract to perform a service, or an employment contract.

- An "express" contract is an actual agreement between parties in which all of the terms are agreed upon and expressed in words, either written or verbal. A verbal contract, once made, can be just as legal and binding as a written contract, but it is much harder to prove and enforce.
- An "implied" contract refers to an agreement where all parties agree to a certain action even though nothing is expressly said or written down. It is a legal narrative which the courts invent in circumstances where no express contract exists, but where it is just that one party should have a right and the other party be a subject to a liability, similar to the rights and liabilities in cases of express contracts (Walter and Richards 1995).
- A "unilateral" involves an action undertaken by one person or group alone. In contract law, unilateral contracts allow only one person to make a promise or agreement. For example, X says to Y, "I promise to pay you $1,000 if you will write a computer program for my system". Accordingly, Y immediately goes to work. This constitutes acceptance of the offer and creates a unilateral contract.
- A "bilateral" contract is a legally binding contract formed by the exchange of mutual or reciprocal promises. Such contracts occur very commonly in everyday life. A bilateral offer may take the form of a promise to do something in return for the agreement of the offeree to do something. It is the most common kind of contract where each party is a promisor to its own word. Both parties are obligated to fulfill their promise to the other party.

3.5.3 Standard form contract

A standard form contract, sometimes referred to as an adhesion contract or boilerplate contract, is a contract between two parties that does not allow for negotiations: for example, take it or leave it. It is an agreement between two parties or more that employ standardized, non-negotiated provisions to do a certain thing, in which one party has all the bargaining power and uses it to write the contract primarily to his or her advantage.

Standard form contracts are known by different names in different countries. In the US, they are called "adhesion contracts" or contracts of adhesion. In the UK, they are called standard form contracts, while in France they are called contracts "d'adhésion".

A standard form contract may be drafted by the party who presents it or by a third party, such as a trade association (Gillette 2009). The evidence on which contract formation is assessed is objective, for example a reasonable person should conclude that an offer and matching acceptance have occurred. In general, every contract should contain the information given in Figure 3.2.

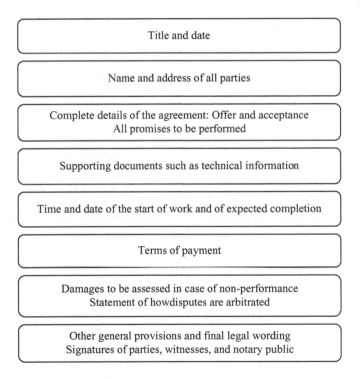

Figure 3.2 Basic content of a contract.

3.5.4   Discharge and breach of contract

Breach means that one party had a duty to execute under the contract, and either did not perform or only partially executed that duty. Failing to perform under the terms and conditions of a contract constitutes a breach of contract. A breach of duty happens when the standard of care is not met. The degree of breach and the results differ according to the type and nature of the term concerned. Most breaches of duty occur due to lack of care, not incompetence. Continuing professional education programs guard against incompetence.

There are two types of breach: minor and material. A breach is minor when, despite the other party's failure to completely perform, the performance is enough that the complaining party really got the advantage of the agreement. Material, or more serious breaches, occur when the complaining party has not received the considerable benefit of the agreement.

The breach of duty required in negligence represents a failure to fulfill the obligation of reasonable care under standards established by society (Nichols 2005). The law provides remedies for discharge and breaches of contracts. A contract may be discharged by performance, agreement, breach, or frustration. Failing to function under the terms and circumstances of a contract forms a breach of contract. A contract is said to be discharged when the agreement has been performed to the satisfaction of both parties. Where a contract is formed by agreement, it may also be discharged or terminated through agreement, subject to the conditions of the contract. The contracting parties can agree at any time that the contract has been discharged. It may be discharged if it becomes impossible to perform due to circumstances beyond the control of the contracting parties.

The contract will be mutually discharged bilaterally when the two parties fail to perform their part of the contract agreement and the parties agree to free one another from any further obligations existing from the original contract. Unilateral discharge happens when one party performs its part, either wholly or partly. It may include novation, accord, and satisfaction. It occurs where one party has completed its part of the bargain and agrees to free the other party from its outstanding obligations under the contract.

A contract is said to be frustrated where the conditions of the contract can no longer be performed due to a change in conditions not provided for in the contract, which occurs after the contract is concluded, and which is beyond the fault of the parties in the contract. In certain cases when a party does not satisfy their own responsibilities, the contract becomes unfulfilled. Where it is impossible to perform the contract, the court will hold that the duties of the parties are ended from the time that the contract was unfulfilled.

There are two general categories of damages that may be awarded if a breach of contract claim is proved (JEC 2018):

- Compensatory damage: Also called "actual damage", it covers the loss the non-breaching party incurred as a result of the breach of contract. The amount awarded is intended to make good or replace the loss caused by the breach. There are two kinds of compensatory damage, general damages, which cover the loss directly and necessarily incurred by the breach of contract; and special damages, also called "consequential damages", which cover any loss incurred by the breach of contract because of special circumstances or conditions that are not ordinarily predictable.
- Punitive damage: Also called "exemplary damage", it is awarded to punish or make an example of a wrongdoer who has acted willfully, maliciously, or fraudulently. Unlike compensatory damages that are intended to cover actual loss, punitive damages are intended to punish the wrongdoer for egregious behavior and to deter others from acting in a similar manner. Punitive damages are awarded in addition to compensatory damages. They are rarely awarded for breach of contract. They arise more often in tort cases to punish deliberate or reckless misconduct that results in personal harm.

3.5.5 Contract liability

Contractual liability, as an area of insurance, involves the financial consequences emanating from liability and not the assumption of the indemnitee's liability itself. It is a very important concept in the domain of risk management and insurance. It means that one party assumes on behalf of another via a contract. Coverages for contractual liability are routinely included in a general liability policy. In this case, a common phrase in contracts should state that one party agrees to hold another party harmless for any injuries, accidents, or losses that occur while the contract is in effect (Nichols 2005).

Damages arising from contract liability are usually calculated from the expectations raised by the contract. For example, if an engineer promises services of a specific quality but is unable to provide it, then the client's damages would include the additional cost of obtaining services of that quality elsewhere (Walter and Richards 1995). For example, suppose an IT business enters into an agreement with a general contractor to set up wiring for a new construction project. The general contractor might ask the IT business to sign an agreement for the work with a "hold harmless" clause. What this means is that if the wiring is faulty in such a way that somebody on the property ends up getting hurt, then the IT business is liable for the damages that result. Even if the injured party sues the general contractor, the IT business is liable for that contractor's attorney fees and any damages awarded to the plaintiff.

3.6   Law of tort

> *Negligence is the rust of the soul that corrodes through all her best resolves.*
>
> **Owen Feltham**

A tort is a civil wrong that comprises damage committed against a person or related property, business, or reputation. This section clearly cannot address the broad fields of torts, but it provides an introduction to the basics of tort law, negligence, and liability.

3.6.1   What is a tort?

The term "tort" is the French equivalent of the English word "wrong" and of the Roman law term "delict". The word tort is derived from the Latin word "tortum", which means twisted or wrong, and is in contrast to the word "rectum", which means straight. The tort is an action that causes harm to someone's health or property. The American Heritage Dictionary defines tort as "a wrong that is committed by someone who is legally obligated to provide a certain amount of carefulness in behavior to another and that causes injury to that person, who may seek compensation in a civil suit for damages".

Torts include assault, battery, false imprisonment, trespass to land or goods, conversion of goods, private and public nuisance, intimidation, deceit, and the very expansive tort of negligence (AG 2018). Generally the tort refers to a private or civil wrong against a person or persons and/or their property that results in a liability for which compensation is justified. Certain torts, such as assault, however, are crimes. The difference between a tort and a crime is that a tort is a civil wrong, while a crime is a wrong against society that threatens the peace and safety of the community. The injured party (plaintiff) files a civil suit against the injuring party (defendant) for definite damages to reimburse for the injury.

Tort law is a body of rights, obligations, and remedies that are applied by civil courts to provide relief for a person who has suffered from the wrongful acts of others. It defines what constitutes a legal injury and establishes the circumstances under which one person may be held responsible for another's injury. Tort law is directed toward the compensation of individuals, rather than the public, for losses which they have suffered within the scope of their legally recognized interests generally rather than one

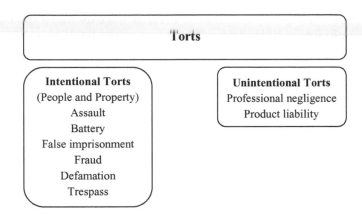

Figure 3.3 Two categories of tort.

interest only, where the law considers that compensation is required. In general, tort law usually fall into one of two main categories, intentional and nonintentional, as shown in Figure 3.3.

3.6.2 Intentional torts

Intentional torts involve harm committed on purpose. For example, assault and battery, trespass, and intentional infliction of emotional distress are all intentional torts. Assault is an intentional tort that occurs from an individual's right to be free from the apprehension of battery. Battery occurs when one party intentionally touches another party without the other party's consent in a way that is harmful or aggressive. False imprisonment occurs as a result of the intentional detention of an individual against consent. Fraud is an intentional tort, which is also known as deceit. Trespass is unauthorized entry onto the property of another person. It is a strict liability tort where the plaintiff is not required to prove purpose or neglect.

3.6.3 Professional negligence

Professionals have a duty to exercise the skill, care, and diligence that may reasonably be expected of a person in a particular discipline of ordinary competence, measured by the professional standards of the time.

Negligence means failure to do something with a lack of ordinary care. It occurs when a person uses less than reasonable care to protect others from compensable harm that is purely economic in nature. Negligence is failure to exercise proper care and provide expertise in accordance with the standards of the profession that result in damage to property or injury to persons. It is the failure to exercise the care that a reasonable person would use in similar circumstances. Product liability is the action whereby an injured party seeks to recover damages for injury to person or property from a manufacturer or seller when the plaintiff alleges that a defective product or design caused the injury.

Professional negligence is an unintentional tort that represents a special case of negligence in which society holds members of a profession responsible for meeting a standard of care and competence (Nichols 2005). It is the term that applies to the care used by members of a profession (law, medicine, architecture, and engineering) in the course of providing professional services. Putting this in an engineering context, negligence is a failure to exercise the care and skill that is ordinarily exercised by other members of the engineering profession in performing professional engineering services under similar circumstances.

In order to establish liability for damage, the courts analyze four elements, including duty, breach, proximate cause, and damages. To be found negligent and in breach of the standard of care, several points have to be proven by the plaintiff:

- The defendant owed a duty of care to the plaintiff.
- The duty of care was breached by the defendant.
- The plaintiff suffered injuries.
- The breach of duty was the actual and legal cause of the injuries suffered by the plaintiff.

In product liability law, the seller is liable for negligence in the manufacture or sale of any product that may reasonably be expected to be capable of inflicting substantial harm if it is defective. Negligence in design is usually based on one of three factors:

- That the manufacturer's design has created a concealed danger
- That the manufacturer has failed to provide needed safety devices as part of the design of the product
- That the design called for materials of inadequate strength or failed to comply with accepted standards

A manufacturer must be reasonable in designing every product. It is not reasonable to manufacture a dangerous product if the same product can reasonably be manufactured with a substantially safe design and reduced risk of injury. Where a plaintiff can show that there was a safer available design at the time of manufacture and that the manufacturer, due to want of reasonable care or skill, failed to use that reasonable alternative design, a claim of negligent design will be proven. However, a manufacturer is not required to use the most advanced design, the safest

design, or the best materials in manufacturing a product. Rather, a manufacturer is only required to use a design that is reasonable in all of the
environments.

3.6.4   Duty of care

"Duty of care" means the responsibility, either of an individual or an
organization, to act with a reasonable standard of care in regards to acts
that could foreseeably cause harm. It is imposed by law to take care to
minimize the risk of harm to another. In tort law, an individual who violates the duty of care by acting negligently is liable for any harm another
person bears as a result of the first individual's failure to be rationally
careful.

Some common relationships where a duty of care exists include manufacturers of products, property owners, and other businesses. Those
who manufacture products owe a duty of care to those who buy them.
Products should also carry warnings about any potential risk that may
result from using the product. This duty toward manufacturers of products makes the product reasonably safe for use and provides warnings
about any dangers the product has. The care extends beyond the original
purchaser of the product to encompass other foreseeable consumers and
users of the product and, in appropriate cases, even others foreseeably in
the vicinity of a product.

The standard that determines the nature of the duty of care is both
objective, adaptable and depends on the specific circumstances of the
damage. Standard of care refers to the degree of attention, caution, and
care that a reasonable person in the circumstances would exercise. The
constraints of the standard are intimately dependent on circumstances.
In certain professions, the standard of care is determined by the standard
that would be implemented by the reasonably careful manufacturer of a
product or the reasonably careful professional in that line of work.

Certain products are inherently dangerous, such that a very high
standard of care should be imposed by courts. In addition to the type
of product, factors which inform the standard of care include the type
of user, the nature of the risk, legal and regulatory standards, industry
codes and practices, the way in which the product is used, the "state-of-
the-art" of the industry at the time of product design and manufacture,
the cost to change the design to ease the defect, and the social utility
of the product.

Professionals, including engineers, owe a tort duty of care to the owner
even if there is no contractual relationship with the owner. An engineer
who prepares specifications owes a duty of care to buyers. Engineers
hired by the owner do not have a duty of care to the contractor, but if the
engineer supervises the work, such duties may occur.

3.6.5   Product liability

Product liability is developed from roots in negligence and warranty causes of action. It refers to a manufacturer or seller being held liable for putting a defective product into the hands of a consumer. It is not limited to manufacturers of final products but rather affects the entire chain of manufacture and distribution. For example, claims for product liability involve express or implied warranties that are part of the contract for the sale of the product and negligence that arises from the breach of contract with respect to the warranty.

In the US, product liability is governed predominately by state law. Accordingly, each state individually adopts its own product liability laws, and the laws that apply in one state may not necessarily apply in another. In Canada, product liability is based on contract liability and under the law of tort (negligence). Increasingly, theories of negligence under tort law are being applied to products.

Product liability lawsuits typically combine a confusing and often redundant array of legal theories, which can include (UK 2018):

- Negligence in the design, manufacture, or marketing of a product
- Strict liability in the design, manufacture, or marketing of a product
- Breach of an express or implied warranty about the product
- Negligent or fraudulent misrepresentations about the product
- Violation of a state consumer protection statute

A manufacturer is negligent if an injury results when the design of a product does not attain a standard of design that the court determines is reasonable. Negligence means that the manufacturer or someone else within the chain of manufacture did not act with reasonable care to ensure the safety of the design and manufacture of the product (Duffy et al. 2014). Negligence also is attributed to failure to provide adequate warnings regarding product usage, hazards, and defects. Once a product defect was proven to have caused injury to the person, damages could be awarded. But, for a negligence case, unreasonable conduct must be proved, and the injury may be merely economic in nature (Abdullah et al. 2009).

3.6.6   Strict liability

In regard to product liability, strict liability applies for a product that is defectively made or designed or does not have proper warnings or instructions. Strict liability means that people injured by defective products may be able to sue the manufacturer without having to prove that the manufacturer was negligent (Peach and Weathers 2017).

In its original form, strict liability spread the costs of the occasional injury caused by an otherwise beneficial product to all the users of the product (Walter and Richards 1995). Strict liability applies to two types of activity: abnormally dangerous (ultra-hazardous) activities and the manufacture/sale of defective or unreasonably dangerous goods/products. It does not require intent, negligence, or anything else. Strict liability makes a manufacturer or vendor responsible for all injuries that might be caused by a defective product that is unreasonably dangerous to the user (Duffy et al. 2014).

Engineering liability could have evolved into a strict liability standard, or it could have settled into a "law of the jungle" kind of justice where there is really no standard and the damaged party can seek some measure of non-judicial redress mainly through some measure of revenge (the engineer gets clubbed in the head to settle up or some similar act) (Pino 2014).

Under a strict liability interpretation in computing, an individual who is harmed in some way by a software failure would have the right to obtain damages either from the manufacturer of the software or the institution operating the software when the error occurred. Under the negligence interpretation of liability, the victim would need to prove that the manufacturer of the software failed to develop and test its product well enough to the point where it was reasonably confident that the product was safe to operate, or that the operator of the software failed to use the software correctly or grossly failed to interpret the software's findings correctly (strict liability versus negligence) (Abdullah et al. 2009). As computer technology evolves, more powerful computer systems and software are available to more individual users and businesses (Gemignani 1980). As a result, software vendors are likely to face increasing exposure to lawsuits alleging that software did not perform as expected. The consequences of such lawsuits to software vendors could be catastrophic.

3.7   Intellectual property (IP)

> *Intellectual property is a key aspect for economic development.*

> **Craig Venter**

The term "IP" generally describes intangible property right, which usually cannot be seen or touched, which is initially created by one's intellectual creative work. The results of this intellectual work, in most cases, is then strengthened with this intangible property right, the fact that gives the creator and/or owner the exclusive right to control, and profit from, the results of the work creativity.

3.7.1 IP law

IP law is that field of law which defines the intellectual creations that are entitled to protection as IP. The goal of IP law is to promote innovation in a competitive marketplace and to provide an incentive for people to develop creative works that advance society by ensuring that they can profit from their works without fear of misuse by others. The law also provides guidance to a competitor who desires to produce a new product or use a new process by designing around, and thus avoiding, the proprietary territory defined by IP rights (Rockman 2004a). Today, the protection of IP by legal means has become a topic of significant interest. Various systems of legal rules exist that empower persons and organizations to exercise such control.

IP is an old concept, although trademarks are thought to date back at least 3,500 years to when potters used them to identify their fired clay pots. The trend of granting patents started in the 15th century with protection for creations of the mind and seems to have originated in Venice, Italy, which is considered the cradle of the IP system; other countries followed in due course. During the 16th century this idea spread rapidly to England, France, Germany, and the Netherlands as governments began to appreciate the benefit of encouraging inventors to create and then to disclose their work and the need to provide an incentive to invest in an invention's business development. The first copyright legislation was passed in England in 1709. This recognized ownership of a literary or artistic creation and granted exclusive rights of use to the author (ESA 2018).

In modern history, the importance of IP was first recognized in the Paris Convention for the Protection of Industrial Property in 1883 and the Berne Convention for the Protection of Literary and Artistic Works in 1886. Both treaties are administered by the World Intellectual Property Organization (WIPO). Most nations have promulgated laws to safeguard IP rights. Besides nurturing creativity of inventors and cascading the usefulness of their inventions, these laws let the inventors' community benefit financially and thus contribute to their country's overall economic development. Usually every country has an agency which issues patents to inventors and businesses for their inventions and trademark registration for product and intellectual property identification.

3.7.2 IP law building blocks

The building blocks of IP law are several IP rights, including patents, copyrights, trademarks, and service marks, as well as anti-cybersquatting laws and trade secret protection laws. Each IP right has particular economic characteristics, terms, and duration of legal protection, mainly depending on the level of development of the technology recipient (UNCTAD 2014).

These are all concepts that were created by legal systems in mostly all of the countries of the world, and although they are merely legal devices, they provide powerful instruments of protection for intellectual creations. These systems of rights are developed to document the existence of IP rights, how they can be protected, and to give the creators the right to exclusively use, own, transfer ownership, or license their rights of IP. The integration of copyright, patent, trademark, and trade secret law into an increasingly combined body of IP law was supported by the development in many jurisdictions of additional types of legal protection for ideas and information. Usually every country has an agency which issues patents to inventors and businesses for their inventions, and trademark registration for product and IP rights. Different types of IPs are protected in different ways as described in Table 3.1.

3.7.3 IP management

Creating, obtaining, protecting, and managing IP is becoming a corporate activity in the same manner as the raising of resources and funds. The current knowledge revolution demands a special platform for IP management (IPM) and treatment in the overall decision-making process (Angell 2000). The term IPM refers to the administration and organization of IP matters in institutions such as companies, public or private research institutions, and any other entity engaged in the creation and commercialization of immaterial rights. IPM has become imperative given that many institutions, including public research entities and universities, have moved away from purely research-oriented policy targets principally based upon generally unremunerated publication of research results towards policies aiming to commercially exploit research results in order to generate additional income (IP4growth 2013). It is obvious that IPM is a multidimensional task that entails many different actions and policies which need to be affiliated with national laws and international treaties and practices.

IP is not a static asset. It is dynamic, requiring ongoing attention and management practices that will allow an institution to protect its value and maximize its utilization. The management of IP is an ongoing task which lasts throughout the life of the IP, until expiry. IP, if it is to be an asset, cannot simply be shelved and left alone, or even licensed and then left alone (Krattiger et al. 2007). Intellectual assets, with patents as a particularly cogent example, must constantly be managed, monitored, maintained, and policed as part of a continual cultivation of IP rights.

Today academic institutions are becoming a powerhouse of knowledge creation and transfer in addition to knowledge sharing, the initial primary motive behind these institutions. Therefore, these institutions started realizing the enormous potential of intellectual capital obtained

Table 3.1 Types of IP rights

Patent	A patent may be considered as a grant of right to exclude others from practicing an invention. A patent does not assure that the patentee can practice the invention. As a requirement, the proposed invention should use the laws of nature, involve a technical concept, be a highly advanced creation, have industrial applicability, be novel, reflect progress, have prior filing, and not violate the public interest (Akakura et al. 2017). The patent is treated like personal property and may be assigned, sold, inherited, mortgaged, or licensed. Patents can be either for a design, utility, or plants.
Copyright	Copyright deals with the rights of intellectual creators in their creation. It is a form of protection given to the authors or creators of original works of authorship. Copyright protection includes only the form of expression used, not the ideas themselves. Thus, the owner of the copyright on a database owns the way the data is compiled but not the data itself (Walter 1986). The author may grant this exclusive right to others (Reynolds 2015). Copyright is obtained automatically without the need for registration, but that is advisable in some cases. Works covered by copyright include, but are not limited to: novels, poems, plays, newspapers, computer programs, databases, films, musical compositions, paintings, drawings, photographs, sculpture, architecture, maps, and technical drawings (WIPO 2018). It is possible to overlap protection between the copyright and patent laws. For example, a computer program may be protectable under both the patent laws and the copyright laws.
Trade Secret	Trade secrets include any valuable business information that derives its value from secrecy. This protection law prevents a competitor or another from misappropriation of valuable and confidential information which is not generally known or available to a competitor or to the public, such as a secret chemical formula or a secret process.
Trademark	A trademark is a specific sign, design, or expression which identifies products or services of a certain source, although trademarks used to identify services in particular are usually called service marks. Trademark and service mark registration laws, as well as the common law, protect the source identity of a product or service, such as the name and/or logo, and sometimes product configuration under which one advertises and markets their goods or services to the trade or public. To avoid the need to register separate applications with each national agency, WIPO administers an international registration system for trademarks.

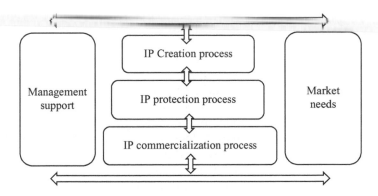

Figure 3.4 Organization of IPM system.

by them and utilizing this strength for their advantage (Jain and Sharma 2006). The academic institutions started developing IPM systems as a managerial and policy tool to cater the needs creation, protection, and commercialization as shown in Figure 3.4.

An IPM can create many benefits for the academic institutions, industry, and the surrounding community, but it requires careful planned and consistent long-term monetary and managerial support. Essentially, one of the roles of an IPM system is to take some IP, de-risk it, advertise it for commercialization and move it out of the academic institution, and then to really do prototyping and proof of concept associated with that IP.

3.8   Technology transfer (TT) practice

> *Successful knowledge transfer involves neither computers nor documents but rather interactions between people.*
>
> **Thomas H. Davenport**
> *[from Davenport and Laurence Prusak's*
> *Working Knowledge: How Organizations*
> *Manage what They Know (1998)]*

TT is often understood to be the transfer of IP. However, there are other means of TT, which is a highly collaborative and mutually beneficial practice. It is the process of transforming scientific findings into meaningful products or services for society. It means the expedition of technological knowledge, skills, and equipment from an originator's environment to a user's environment (Ruimy 2017). It refers to transactions in which knowledge developed within academic institutions is transferred to the industry for development and commercial purposes.

3.8.1   TT policy

The goal of TT policy is not only to commercialize academic IP but also to build the innovative capacities of academic institutions, small and medium enterprises (SMEs), and entrepreneurs by facilitating collaborative ventures (Ruimy 2017). As such, TT constitutes a part of knowledge transfer. Knowledge can be transferred through multiple means, including collaborative research, publishing, consulting, standardization, hiring of graduates, etc., the use of which depends on circumstances, available resources, and objectives of the involved parties (OECD 2013).

IP law plays an important role in facilitating TT. Transactions of and speculation on IP can serve as a focal point for further knowledge transfer, for example by facilitating the transfer of tacit knowledge to licensees through contact with the inventor (Ruimy 2017). The aim is to have a significant, positive impact on the economy. TT begins when research performed at academic institutions leads to a potential new product or service, followed by its commercialization by a "spin-off" firm or an existing one. IP law and policy-making aspire to maintain a balance between protecting innovators against anticompetitive practices on one hand and fostering a rich public domain for the benefit of future innovators and the general public on the other.

3.8.2   TT process

The initial step in the transfer of technology process starts with the recognition of an economic need and, accordingly, a business idea. If the transferred technology goes on to be developed and adopted, it becomes an innovation. Patents can play a prominent role in the entire technology life cycle, from initial R&D to the market introduction stages, where competitive technologies can be protected with patents and licensed out to third parties to expand financial opportunity. It may be useful to examine the distinction between TT and technology diffusion, where the later means the spreading, often passively within a certain technological population, of knowledge linked to a specific innovation of interest. Figure 3.5 describes the major steps of the TT process and innovation as its outcome.

There is no doubt that IP in general, and patenting and licensing in particular, can be feasible strategies for TT. Patents serve as markers of achievement for academic institutions and provide incentives to commercialize the fruits of academic research, which is often at the cutting edge of technological development (Ruimy 2017). Patent protection is usually sought at the R&D stage of the technology life cycle. A patent may be a powerful business tool, allowing innovators to gain exclusivity over a new product or process, develop a strong market position, and earn additional revenues through licensing (Isaka 2018). A patent provides rights

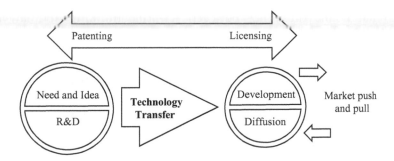

Figure 3.5 Patenting and licensing as a TT outcome.

to exclude others from making, using, selling, or importing the patented invention for a limited time (limited monopoly); the rights are given in exchange for full disclosure of the details of the invention, they are not assenting.

Licensing is the only mode of disembodied TT that can be measured. Under licensing agreement, the licensor (technology owner or rights holder) continues to own the technology and gives a defined right to the licensee for the use of the technology. IP law plays an important role in facilitating TT. The licensee, by the terms of the license, is permitted to exploit the IP. There are two main types of licenses: one which grants an exclusive right to use the technology; another with non-exclusive rights, which implies that the patent owner may transfer the right to use the technology to other companies in the same area. Additionally, the licensing agreement could include a sublicensing clause which permits the licensee to grant to someone else the right to use the technology.

The main challenge to the commercialization of IP and TT is the period between the creation of an invention and its commercialization. In the past, obtaining a patent was enough to attract attention and private-sector investment. Today, firms are reluctant to take on the risk of commercializing unproven inventions (Ruimy 2017). Therefore, academic institutions that hold patents have to invest increasing amounts of effort and money to bring inventions to the commercialization stage by developing prototypes, proving the invention's technical effectiveness and conducting market research.

3.9   Knowledge acquisition

Attempting to answer the following questions involves acquisition of knowledge from this book and other books, documents, and the Internet.

- Should law be introduced into the engineering curriculum?
- What types of law do engineers need to know?

- What is the difference between scientific thinking and lawyer thinking?
- Differentiate between law and ethics.
- Explain what contract liability entails and why it is important.
- What is the difference between a contractual liability and tortious liability?
- When does a contract become frustrated? What can the parties do to remedy the situation?
- What is a tort?
- What does the term IP encompass, and why are organizations so concerned about protecting IP?
- Explain the nature of a tortious liability.
- Distinguish between a tortious liability and a contractual liability.
- What must be present for negligence to occur?
- What is strict liability and when does it apply?
- Explain the role of culture as it applies to ethics in IT security.
- Why is IP protection important?
- What are the ethical implications of AI that organizations need to consider and why?
- What is TT?
- What is the proper definition of a start-up?
- What is the difference between adoption and diffusion of technology?
- Why should one patent something? What kinds of things are patentable?
- What kind of protection do patents offer?
- What is copyright? What are the benefits of protecting copyright?
- What is WIPO's role in IP rights?

3.10   Knowledge creation

Collaborate with peers on learning or work with others outside the class to narrow down the objectives of each activity. You may access class and online resources and analyze data and information to create new ideas and balanced solutions. High-level digital tools may be used to develop multimedia presentations, simulations or animations, videos and visual displays, digital portfolios, reflective practice (online publishing and blogging), or well-researched and up-to date reports.

3.10.1   IP for software

IP is defined as the commercial application of imaginative thought to solving a technical or artistic challenge. Software is one of the many manifestations of IP, and it is usually protected using IP legislation. Laws keep evolving and changing, trying to cope with the evolution of technology and, at the same time, trying to provide a good framework in which businesses can grow and compete. Software engineers and researchers need to understand the laws that govern software and how they can affect their daily work. This is particularly true for researchers who are interested in reverse engineering or those interested in incorporating free and open-source software into their own projects. For this task, develop and deliver a 15-minute tutorial presenting the following topics: software as IP; IP and the reverse engineering of software; reverse engineering legislation around the world and how software is protected; types of licenses; based upon copyright law, licenses as contracts; and software patents. This tutorial is intended for people who are involved in software engineering. It does not assume any previous knowledge of IP. You may use Idris (2005) as a reference.

3.10.2   Engineering trade secret

An engineer (X) was employed by a company (Y). Y licensed technology from another company (Z) explicitly to enable Y to make a mechatronics device based on the Z technology. The Y/Z license included a provision prohibiting the disclosure of the technology by Y or its employees. Subsequently, Y reduced the number of its employees and X lost his career after having worked with the new technology at Y for two years. X started a small company to build mechatronics products. X bought one of Y's devices and, by reverse engineering, supplemented what he knew about the underlying technology, and then manufactured a much cheaper version of the device. Y sued Z, and both sued X, who argued that he created his own version of the device through years of expertise and reverse engineering. Give an opinion about this case and see if X may be liable in stealing the trade secret.

3.10.3   Website or blog design

Consider the following link: https://blog.feedspot.com/intellectual_p roperty_blogs/. It shows the best IP blogs from thousands of top IP blogs in its index using search and social metrics. For this task, build a website or a blog on IP that includes links to the following: key topics for engineers and computing specialists; IP key information links; IP law links (legal resources); and links to resources of activities, including possibly other important sites.

3.10.4   IP guaranties the continuing process of
renewable energy innovation

Innovation is essential for the accelerated deployment of renewable energy technologies that will play a key role in addressing the issues of energy security, energy access, and climate change. Technological innovation is achieved through a mix of various demand factors and technology supply factors. Various modes of innovation operate within different contexts at different stages of technology development, involving various players over different timescales (Isaka 2013). For this task, investigate the above topic with a focus on patents related to solar and wind farms. Include the basics of what patents are and how they work, and present some ideas of how patents and their information can be used to encourage renewable energy innovation. Some examples of the use of patent information to indicate the trends of TT and knowledge generation may be presented. The results of the investigation may be presented in a several-page e-Portfolio.

3.10.5　Debate on IP and information age

There are two conflicting motivations for IP rights: (1) creations of the mind are becoming more valuable in the information age, and (2) modern computing makes it easy to transfer and copy such information. It is realized in Section 3.7 that IP is protected by patents, copyrights, trademarks, and trade secrets. These entities fall within the area of IP law, and as such they can be sold or leased just like other forms of property (Rockman 2004b). Two students may debate the above conflicting motivations in the class, each defending a fact.

References

Abdullah, F., K. Jusoff, H. Mohamed, and R. Setia. 2009. Strict versus negligence software product liability. *Computer and Information Science* 2(4): 81–88.

AG. 2018. Immunity from civil liability. https://www.alrc.gov.au/publications/what-tort.

Akakura, T., T. Kawamata, and K. Kato. 2017. Development of a blended learning system for engineering students studying intellectual property law, and an analysis of the relationship between system usage and the knowledge acquisition process. IEEE International Conference on Teaching, Assessment, and Learning for Engineering (TALE), December 12–14, The Education University of Hong Kong.

Angell, M. 2000. The pharmaceutical industry: To whom is it accountable? *North England Journal of Medicine* 342: 1902–1904.

Bond, J. 2004. The professional engineer and his enhanced duty of care. https://www.icheme.org/communities/subject_groups/safety%20and%20loss%20prevention/resources/hazards%20archive/~/media/Documents/Subject%20Groups/Safety_Loss_Prevention/Hazards%20Archive/XVIII/XVIII-Paper-57.pdf.

Bruce, S. 2013. European employment law 101: Employment at-will is truly a foreign concept. https://hrdailyadvisor.blr.com/2013/04/07/european-employment-law-101-employment-at-will-is-truly-a-foreign-concept/.

Buckland, T. 2012. How a lawyer approaches the problems of physicians, scientists, and engineers: Exclusive with attorney Anthony Wicht. https://www.medgadget.com/2012/11/how-a-lawyer-approaches-the-problems-of-physicians-scientists-and-engineers.html.

Duffy, P. J., P. Flagel, and J. Hagenkötter. 2014. Product liability law in the United States of America. https://www.gibbonslaw.com/product-liability-law-in-the-united-states-of-america-06-11-2014/.

Dupuis, C. 2010. Engineers and their employers: What becomes of professional independence? Ethics and Professional Conduct. https://www.oiq.qc.ca/Documents/DCAP/chroniques_PLAN/ethique_deontologie/Professional Independence.pdf.

ESA. 2018. Intellectual property. http://www.esa.int/About_Us/Law:at_ESA/Intellectual_Property_Rights/Intellectual_Property.

Gemignani, M. C. 1980. Product liability and software. *Rutgers Computer and Technology Law Journal* 8: 173.

Gillette, C. P. 2009. Standard form contracts. NELLCO Legal Scholarship Repository. https://lsr.nellco.org/cgi/viewcontent.cgi?referer=https://www.google.ca/&httpsredir=1&article=1185&context=nyu_lewp.

Idris, K. 2005. Intellectual property, a power tool for economic growth. World Intellectual Property Organization. ftp://ftp.wipo.int/pub/library/ebooks/wipopublications/wipo_pub_888e.pdf.

Isaks, M. 2013. Intellectual property rights. The role of patents in renewable energy technology innovation. https://www.irena.org/-/media/Files/IRENA/Inspire/Intellectual_Property_Rights.pdf?la=en&hash=5B7B01F9B4927DF4817858ACF487BF788E16E9D8.

IP4growth. 2013. Intellectual property management a guide to relevant aspects. http://www.cires-ci.com/pdf/IP4GROWTH/IP4GROWTH%20-%20Intellectual%20Property%20Management.pdf.

JEC. 2018. Remedies for breach of contract. http://jec.unm.edu/education/online-training/contract-law-tutorial/remedies-for-breach-of-.

Krattiger, A., R. T. Mahoney, L. Nelsen, J. A. Thomson, A. B. Bennett, K. Satyanarayana, G. D. Graff, C. Fernandez, and S. P. Kowalski. 2007. *Intellectual Property Management in Health and Agricultural Innovation: A Handbook of Best Practices.* Oxford, UK: Centre for the Management of Intellectual Property in Health Research and Development.

Laukyte, M. 2012. Artificial and autonomous: A person? Social computing, social cognition, social networks and multiagent systems social turn. http://events.cs.bham.ac.uk/turing12/proceedings/11.pdf.

LEG. 2004. *Employment Law in British Columbia.* Vancouver, BC: Bull, Housser and Tupper.

McCarthy, T. 2012. Five key differences between Canadian and U.S. employment law. https://www.mccarthy.ca/en/insights/articles/five-key-differences-between-canadian-and-us-employment-law.

McMillan. 2011. Employment law in Canada: Provincially regulated employers. https://mcmillan.ca/files/Employment%20Law%20in%20Canada%20-%20provincially%20regulated%20employers.pdf.

Monkhouse, A. 2018. American vs. Canadian employment laws. https://www.monkhouselaw.com/canadian-vs-american-employment-laws/.

Nichols, S. P. 2005. A design engineer's view of liability in engineering practice: Negligence and other potential liabilities. *International Journal of Engineering Education* 21(3): 384–390.

Ng, J. 1997. Should law be introduced into the engineering curriculum? *International Journal of Engineering Education* 13(1): 72–78.

OECD. 2013. *Commercializing Public: New Trends and Strategies.* Paris: Organization for Economic Co-operation and Development, pp. 18–21.

Ottino, J. M. 2016. Law and engineering should share curriculum. https://news.no rthwestern.edu/stories/2016/05/opinion-chronicle-engineering-law/.

Pino, J. D. 2014. Do you know the standard of care? https://docs.acec.org/pub /18803059-a2fd-2d06-cc39-a6d1dd575265.

Rockman, H. B. 2004a. *Intellectual Property Law for Engineers and Scientists.* Hoboken, NJ: John Wiley and Sons.

Rockman, H. B. 2004b. Overview of intellectual property law. In Whitney, E. (ed.). *Inventors and Inventions.* Wiley-IEEE Press eBook Chapters. https://ieeexpl ore.ieee.org/xpl/ebooks/bookPdfWithBanner.jsp?fileName=5237403.pd f&bkn=5237401&pdfType=chapter.

Ruimy, D. 2017. Intellectual property and technology transfer: Promoting best answers: Report of the Standing Committee on Industry, Science and Technology. House of Commons, Canada. http://www.ourcommons.ca/ Content/Committee/421/INDU/Reports/RP9261888/indurp08/indurp 08-e.pdf.

Sharma, K., and V. Sharma 2006. Intellectual property management system: An organizational perspective. *Journal of Intellectual Property Rights* 11: 330–333.

UK. 2018. US product liability law. https://assets.publishing.service.gov.uk/gove rnment/uploads/system/uploads/attachment_data/file/301340/US_Prod uct_Liability_Law.pdf.

UNCTAD. 2014. Transfer of technology and knowledge sharing for development science, technology and innovation issues for developing countries. United Nations Conference on Trade and Development. http://unctad.org/en/Publ icationsLibrary/dtlstict2013d8_en.pdf.

Walter, C. 1986. Engineering and the law: Part I: About intellectual property. *IEEE Engineering and Medicine and Biology* 5(2): 34–45.

Walter, C., and E. P. Richards. 1995. Employment obligations. https://biotech.law. lsu.edu/ieee/duties.htm.

Willey, B. 2012. *Employment Law in Context: An Introduction to HR Professionals.* London, UK: Pearson Longman.

Williams, K. 2013. Intellectual property: The intersection of law and innovation. *IEEE Women in Engineering Magazine* 7(2): 17–19.

WIPO. 2018. What is intellectual property? http://www.zis.gov.rs/upload/ documents/pdf_en/pdf/What%20is%20IP_WIPO.pdf.

Professional practice leadership

4.1 Knowledge and understanding

Having successfully completed this module, you should be able to demonstrate knowledge and understanding of:

- The concept of leadership and the three circles approach to leadership
- Leadership theories, including early theories that focus on character and personality and recent ones that focus on what leaders do
- Leadership theories of motivation and management including theories X, Y, Z, Maslow's hierarchy of needs, and the Hawthorne effect
- Emotional intelligence and its value to leadership development
- Effective leadership and its three overlapping areas: individual, team, and task
- The concepts of positive psychology and positive leadership and their impact on innovation
- Authentic leadership practice, its four major tasks, and its strong relevance to effective management
- Innovation leadership practice and its two-tiered approach
- Impact of leadership on engineering practice
- Design thinking leadership, which is about building a questioning mindset
- Path towards practice systems thinking and why leaders should embrace it
- Lean leadership, its principles and behaviors, and the Toyota model
- Community of practice as an informal group of practitioners that shares knowledge on common development problems while pursuing collaborative solutions

4.2 Understanding leadership

> *Leadership consists not in degrees of technique but in traits of character.*
>
> **Lewis H. Lapham**

Leadership, in the sense perceived in the quotation above, integrates several traits as mutually-reinforcing concepts (Figure 4.1). Leadership can be defined as collective ethical actions which influence and direct the performance of others towards the achievement of common goals.

The concept of leadership has evolved over the years. The term was once confused with management, but today the two are distinct roles, each with its own characteristics. Rather than debate a definition of leadership, it is advantageous to discuss what leaders do (Kleim and Ludin 1998). There are numerous definitions and theories of leadership; however, there are enough similarities in the definitions to conclude that leadership is an effort of influence and the power to induce compliance (Wren 1995). Leadership is a quality that everyone can relate to, but it is difficult to describe it in a way that is applicable to all professionals at all levels. The whole concept of leadership means creating change as contrasted to maintaining the status quo. It implies thinking of the future, influencing, persuading, changing minds, doing what those above and below may consider unacceptable, sticking your neck out, taking calculated risks, risking yourself as a person in championing a controversial point of view or approach, and having the confidence and ability to speak out and support unpopular but necessary issues Gaynor 1993). Leadership is a skill comprised of many traits and qualities. Some of these qualities include vision, mission, values, commitment, motivation, and consensus building. An important purpose of leadership is to provide vision, direction, and motivation for a team of individuals to accomplish a mission that otherwise could not be accomplished by a single individual. It is about creating change and thinking about the imaginable and the unimaginable.

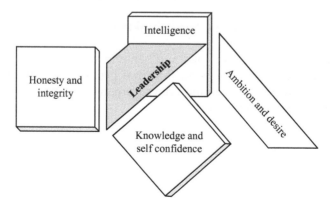

Figure 4.1 Several traits of leadership.

4.3   Leadership theories

Service-based leadership is a mindset: you work for your people. It is not complex; often it's the small acts of service that have the greatest impact on morale and camaraderie.

Courtney Lynch

The subject of leadership has been studied and evolved for hundreds of years and generated a succession of theories. Leadership theories try to explain how and why certain people become leaders. The earliest theories focused mainly on character and personality of successful leaders. The more recent theories focus on what leaders really do rather than their distinctive qualities or traits (Team FME 2015).

Trait and character theories of leadership represent an early belief that leaders are born, and due to this belief, those that possess the correct qualities and traits are better fitted to leadership. Early theories attempted to create lists of leadership qualities that make a leader. These include charisma, initiative, honesty and integrity, flexibility, creativity, drive and motivation, emotional maturity, confidence, cognitive ability, and achievement drive. Table 4.1 summarizes three major leadership theories that focus on the above characters and traits. Advocates to the above theories, which are now considered mostly out of date, believe that leadership development entails recognizing and measuring leadership qualities and then training those with aptitude.

Modern thinking suggests that the above traits are little more than characteristics, which although some people may possess them naturally, can be learned and built into one's behaviors and thinking, thus affecting their leadership potential (Eba 2018). Today, a majority of modern leadership theories are centered on the levels of skill, as well as the situational adaptability of the individual leading (Mabugat 2018). In accord with modern-day thinking, and due to the need for effective leaders, this has led to theories and methodologies that rely on behaviors that can be learned, the good tasks to meet certain goals or to achieve a particular performance standard with focus on meeting the needs of everyone involved, rather than traits only. Table 4.2 summarizes major leadership theories that focus on what leaders learn and do and achieve.

4.4   Theories of management and motivation

At the end of the day, man-management is all about managing people's sense and sensitivity.

Sandhya Jane

Table 4.1 Major leadership theories that focus on character and personality

Theory	Summary
Great Man	Proposed by historian Thomas Carlyle, some argued that great men, such as Alexander the Great, Abraham Lincoln, and Martin Luther King Jr., provided validity for this theory, with great men emerging from what looks like nowhere to lead and influence the world (Mabugat 2018). This theory states that leadership is directly dependent on who an individual is rather than what he knows or what he can do, therefore basing leadership on inherited features.
Trait	This is one of the first academic theories of leadership that attempts to answer why some people are good leaders and others are not. It is similar to the great man theory, which is based on the assumption that people are born with particular traits that make them better suited to become leaders. The basic premise behind trait theory is that effective leaders have certain characteristics that are utilized to enhance organizational performance and leader prestige. A major argument in this theory is the problem of how two individuals with similar traits could end up in completely divergent leadership positions, one becoming a great leader while the other becomes a failed leader, despite the similarity in traits.
Charismatic	Charisma is a Greek word meaning "divinely inspired gift", which imparts an extraordinary quality to charismatic individuals by which they can influence hearts and souls of others, perform miracles, or predict the future.

Several theories help explain how workers are motivated and provide ideas for how to increase motivation in the workplace. Understanding which theory is the best may help improve management of organizations by increasing employee retention rates and improving worker productivity. Four management theorems at the workplace are discussed in this section.

4.4.1　Theory X and Theory Y

Theory X and Theory Y are theories of human motivation and management. Douglas McGregor of the Massachusetts Institute of Technology (MIT), an American social psychologist, proposed his famous XY theories in his 1960 book *The Human Side of Enterprise*. They are still referred as two contrasting theories in the field of management and motivation. Whilst more recent studies have questioned the rigidity of the model, McGregor's XY theories remain a valid basic principle from which to develop positive management style and techniques. They are central to organizational development and to improving organizational culture.

Table 4.2 Major leadership theories that focus on what leaders learn, do, and achieve

Contingency	This theory claims that there is no single style of leadership that is universally effective, and that one style of leadership may work better under particular circumstances than another style of leadership (Mabugat 2018). It recommends focusing on particular variables related to the environment that might determine which particular style of leadership is best suited for the situation.
Situational	Developed by Dr. Paul Hersey in the late 1960s, this model is a powerful yet flexible tool that enables leaders of all kinds, including managers, salespeople, peer leaders, teachers, or parents to more effectively influence others. Situational theory claims that leaders should not utilize a single style of leadership but should rather lead according to social and environmental factors such as the capabilities of those who follow (Mabugat 2018). This, among a number of other factors, will affect what the leader eventually does.
Transactional	Also known as management theory. The underlying theory of this leadership model is that leaders exchange rewards for employees' compliance, a concept based in bureaucratic authority and a leader's legitimacy within an organization.
Transformational	This theory focuses on the exchanges that happen between leaders and followers. It is based in the notion that a leader's job is to create structures that make it abundantly clear what is expected of followers and also the consequences (for example, rewards and punishments) for meeting or not meeting these expectations.

Theory X assumes that the primary source of employee motivation is monetary, with security as a strong second. It assumes that people are naturally lazy, try to avoid work as much as possible, attempt no responsibility, and prefer to be supervised. It is more suitable for an organization in which the employees do not like their work situation and will avoid work whenever possible. In such cases the employees have to be forced, controlled, or reminded in order for the organization to meets its objectives (Habash 2017). In brief, Theory X is an authoritarian style where the emphasis is on "productivity", on the concept of a fair day's work.

Theory Y is a participative style of management which assumes that people will exercise self-direction and self-control in the achievement of organizational objectives to the degree that they are committed to those objectives (Mohamed and Nor 2013). Enlightened managers use Theory Y, which produces better performance and results and allows people to grow and develop. Theory Y is appropriate for an organization in which the employees like their jobs and tend to be self-directed. Theory Y is indeed a democratic form of leadership, where people will apply self-control and self-direction in the pursuit of organizational objectives without external control or the threat of punishment. Theory Y is a participative style of management which assumes that people will exercise self-direction and self-control in the achievement of organizational objectives to the degree that they are committed to those objectives. It is management's main task in such a system to maximize that commitment.

Many managers will find that Theory Y is the most difficult management approach to implement at work, while Theory X is simple, and its communication style is mainly in one direction. In both theories, managers are still accountable for the planning process, getting workers on board, and approaching goals.

4.4.2   Theory Z approach to management

Theory Z was developed by William Ouchi of UCLA, Los Angeles, in his 1991 book *Theory Z: How American management can meet the Japanese challenge*. Theory Z is often referred to as the Japanese management style, which is essentially what it is. Ouchi chose to name his model "Theory Z", which apart from anything else tends to give the impression that it is a McGregor idea. For Ouchi, Theory Z focused on increasing employee loyalty to the company by providing a job for life with a strong focus on the well-being of the employee, both on and off the job. Theory Z presumes that given the right management support, workers can be trusted to do their jobs to their highest capacity and look after for their own and others' happiness.

As a management concept, Theory Z looks at motivating workers. It emphasizes the need to help workers become generalists rather than specialists. It essentially advocates a combination of all that is best about Theory Y and modern Japanese management, which places a large amount of freedom and trust with workers and assumes that workers have a strong loyalty and interest in team-working and the organization (Habash 2017).

4.4.3   Maslow's hierarchy of needs

The Maslow's hierarchy of needs is one of the best-known theories of motivation. It contains five levels that often shape motivation styles in an organization as shown in Figure 4.2. Maslow believed that these needs are similar to instincts and play a major role in motivating behavior (Cherry 2018). To motivate employees, an organization must move up the pyramid of needs to ensure all of an employee's needs are met.

The bottom of the pyramid contains physiological needs such as food, sleep, and shelter. Safety makes up the second level, where security and safety become primary, including financial, health, and safety

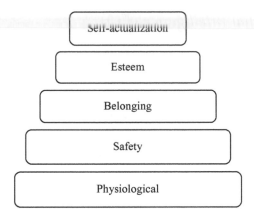

Figure 4.2 Maslow's hierarchy of needs.

against accidents and injury. The social needs in Maslow's hierarchy include such things as love, acceptance, and belonging. At this level, the need for emotional relationships drives human behavior, including family and friendship. The top two levels of the pyramid include esteem and self-actualization. Successful organizations focus on the top two levels of the pyramid by providing employees with the necessary recognition and developing opportunities for employees to feel they are doing valuable work and reaching their potential and personal worth within the organization (Zeiger 2018). Maslow's theory is popular both in and out of psychology. The fields of education and business have been very influenced by this theory.

4.4.4   The Hawthorne effect

The Hawthorne effect is a term referring to the tendency of some people to work harder and perform better when they are participants in an experiment (Cherry 2017). Through a series of experiments in the late 1920s, Elton Mayo (1880–1949) developed the Hawthorne effect, later described in the 1950s by researcher Henry A. Landsberger. The Hawthorne effect refers to the fact that workers will adapt their behavior simply because they are being observed.

This effect theorizes that employees are more productive when they know their work is being measured and studied. In addition to this, Mayo realized that employees were more productive when provided with feedback related to the studies and allowed to provide input into the work process (Zeiger 2018). Workers need recognition for a job well done and reassurance that their opinion matters in the workplace to be motivated to perform.

4.5   Emotional intelligence (EQ)

As more and more artificial intelligence is entering into the world, more and more emotional intelligence must enter into leadership.

Amit Ray
[from Mindfulness Meditation for Corporate Leadership and Management (2017)]

Emotions are important pieces of information that tell us about ourselves and others. The ability to express and manage emotions is critical, but so is the ability to understand, interpret, and respond to the emotions of others. However, emotions can be constructive or destructive, as shown in Figure 4.3.

4.5.1   The term EQ

The term EQ was first defined in 1990 by Salovey and Meyer (1998). Their work has since been significantly expanded by Daniel Goleman, an American psychologist (in his role as a science reporter at *The New York Times*), who helped to popularize EQ (Goleman 1995, 1998). Those were times when the notion of intelligence quotient (IQ) as the standard of excellence in life was unquestioned; a debate raged over whether it was set in our genes or due to experience. Goleman identified that IQ is actually less important for success in life and work than EQ, a set of skills that are not directly related to academic ability. Goleman has asserted that EQ abilities were about four times more important than IQ in determining professional success and prestige, even for those with a scientific background.

EQ is the ability to understand and manage one's own emotions and those of others. EQ differs from what people think of intellectual ability, in that EQ is learned, not acquired. EQ is the ability to identify, use, understand, and manage emotions in positive ways to relieve stress,

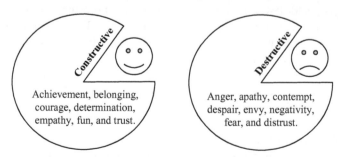

Figure 4.3 Elements of constructive and destructive emotions.

communicate effectively, empathize with others, overcome challenges, and defuse conflict. It is the ability used in handling conflicts or the capability of resolving problems. Individuals who have a high EQ level should be able to walk and think calmly even when tested with various problems (Habash 2017).

It has been stated that in industry, IQ gets you hired, but EQ gets you promoted (Gibbs 1995). For example, a manager at AT&T Bell Labs was asked to rank his top performing engineers. High IQ was not the deciding factor, but instead how the person performed regarding answering emails, how good they were at collaborating and networking with colleagues (rather than lone wolf), and their popularity with others (rather than socially awkward) in order to achieve the cooperation required to attain the goals.

4.5.2   EQ competencies

For leaders, EQ is important to success. Several attributes and competencies of EQ along two major domains, including self-mastery and social mastery skills, determine leader effectiveness, as shown in Table 4.3.

Good leaders must be self-aware and understand how their verbal and non-verbal communication skills can affect their performance. Self-regulation, known also as discipline, involves controlling disruptive emotions and adapting to change circumstances in order to keep the involved team moving in a positive direction. EQ also includes the ability to harness

Table 4.3 EQ attributes and domains

Self-Mastery	
Self-awareness	Ability to identify one's own emotions and their impact. Being emotionally aware is just the first step to emotional management.
Self-regulation	Ability to control emotions and behavior. Exert greater self-control: like a traffic signal, stop (red)/think (yellow)/act (green).
Self-motivation	Stay positively self-motivated with a desire to do things by an interest in learning. It is also self-improvement versus the pursuit of wealth and status.
Social Mastery	
This is feasible when one has achieved self-mastery	
Empathy	Ability to understand and share in others' experiences and emotions. It is about compassion and caring. Empathy is a matter of projecting outside of oneself to appreciate what other people are going through.
Social skills	Ability to recognize and understand the emotions of others and connect with them.

emotions and apply them to tasks like thinking and problem-solving; the ability to manage emotions, including the ability to regulate emotions; and the ability to cheer up others or calm them down (Glesson 2018). Practicing empathy leads to understanding and treating one another better. It is critical management approach to creating the kind of conditions in which real learning can take place. In EQ, as part of leadership, social skills refer to the skills needed to handle other people's emotions effectively by understanding and managing self-emotions first.

Given the attributes stated above, it becomes quite apparent that encouraging EQ abilities should be a component of education. This becomes especially relevant given that the skills that employers value include a willingness to learn, flexibility, communication skills, teamwork, and other forms of working with others (Riemer 2003). Because such skills fall into the category of EQ, academic institutions need to be aware of industry demands on graduates.

4.6   *Effective leadership*

> *An effective boss is someone who doesn't have to boss around to be effective.*

> **Jag Randhawa**

John Adair developed his action-centered leadership, presented by the three-circle model, at the Royal Military Academy at Sandhurst in 1973. He observed what effective leaders did to gain the support and commitment of their followers. Adair found that effective leaders pay attention to three balanced areas of need: task, need, and individual, as shown in Figure 4.4 (Thomas 2004; Team FME 2015). The emphasis on each circle may vary at each period of time, but all are interdependent and play a role in the leadership picture, therefore the leader must recognize all three equally.

Leadership in general is concerned with the interaction of the three areas: task, including goal-setting, achieving, methods, and process; team, including building and maintaining, effective interaction and communication, clarifying roles, and team morale; and individual, including attention to development, behavior, and feelings. An effective leader pays equal attention to all three areas rather than focusing on, for example, just getting the job done and building the team. No matter what the goal is, the task is what will guide the leadership that has to be provided to the team.

An effective leader in teambuilding must act as encourager, harmonizer, compromiser, gatekeeper, standard setter, group observer, and follower (Thomas 2004). Effective leaders are able to create an environment that will encourage all the members of their team to develop their skills

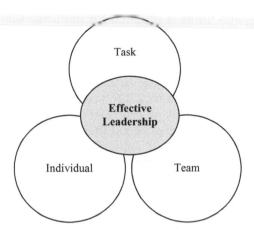

Figure 4.4 Three overlapping areas of effective leadership.

and imagination so that they can contribute to the common goal and vision of the organization. Only a demanding leader will achieve great results. In addition to thoroughness, an effective leader must know how to listen in order to know the needs of the individuals in the team. Placing team members in the roles that are best for their skills provides the necessary time and resources for them to do their job properly and therefore meet what is demanded of them. Effective leaders must be at the forefront to lead and guide teams throughout the whole process until the goal is reached. The leader is the one responsible for taking the risks that others are not willing to take. Through motivation, the effective leader channels the energy and professional potential of coworkers in order to achieve the objectives.

4.7   Positive psychology and leadership

> *If the only tool you have is a hammer, you tend to see every problem as a nail.*

Abraham Maslow
[from Toward a Psychology of Being (1962) and Maslow's article "The psychology of science" (1966)]

According to the American Psychological Association (APA), "Psychology is the study of the mind and behavior. The discipline embraces all aspects of the human experience in every conceivable setting … the understanding of behavior is the enterprise of psychologists" (APA 2013). Psychological knowledge is essential to scientific and technological innovation. Technology requires the use of human operators, and understanding human capacities and limits is essential for implementing technological advances.

The subfield of positive psychology, a relatively new branch within the field of psychology, focuses on helping people and organizations create well-being and meaning in their lives in order to understand and enhance their human experiences (Adams 2012). Positive psychology focuses on thriving individuals, especially on their strengths and virtues, their subjective experiences, and on living a good life.

When positive psychology is applied in the workplace, the result is a positive organizational behavior, which leads to increased hope, optimism, resiliency, and efficacy. Positive emotions have been found to predict happiness, well-being, better outcomes, satisfaction, and success at work. Managers who infuse positive psychology into their leadership style can create a positive psychological work culture within the employee base and allow employees to begin to innately practice antecedents of innovation, such as creativity and engagement, that lead to innovation itself. One way for leaders to infuse their leadership style with positive psychology is to cultivate the use of their innate character strengths. Leaders can use positive psychology to create and support a more positive organizational culture that in turn creates positive psychological states within the employees of an organization. Within this new psychological paradigm, employees are not merely products of cultural events and experiences; they become invested in or take psychological ownership of their work (Avey et al. 2009), working from a more innovative mindset.

On the other hand, positive leadership can be defined as the application of character strengths to leadership and management situations in order to create a virtuous organization where employees can flourish. Virtues are values that have been identified by various philosophical systems. Positive psychology's framework encompasses six virtues, which include wisdom and knowledge, courage, humanity, justice, temperance, and transcendence (Peterson and Seligman 2004). Positive organizations always make the managers concentrate on people's strengths rather than weaknesses (Gardner et al. 2004). Positive leaders fuel positive emotions within themselves and their followers, and this can lead to more job satisfaction, greater engagement in their work, increased performance, and better moods.

4.8 Authentic leadership practice

> *Telling people what to do is showmanship. Showing people how to do it is leadership.*
>
> **Janna Cachola**

Of all principles that support sustainable leadership, Authenticity is one of the most important. Authenticity means genuine and original. Authentic leadership brings together the concept of authenticity with positive psychology; it focuses on whether leadership is genuine. It is one of the challenges to practice. Luthans and Avolio (2003) defined authentic leadership as "a process that draws from both positive psychological capacities and a highly developed organizational context, which results in both greater self-awareness and self-regulated positive behaviors on the part of leaders and associates, fostering positive self-development".

As conceptualized within the emerging field of positive psychology (Seligman 2002), authenticity can be understood as "owning one's personal experiences, be they thoughts, emotions, needs, preferences, or beliefs, processes captured by the injunction to know oneself", and behaving in accordance with the true self (Harter et al. 2002). Authentic leaders have insight, sometimes referred to as vision, but that usually has exclusive reference to the future; they demonstrate initiative; they go first and do not sit on the sidelines. Such leadership involves insight, initiative, impact, influence, and integrity. The most important skill a leader can master is the ability to listen in a way that surfaces the underlying concerns of another and finds the intersections between seemingly opposing points of view (George and Jones 2008). Real leaders spend more time listening than they do talking.

The essence of authentic leadership is EQ. People with high IQs and low EQs can hardly be called authentic leaders. In contrast to IQ, which basically does not change in one's life, EQ can be developed. The first and most important step on this journey is gaining self-awareness (George 2016). Authentic leadership is not about showing dominance of knowledge and competence over others but about exercising and executing. The traits of authenticity emerge in an individual from the inside out and take time, courage, and practice. Then that individual may become an authentic leader and can be a role model for the organization's values. It is realizable and tangible: first selecting, developing, and training the talent and then placing the talent into the right practice (Habash 2017). In general, practicing authenticity requires four major tasks within an organization in order to make the difference, as shown in Figure 4.5.

According to Stajkovic and Luthans (1998), confidence is strongly linked to work performance in terms of job satisfaction, goal settings, conscientiousness, feedback, etc. Hope is the combination of two things, agency (the will) and the pathways (the ways), like goal-directing and the plan for reaching this goal. The third task of authentic leaders is to raise optimism. Optimists usually attribute the success to their internal, stable, or global causes, such as their own abilities. The fourth task of authentic leaders is strengthening resilience. The individual facing hardships and difficulties should be able to withstand or recover quickly from difficult

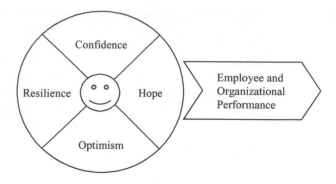

Figure 4.5 Four tasks of authentic leadership.

conditions and emerge with new improved leadership skills (Khan 2010). Similarly, authenticity concentrates on one's inner thoughts, beliefs, and emotions and acting in such a way that reflects one's true self.

4.9   Systems thinking (ST) practice

> *Systems thinking provides the more holistic way to view the problems.*
>
> **Pearl Zhu**
> *[from Thinkingaire: 100 Game Changing Digital Mindsets to Compete for the Future (2016)]*

The concept of ST was developed by Professor Jay W. Forrester at the MIT Sloan School of Management. It was popularized by Peter Senge in his book *The Fifth Discipline* (1994), where he describes ST as a discipline for seeing wholes. ST is a framework for seeing interrelationships rather than things, for seeing patterns of change rather than static snapshots (Ambler 2013).

4.9.1   Why ST?

ST is a perspective, a language, and a set of tools (Monat and Gannon 2015). It is a thinking approach that may help leaders identify and remedy complex problems by understanding not only the full extent of the problem but the reasons of the problem. ST is a management discipline that concerns an understanding of a system by assessing the linkages and interactions between the components that encompass the wholeness of that defined system. It is useful for seeing and understanding wholes, interrelations, and change patterns. The practice of ST helps to observe the underlying interrelationships and connections which make the events occur in organization. ST is an effective approach to managing organizations. It sees complex systems as a series of components that make up the whole, each part interacting with and influencing the rest.

Recent theories of leadership stress the significance of holism, intuition, and creativeness and a systems conception of the world for a successful application of the leader's potential. Leadership is a process and there is a two-way relationship between the leader and the team (Skaržauskienė 2009). Leaders today should become fluent in ST because, in various ways, ST is the essence of leadership. Through practicing ST, leaders can inspire and influence teams to accomplish things that they otherwise would not have done on their own.

4.9.2   How to practice ST?

According to Peter Senge (2006), the three characteristics of ST include:

- A consistent and strong commitment to learning
- A willingness to challenge one's own mental model; accepting one's own role in problems and being open to different ways of seeing and doing
- Always including multiple perspectives when looking at a phenomenon

Based on the above, leaders may practice ST by following the path shown in Figure 4.6. Organizational complexity involves four levels, including the external world (environment, competitors, and customers);

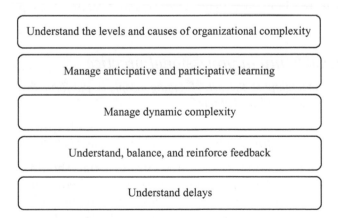

Figure 4.6 Path towards ST.

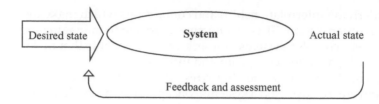

Figure 4.7 ST feedback loop.

the organization's and manager's own actions, such as strategies, management practices, and policies and procedures; the organization's and manager's own problems and problem-solving processes, like culture, expertise, and functional orientation; and organizational consciousness that is the experience of all of the above.

ST skills are best developed through a combination of formal training and experiential, on-the-job development. Training is important for learning specific tools and processes for mapping out complex systems, while on-the-job experiences provide opportunities for building expertise and confidence (Bullock 2013). In addition, leaders should manage anticipative learning by helping employees and the organization to forecast future needs. They should provide the conditions for employees to work together, participate in dialogues, and empathize with each other so that participative learning can exist and flourish.

The practice of ST starts with the concept of "feedback" (Figure 4.7), that illustrates how actions can reinforce or balance each other. In this contest, feedback means a reciprocal flow of influence. In ST every influence is both cause and effect. In all feedback processes, there are delays, which are either unrecognized or not well understood (Akay 2015). ST is related with the long-term view, so delays and feedback loops are very significant.

4.10   Leadership in professional practice

> Leadership is the art of giving people a platform for
> spreading ideas that work.
>
> **Seth Godin**
> [from Tribes: We Need You to Lead Us (2008)]

In preparation for leading opportunities, professionals should understand the principles of leadership and be able to practice them in growing proportions as their careers advance. In addition to the necessity for strong leadership ability is the need to also acquire a working framework upon which high ethical standards and a strong meaning of professionalism can be developed.

4.10.1   Practices and relations

Leadership first comes from the human heart and second from the mind. It is a human experience and process both emotional and intellectual. A profession as a specific form of collective organization of humans is inseparable from two aspects, an articulation of a vision and an appropriate set of practices and relations (Habash 2017). Some comments from Robert Lutz (Tobia 1999), then former president and vice chair of Chrysler Corporation and now retired General Motors vice chair, noted in an IEEE-USA's *Today's engineer* article, "Robert Lutz gives engineers the nod": "Engineers need to be, like anybody else in business, proactive and somewhat outgoing. And they need to reach outside technical areas. Mainly, engineers need to be good communicators, because there is no point in achieving an engineering breakthrough; having a new idea; or coming up with a new material, if you cannot get your colleagues excited about it".

For engineering education, leadership development is a recent topic; learning leadership requires both formal and informal education that goes beyond the traditions of academic experience and the engineer-in-training program (MacIntyre 2016). However, the education system may contribute actively to the process by enriching the typical curriculum with some elements of leadership education including courses, workshops, internships, and other exercises. Figure 4.8 shows a framework for such education enhancement.

In an engineering and computing context, leadership integrates a number of capabilities which are critical in order to function at a professional level. These capabilities include the ability to assess risk and take initiative, the willingness to make decisions in the face of uncertainty, a sense of urgency, and the will to deliver on time in the face of limitations or difficulties, resourcefulness and flexibility, trust and loyalty in a team setting, and the ability to relate to others (Habash 2017).

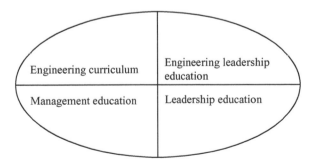

Figure 4.8 Engineering leadership framework.

4.10.2   Leadership for technical managers

Engineers and computing specialists are no longer only involved with the technical project details but must also understand the broader picture, as they are often acting as team leaders. Effective leadership consists of capabilities and values that transform technical people from individual contributors into those who can lead teams to manage a complex multi-disciplinary product. Many managers came to management through the technical ranks. Although they may have had enough of training and mentoring, they frequently learn management skills the hard way, through trial and error (Rothman 1999). Effective managers are capable of employing a blend of supervisory and technical skills in the direction and wrap-up of complex projects. This always demands that they are able to work well within teams and have the strength of character to lead a team of engineers who may come from a range of various disciplines.

Some would define management as an art, while others would define it as a science. Whether management is an art or a science is not what is most important. Management is a process that is used to accomplish organizational goals. Leaders, on the other hand, set a direction, align people, motivate, and inspire (Kotter 2001). Sometimes, it is useful to distinguish between management and leadership behaviors. Both must go hand in hand. They are not the same thing. But they are necessarily linked, and complementary. Any effort to separate the two is likely to cause more problems than it solves. Still, significant differences exist. The manager's job is to plan, organize, and coordinate. The leader's job is to inspire and motivate. Figure 4.9 shows the difference between a manager and a leader.

4.10.3   Leadership and design thinking

The notion of "design" as a "way of thinking" was introduced in 1969 and adopted for business process in the 1990s. Design thinking is about

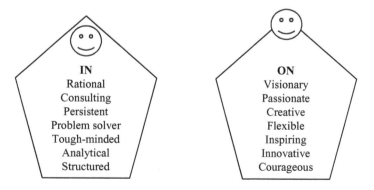

IN
Rational
Consulting
Persistent
Problem solver
Tough-minded
Analytical
Structured

ON
Visionary
Passionate
Creative
Flexible
Inspiring
Innovative
Courageous

Figure 4.9 Elements of both management and leadership.

building a questioning mindset to grow conversation and challenge assumptions between designers and leaders. Designers face tough problems every day, problems that require them to find design solutions that deal with business and technical constraints while also addressing user needs. Questioning is vital to almost every aspect of learning, and so questioning is central to good design. In a design environment, for example, designers always ask open-ended questions related to technical and operational details, while leaders ask questions related to planning, accomplishment, and resources. Questioning is a powerful tool that every designer should be able to use smoothly. As part of a design thinking process, questions can help one understand a situation and get beneficial insights. They can also foster creativity and innovation within an organization and can help teams unite and connect. A combination of questions from both sides of the design team makes a good questioning mindset. Table 4.4 summarizes a simple example of such a mindset.

Design thinking consists of several steps, including "empathize", "define", "ideate", "prototype", and "test". Communications with end users are very important, since observations of the responses of individuals yield valuable signs for new products and services. In the "empathizing" process, an approach based on field work is adopted in order to get insights into potential needs. In the "test" process, simple prototypes are utilized to verify business hypotheses through communications with users. It is rational to communicate with customers in the early stage of business development since ideas do not often meet the true needs of customers.

Design thinking is undoubtedly emerging as an important topic, gaining wider awareness and adoption. It is a way of thinking based on cognitive processes typically employed by designers Brown 2008). Successful companies such as Tesla, Apple, Microsoft, Amazon, and Google innovate continuously, enabled by design practice, design culture, and design leadership. These firms connect with customer needs and emotions to create exciting products and services through collaborative team design and development processes.

Table 4.4 A sample of questioning mindset

Designer	Design leader
How do we make something good and usable?	What is the goal and how to achieve it?
What are the goals of the project?	How do we accomplish the milestones?
How does it go together?	What people and resources are needed to make the project happen?
How do we reflect the brand?	What successes have been achieved recently?

4.10.4   *Innovation leadership practice*

Innovative leadership is the ability to think differently and motivate others to create new and better ideas to move towards positive results. It has two approaches, as shown in Figure 4.10. First is to bring new thinking and different actions to how to lead, manage, and go about work. Second is about leadership for innovation, where leaders must learn how to create an organizational climate where others apply innovative thinking to solve problems and develop new products and services. It is about growing a culture of innovation, not just hiring a few creative outliers (Horth and Buchner 2014). This two-tiered approach generates the kind of innovation that can produce the next new product or design, but it goes well beyond (Horth and Buchner 2014).

The innovative leader ignores the conventional order and tries new things. Such a leader rallies the entrepreneurial energy, champions innovation, and, if required, pushes past the drives of negativity. Innovative leaders may not always be successful each time they try something, but they set up a direction, and they often cause large changes. Innovation leadership in organizations is not about micromanagement, it is about the big picture and works well with creative thinking that adds to the vision and makes it greater rather than focusing far too much on details. Today, innovation leaders are generally required in technology-based organizations that evolve rapidly. Therefore, such leaders must have the required skills and knowledge to communicate effectively with their teams, deliver a cohesive vision, and realize the inherent risks and benefits of creativity and innovation (Habash 2017).

Many of today's leadership problems are critical and pressing; they demand quick and decisive action; but, they are complex. Because the organization, team, or individual does not know how to act, there is a need to slow down, reflect, and approach the situation in an unconventional

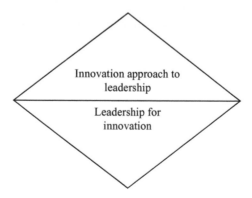

Figure 4.10 Two-tiered approach to innovation leadership.

way using innovative thinking (intuition), which is a crucial addition
to traditional business thinking (logic) (Horth and Buchner 2014). This
thinking allows enterprises to bring new ideas and energy to leaders and
to solve challenges. It also paves the way to bring more innovation into
organizations.

4.11   Lean leadership

Lean is about constant ticking, not occasional kicking.

Alex Miller

"Lean", as a business philosophy, refers to stripping out the wasteful
aspects of processes and maximizing the value to customers (Hines et al.
2004). Lean leadership is a leadership model focused on cultural transformation enabling people to identify and deal with quality issues where
work happens. It is all about commitment to employees, systems, and
effectively making changes towards organizational improvement opportunities. The model teaches leaders about the importance of three core
principles: go see, ask why, and show respect. A Lean environment needs
leaders to succeed at communication skills in order to realize the problems that their people are facing.

4.11.1   The Toyota model

The concept of "Lean" was developed by the Toyota executive, Taiichi
Ohno (1912–1990), who first identified the seven types of Muda (waste).
Ohno's beliefs were shaped by his study of the Model T Ford's (1913) continuous flow in final assembly. In 1913, Henry Ford designed the Model T
assembly line so that all the processes were in the same sequence as the
build. Prior to this, all manufacturing processes were grouped together
creating batch manufacturing (Epply and Nagengast 2018).

Lean, which has its roots in the Toyota Production System (TPS),
became a "buzz" word in the early 1990s. The Toyota model contains
four layers: philosophy, process, people and partners, and problem-
solving (Figure 4.11). The "people" layer is placed above the "process"
layer, reflecting that the roles of leadership, employees, and partners as a
combination are more important than the operational or tactical lean tools
(Shang 2014).

The philosophy is the base of the pyramid, which is long-term and
integrated in the whole organization. The next level is the processes and
refers to eliminating waste. The third level in the pyramid is the people, which includes both employees and partners. The people should
be challenged, treated with respect, and grow. The top of the pyramid

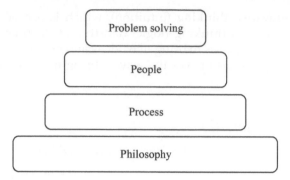

Figure 4.11 The 4Ps model according to Toyota.

includes problem-solving and continuous improvements (Andersson and Andersson 2014).

The manufacturing industry started to become curious and eventually even familiar with Toyota's unique practices (Liker 2009). Toyota's management principles include names like TPS, Toyota Management System (TMS), and different Lean combinations (Emiliani and Stec 2005). The Lean management system is rooted in two key principles: continuous improvement and respect for people, and both strive to eliminate waste while adding value to customers/stakeholders. Essentially, the principle, respect for people, includes leadership behaviors (Bass 1990).

4.11.2   Lean principles and behaviors

There are five fundamental concepts in Lean philosophy: specify value, value stream, flow, pull, and perfection. Lean leadership behaviors are analogous to Lean principals and are defined "simply as behaviors that add or create value". Successful Lean leaders know that they need to be consistent; "if they tell the employees to eliminate process waste", then the leaders must not behave in wasteful ways (Emiliani 2008).

The Lean principles of continuous improvement, respect for people, and a relentless focus on delivering customer value are making teams and organizations rethink the practices that might have guided them for decades. A new, transformative approach to working requires a transformation in leadership as well. For Lean to be truly effective, it needs effective Lean management to champion Lean principles, offer guidance, and ensure that Lean is being used to optimize the entire organizational system for value delivery (LeanKit 2018).

Lean behaviors are those that add or create value, such as trust, generosity, patience, objectivity, discipline, and reflection. People using those value-creating behaviors are often seen as role models. The opposite of

Table 1.5 Examples of Lean behaviors (Emiliani 2008)

Value-added Behaviors	Necessary Behaviors	Behavioral waste
Humility	Gossip	Blame
Calmness	Short-term thinking	Office politics
Wisdom	Ignorance	Confusion
Patience	Inconstancy	Inconstancy
Objectivity	Negative thoughts	Unknown expectations
Balance	Bias	Revenge
Trust	Stereotypes	Elitism

behaviors that create value are waste behaviors, which are behaviors that inhibit work flow. Waste behaviors are also called fat behaviors. Fat behaviors can also be recognizable as talking but no action, creativity waste, underutilizing workers' talents, or mismanagement of people. Table 4.5 illustrates some examples of the differences between the three types of behaviors.

4.12   Leadership community of practice (CoP)

Coming together is a beginning; keeping together is progress; working together is success.

Edward Everett Hale

Lave and Wenger (1991) coined the phrase CoP to describe a natural kind of learning that is social and context-dependent (situated). They define CoP as groups of people who share a concern or a passion for something they do and learn how to do it better as they interact regularly (Wenger 1998). CoP is focused on collective responsibility for learning and translating this to performance.

4.12.1   CoP: Leadership in practice

CoPs were common as far back as ancient times. In Greece, for instance, corporations of metalworkers, potters, masons, and other craftsmen had both a social purpose and a business function (members trained apprentices and spread innovations). In the Middle Ages, guilds played similar roles for artisans throughout Europe. Today's CoPs are different in one important respect: instead of being composed primarily of people working on their own, they often exist within large organizations (Wenger and Snyder 2000).

Practice is considered to be a set of frameworks, ideas, tools, and information. It is meaningful performance governed by social rules and norms. Wenger et al. (2002) presented a structure that can be represented by three concentric triangles, as shown in Figure 4.12. The inner triangle represents the CoP's core group. These are the members who lead and help to define the direction of the community, and also determine specific actions and processes with the CoP. Within the core, one person (champion) or a small group assumes the role of community coordinator, who takes responsibility for the growth of the community. The second triangle is comprised of the active members, who share information, insights, and experiences; participate in discussions; and raise issues and concerns regarding needs and requirements. The outermost triangle is comprised of the peripheral group. These are members who pop in and out of the community and who interact less regularly. And finally, outside the triangles are outsiders, those who are not yet in the CoP. In addition, CoP must have three traits, including domain (shared area of interest), community (group of individuals who care about the domain to participate in regular interaction), and practice (shared knowledge, experience, and techniques).

At its core, the social construction of learning means learning by doing. In CoP, individuals come together based on a common interest or passion in a disseminated leadership model. In the CoP and distributed leadership literature, leadership is process-oriented, shared, situated, and dependent on a positional or key leader, termed the community coordinator (Lester and Kezar 2017).

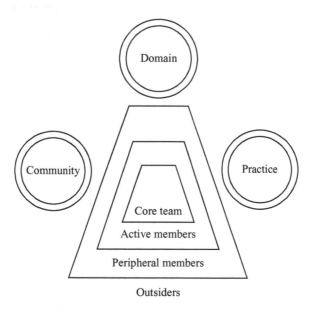

Figure 4.12 Structure of CoP.

In order to have a vibrant community, the membership of the three levels needs to be dynamic. Outsiders need to keep coming into the community, and the core, active, and peripheral membership needs to keep changing. Wenger stressed that there needs to be a conscious effort on the part of the old-timers – members who have been around a long time at the core or active levels – to welcome in newcomers, those who are just entering the community. This is an essential mechanism for revitalizing the community.

There are a few roles to be played in the CoP, the key role being the community leader, the person who is accountable for ensuring the community functions as a knowledge-sharing community. This person is involved in the start-up and growth of the community, and in developing and maintaining the CoP processes. The choice of a good leader is crucial to the effective operation of the community. In CoPs, learning is portrayed as a social formation of a person rather than as only the acquisition of knowledge. Learning entails change in one's identity, as well as the re-negotiation of meaning of experience. In the original formulation of CoPs, the main focus is on the person becoming more competent in the context of idiosyncratic practice (Lave and Wenger 1991). The strength of communities of practice is self-perpetuating. As they generate knowledge, they reinforce and renew themselves.

Organizations often consider professional development as an individual activity and promote it with personal training budgets or solo learning objectives. While it is useful to think about professional development for individuals, it is also valuable to think about the professional development of a group of people and the organizational capability it may bring.

CoPs can be an essential part of any Agile organization. In such organizations, Lean-Agile frameworks champion the multidisciplinary team, which is a great way to focus people on a specific outcome as that of CoPs. This is different from the traditional role-based-team setup where people performing the same role sit together (Webber 2016).

4.12.2   Entrepreneurial CoP

At the inter-organizational level, CoPs represent an area in which entrepreneurs can face the challenges collectively and carry out managerial and innovation actions related to their own businesses (Guimarães 2016). From this perspective, Dibiaggio and Ferrari (2003) observed the formation of different CoP into the ecosystem of innovation in Silicon Valley. The cooperation between peers has created commonsense deals with ambiguities and discrepancies related in particular to new social links between partners. This vision provides an understanding of tensions between the simple reproduction of knowledge and routines and the emergence of new practices to solve problems. Thus, for innovative entrepreneurs, engagement in a community can support the operation of technological ambiguities, partnerships, and commercially-related innovation. The cooperation practices in CoP can be a learning source of multiple behaviors and activities that entrepreneurs must develop to survive (Burger-Helmchen 2008). They can also be an exploration process or a knowledge creation related to the new products and services (Harvey et al. 2015). The common field of knowledge, the intensity of relations, the voluntary commitment of members, the share norms, and the values of CoP foster trust between their members (Wenger 1998). These protected areas of cooperation constitute an intermediate level between the individual and the organization and create conditions for new knowledge and technologies.

CoPs are emerging in organizations that thrive on knowledge. The first step for leaders, whether schoolteachers, company managers, or community organizers, is to understand what these communities are and how they work. The second step is to realize that they are the hidden source of knowledge development and therefore the key to the challenge of the knowledge economy. The third step is to appreciate the irony that these informal arrangements require specific managerial efforts to develop them and to integrate them into the organization so that their full power can be leveraged (Wenger and Snyder 2000).

4.12.3   Experiential learning CoPs

CoPs are social, powerful learning organizations at the plainest level. They are rich learning spaces that support knowledge creation, social engagement, practice improvement, and connection through networks (Wenger 1998). They generally evolve naturally to address commonly shared interests and problems. By their nature, they tend to exist outside formal educational organizations. In some university settings, there is a resilient interest in engaging students in experiential learning outside their classrooms by creating and supporting interdisciplinary knowledge and practice, leadership skills, and initiatives to be professional members of the workforce and to lead social change.

CoP learning is one form of experiential education and is meant to be a purposeful effort to connect real-world experiences to the content and theory being learned in the specific course. It may take many forms and varies in size and required effort for planning and implementation. CoP can provide an education that attends in some balanced way to the student's need to advance both knowledge acquisition and creation to critical judgment; both thinking and acting; reflection and engagement; growth as an individual; and greater connectivity with the larger community.

Educators and instructional designers may capitalize on the CoP model by trying to instantiate or support communities in which desired practices reside, and allowing learners to engage through the process of legitimate peripheral participation. Such communities can be supported or fostered through a variety of means, many of which involve providing technologies that support the community. Technology has affordances that allow it to represent content, scaffold processes, and shift the user's social context (Hoadley and Kilner 2005).

4.13   Knowledge acquisition

Attempting to answer the following questions involves acquisition of knowledge from this book and other books, documents, and the Internet.

- What is leadership? What are leadership skills?
- What qualities make an effective leader?
- What is the relationship between leaders and followers?
- What is the difference between leadership and power?
- What advice would you give someone going into a leadership position for the first time?
- Is leadership about showing how much you know?
- Differentiate between Theory X, Theory Y, and Theory Z.
- What is Maslow's hierarchy of needs?
- Who are innovative leaders and what are their qualities?
- What is the difference between a manager and a leader?
- What is EQ, compared with regular intelligence? What does it measure?
- What is ST? Are there different types of ST? What are the main concepts?
- Why should leaders practice ST?
- Give examples of effective methods to support the attempts of improving leadership.
- What is design thinking? How should leaders practice ST?
- How do you handle resistance to ideas and policies that you propose to others?
- Does every manager need to be a leader?
- What should leaders keep in mind about success and failure?
- Discuss examples you may have come across of strong and weak leadership. You may use examples from academia or from the community (keep anonymous).
- In which way do you see that new technologies will affect leadership?
- Identify an economic, environmental, or social problem, which currently exists that impacts one as an effective leader.
- In terms of EQ self-control, how do you slow down your response through active listening?

- A true leader speaks from experience, not theory. Comment on the statement.
- What is Lean? Where does Lean come from?
- In what way is leadership a critical link to succeed with a Lean strategy?
- What are the four cornerstones (leadership principles) in leading towards Lean?
- Why are CoPs important? What is the role of technology in CoPs?
- What are the common approaches to support and develop leaders in CoP?

4.14   Knowledge creation

Collaborate with peers on learning or work with others outside the class to narrow down the objectives of each activity. You may access class and online resources and analyze data and information to create new ideas and balanced solutions. High-level digital tools may be used to develop multimedia presentations, simulations or animations, videos and visual displays, digital portfolios, reflective practice (online publishing and blogging), or well-researched and up-to-date reports.

4.14.1   Leadership portfolio

The leadership portfolio is a communication task of where you have come from, where you are currently, and where you are headed on your leadership route. It expresses your story and documents your development in the career leadership path. The portfolio is your opportunity to pose yourself as a leader with knowledge, insight, and experience.

For this task, prepare your leadership portfolio, which summarizes your leadership style, including key qualities you possess; your strengths; and areas for improvement. Specify examples of your leadership experience in class, projects, sports, community, etc., and how you have exhibited specific leadership qualities in each. Finally, what do you see as your unique advantage over others? Develop the portfolio using high-level digital tools of your preference.

4.14.2   Leadership as high EQ

Communication and leadership skills are no longer just nice to have. They are must-haves. The industry is going toward more collaboration-integrated project delivery (Walpole 2016). Many elements of EQ might be more familiar to us as "soft skills" and "people skills" (Kumar and Hsiao 2007). While talking about those terms, they do not sound as important, but while thinking of them as intelligence traits, they look like a set of competencies that can bring the job to life (Platt 2015). Investigate this topic and reflect the outcomes, and answer the following questions in a poster format.

- Do you think that engineers and computing professionals tend not to concern themselves with emotions while being more interested in technical ideas, problems, and solutions?
- Do you think improving one's EQ comes easily?
- What drives and motivates you?

4.14.3 Critical evaluation of management and leadership

Leadership and management are two distinct but complementary systems. While managers promote stability, leaders press for change. Only organizations that can embrace both sides of that contradiction can thrive in turbulent times (Kotter 1995). Make a list of what you believe are leadership tasks and what are management tasks. Then critically evaluate the above quotation. Reflect the outcome in a piece of art.

4.14.4 Designing a CoP

The idea of CoP is that learning occurs in social contexts that emerge and evolve when people who have common goals interact as they strive towards goals. For this task, design a virtual CoP in your domain that provides a "sense of place" in the minds of community members through an integrated, caring combination of live online events and collaboration over time within a continual Web environment. Investigate this topic and reflect the outcome as well as answers to the following questions in a portfolio format.

- Identify the audience, purpose, goals, and vision for the community.
- What are the critical building blocks of the proposed CoP?
- Define the activities, technologies, processes, and roles that will support the community's goals.
- What kind of knowledge do CoPs create?

4.14.5 CoP: ST to co-create a sustainable place

How can you connect architects, engineers, scientists, and city planners who believe that wood is the best material to build homes and cities with communities who harvest it sustainably and scientists who study how to do this best? How can you accomplish this? That's where CoP comes in.

It is about co-creating ideas and solutions that would never come about without active participation of people from many disciplines, field experience, and study. In a team of three to four students, reflect this ill-defined problem in a design leadership portfolio. You should involve ST as an approach to solving problems holistically.

References

Adams, N. 2012. Skinner's Walden two: An anticipation of positive psychology? *Review of General Psychology* 16(1): 1–9.

Akay, E. 2015. Why and how should leaders practice systems thinking? https://www.linkedin.com/pulse/why-how-should-leaders-practice-systems-thinking-esin-akay/.

Ambler, G. 2013. Systems thinking as a leadership practice. http://www.georgeambler.com/systems-thinking-as-a-leadership-practice/.

Andersson, C., and H. Andersson. 2014. Lean leadership: The Toyota way in agricultural firms. Master's Thesis, Swedish University of Agricultural Sciences, Department of Economics.

APA. 2013. How does the APA define psychology? http://www.apa.org/support/about/apa/psychology.aspx#answer.

Avey, J. B., B. J. Avolio, C. D. Crossley, and F. Luthans. 2009. Psychological ownership: Theoretical extensions, measurement and relation to work outcomes. *Journal of Organizational Behavior* 30(2): 173–191.

Bass, B. M. 1990. *Bass and Stogdill's Handbook of Leadership: Theory, Research, and Managerial Applications*. New York, NY: Free Press.

Brown, T. 2008. *Design Thinking*. Boston, MA: Harvard Business Review.

Bullock, R. 2013. Systems thinking: How to lead in complex environments. http://www.scontrino-powell.com/2013/systems-thinking/.

Burger-Helmchen, T. 2008. Plural-entrepreneurial activity for a single start-up. *Journal of High Technology Management Research* 19(2): 94.

Cherry, K. 2017. What is the Hawthorne effect? https://www.verywellmind.com/what-is-the-hawthorne-effect-2795234.

Cherry, K. 2018. The five levels of Maslow's hierarchy of needs. How Maslow's famous hierarchy explains human motivation. https://www.verywellmind.com/what-is-maslows-hierarchy-of-needs-4136760.

Dibiaggio, L., and M. Ferrary. 2003. Communities of practice and social networks in the dynamics of functioning of high technology clusters. *Journal of Industrial Economics* 103(2 and 3): 111–130.

Eba. 2018. Trait theory of leadership and its key characteristics. https://www.educational-business-articles.com/trait-theory-of-leadership/.

Emiliani, B. 2008. Practical Lean leadership. A strategic leadership guide for executives. The Center for Lean Business Management, LLC, Wethersfield.

Emiliani, M. L., and D. J. Stec. 2005. Leaders lost in transformation. *Leadership and Organization Development Journal* 26(5): 370–387.

Epply, T., and H. Nagengast. 2018. How was Lean manufacturing developed? http://www.continental-design.com/lean-manufacturing/handbook-3.html.

Gardner, W. L., R. John, and J. R. Schermerhorn. 2004. Unleashing individual potential: Performance gains through positive organizational behavior and authentic leadership. *Organizational Dynamics* 33(3): 270–281.

Gaynor, G. H. 1993. *Exploiting Cycle Time in Technology Management*. New York, NY: McGraw-Hill.

George, B. 2016. HBS: The truth about authentic leadership. http://www.billgeorg e.org/page/hbs-the-truth-about-authentic-leaders.

George, J. M., and G. R. Jones. 2008. *Understanding and Managing Organisational Behavior*. Upper Saddle River, NJ: Prentice Hall.

Gibbs, N. 1995. The EQ factor. *Time* 146: 60–68.

Glesson, B. 2018. 5 Aspects of emotional intelligence required for effective leadership. https://www.inc.com/brent-gleeson/5-aspects-of-emotional-intellig ence-required-for-effective-leadership.html.

Goleman, D. 1995. *Emotional Intelligence: Why It Can Matter More Than IQ?* New York, NY: Bantam Books.

Goleman, D. 1998. *Working with Emotional Intelligence*. London, UK: Bloomsbury Publishing.

Guimarães, T. 2016. Communities of practice of innovative startups Cooperation or competition: Is this the question? https://hal.archives-ouvertes.fr/ha l-01345645/document.

Habash, R. 2017. *Green Engineering: Innovation, Entrepreneurship, and Design*. Boca Raton, FL: CRC Taylor and Francis.

Harter, J. K., F. L. Schmidt, and T. L. Hayes. 2002. Business-unit-level relationship between employee satisfaction, employee engagement, and business outcomes: A meta-analysis. *Journal of Applied Psychology* 87: 268–279.

Harvey, J., P. Cohendet, L. Simon, and S. Borzillo. 2015. Knowing communities in the front end of innovation. *Research Technology Management* 58(1): 46–54.

Hines, P., M. Holweg, and N. Rich. 2004. Learning to evolve: A review of contemporary Lean thinking. *International Journal of Operations and Production Management* 24(10): 994–1011.

Hoadley, C., and P. G. Kilner. 2005. Using technology to transform communities of practice into knowledge-building communities. *SIGGROUP Bulletin* 25(1): 31–40.

Horth, D., and D. Buchner. 2014. Innovation leadership: How to use innovation to lead effectively, work collaboratively, and drive results. Centre for Creative Leadership. White Paper. http://www.ccl.org/wp-content/uploads/2015/04 /InnovationLeadership.pdf.

Khan, S. N. 2010. Impact of authentic leaders on organization performance. *International Journal of Business and Management* 5(12): 167–172.

Kleim, R. L., and I. S. Ludin. 1998. *Project Management Practitioner's Handbook*. New York, NY: AMACOM.

Kotter, J. P. 1996. *Leading Change*. Boston, MA: Harvard Business School Press.

Kotter, J. P. 2001. What leaders really do? *Harvard Business Review* 79(11): 85–96.

Kumar, S., and J. K. Hsiao. 2007. Engineers learn 'soft skills the hard way': Planting a seed of leadership in engineering classes. *Leadership and Management in Engineering* 7(1): 18–24.

Lave, J., and E. Wenger. 1991. *Situated Learning: Legitimate Peripheral Participation*. New York, NY: Cambridge University Press.

Leankit. 2018. Lean management: The role of Lean leaders. https://leankit.com/ learn/lean/lean-management/.

Lester, J., and A. Kezar. 2017. Strategies and challenges for distributing leadership in communities of practice. *Journal of Leadership Studies* 10(4): 17–34.

Liker, J. K. 2009. The Toyota way. http://gtu.ge/Agro-Lib/%5BJeffrey_Liker%5D_
The_Toyota_Way_-_14_Management_Pri(BookFi.or.pdf.

Luthans, F., and B. J. Avolio. 2003. Authentic leadership development. In Cameron,
K. S., J. E. Dutton, and R. E. Quinn (Eds.). *Positive Organizational Scholarship.*
San Francisco, CA: Berrett-Koehler, pp. 241–258.

Mabugat, M. 2018. Just what makes a leader? https://psych2go.net/modern-th
eories-on-leadership-just-what-makes-a-leader/.

MacIntyre, P. 2016. Advancing leaders in engineering: Ways of learning leadership. https://www.kpu.ca/sites/default/files/Transformative%20Dialogues
/TD.8.3.6_MacIntyre_Ways_of_Learning_Leadership.pdf.

Mohamed, R. K. M., and C. S. M. Nor. 2013. The relationship between McGregor's
X-Y theory management style and fulfillment of psychological contract: A
literature review. *International Journal of Academic Research in Business and
Social Science*s 3(5): 715–720.

Monat, J. P., and T. F. Gannon. 2015. What is systems thinking? A review of selected
literature plus recommendations. *American Journal of Systems Scienc*e 4(1):
11–26.

Peterson, C., and M. E. P. Seligman. 2004. *Character Strengths and Virtues: A
Handbook and Classification.* New York, NY: Oxford University Press.

Platt, J. R. 2015. Why emotional intelligence is key to your success? The Institute.
http://theinstitute.ieee.org/career-and-education/career-guidance/why-
emotional-intelligence-is-key-to-your-success.

Riemer, M. J. 2003. Integrating emotional intelligence into engineering education.
World Transactions on Engineering and Technology Education 2(2): 189–194.

Rothman, J. 1999. Successful engineering management: 7 lessons learned. http:
//www.jrothman.com/articles/1999/01/successful-engineering-manage
ment-7-lessons-learned/.

Salovey, P., and J. M. Meyer. 1998. Emotional intelligence. In Jenkins, J. M., K.
Oatley, and N. L. Stein (Eds.). *Human Emotions: A Reader.* Malden, MA:
Blackwell.

Seligman, M. E. P. 2002. *Authentic Happiness: Using the New Positive Psychology to
Realize Your Potential for Lasting Fulfillment.* New York, NY: Free Press.

Senge, P. M. 1994. *The Fifth Discipline: The Art and Practice of the Learning Organization,
Currency.* New York, NY: Crown Business.

Senge, P. M. 2006. *The Fifth Discipline: The Art and Practice of the Learning Organization.*
New York, NY: Random House.

Shang, G. 2014. Toyota way Lean leadership: Some preliminary findings from the
Chinese construction industry. *Proceedings IGLC-22* June: 1145–1156.

Skaržauskienė, A. 2009. System thinking as a competence in leadership paradigm. *Management Theory and Studies for Rural Business and Infrastructure
Development* 16(1): 97–105.

Stajkovic, A. D., and F. Luthans. 1998. Social cognitive theory and self-efficacy: Going beyond traditional motivational and behavioral approaches.
Organizational Dynamics 26: 62–74.

Team FME. 2015. *Leadership Theories. Leadership Skills.* Free Management e-Books.
http://www.free-management-ebooks.com/dldebk-pdf/fme-leadership-
theories.pdf.

Thomas, N. 2004. *The John Adair Handbook of Management and Leadership.* London,
UK: Thorogood.

Tobia, P. M. 1999. Robert Lutz gives engineers the nod. *IEEE Today's Engineer* 2(1): 6–11.

Walpole, B. 2016. Leadership is communication, rising engineers told. ASCE. http://news.asce.org/leadership-is-communication-rising-engineers-told/.

Webber, E. 2016. Communities of practice: The missing piece of your Agile organization. https://www.infoq.com/articles/communities-of-practice-agile-organisation.

Wenger, E. 1998. *Communities of Practice: Learning, Meaning and Identity*. New York, NY: Cambridge University Press.

Wenger, E., and W. M. Snyder. 2000. Communities of practice: The organizational frontier. Harvard Business Review. https://hbr.org/2000/01/communities-of-practice-the-organizational-frontier.

Wenger, E., R. A. McDermott, and W. Snyder. 2002. *Cultivating Communities of Practice: A Guide to Managing Knowledge*. Brighton, MA: Harvard Business Press.

Wren, J. T. 1995. *The Leader's Companion: Insights on Leadership through the Ages*. New York, NY: The Free Press.

Zeiger, S. 2018. Theories on motivation in organizations and management. https://smallbusiness.chron.com/theories-motivation-organizations-management-25221.html.

part two

Communication skills and reflective practice

Communication skills in practice

5.1 Knowledge and understanding

Having successfully completed this module, you should be able to demonstrate knowledge and understanding of:

- Communication skills for professional effectiveness
- Communicating ethically, and real-world skills
- Impact of emotional intelligence on communication skills and leadership
- Various arenas for communicating in groups: speaking, listening, writing, presenting, and meeting
- Active listening, reflective listening, critical listening, and ethical listening
- Effective speaking skills, including ethical speaking, public speaking, debates, and interviews
- Viewing and representing using digital media for knowledge creation
- Non-verbal communication including facial expressions, body movements and posture, gestures, eye contact, touch, personal space, and voice
- Types of writing including journaling, technical reports, and project proposals
- Preparing phases of effective presentations including planning, researching, developing, and writing
- Basic structure of a professional meeting plan
- Intercultural competence in practice

5.2 Communicating as a professional

> *The most important thing in communication is hearing what isn't said.*

Peter Drucker

An effective professional needs a list of critical soft skills. These are skills key to effective performance across all professional career categories. A strong soft skill that features towards the top of the list is good communication (Atre et al. 2013). Communication skills, in the sense perceived in the quotation above, are not just about verbal (explicit) communication. However, this emerges as the single most important topic that encompasses many media (written, spoken) and may be expressed non-verbally (implicitly), independent of a formal language, for example with the use of gestures, body movements, facial expressions, and much more (Figure 5.1). According to Leathers (1992), 93% of all communication that occurs face-to-face is nonverbal.

The term "communication" refers to the various forms of listening, speaking, writing, and non-verbal cues. Effective communication occurs when a whole message is sent and completely received and understood. It is about getting the correct message to the accurate person in the appropriate medium at the right time. The ability to communicate effectively is one of the most valuable professional skills that creates a positive and encouraging atmosphere in the workplace.

Communicating with others is part of everyday life. Largely, communication is about explicit language, speaking, and writing words; however, communication is also about implicit messages, sent via tone or eye contact. Learning to communicate effectively both implicitly and explicitly is a valuable skill for any professional (ESF 2008).

To be professional is to behave appropriately and competently. Communication is multifaceted and incorporates various elements, such as verbal, nonverbal, written, listening, visual, intercultural, interdisciplinary, etc. Communication skills development can be enhanced and demonstrated through the use of various methods, such as class discussions

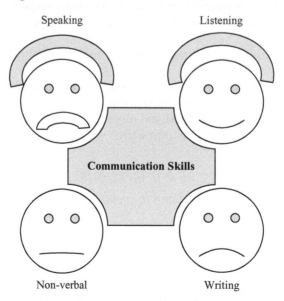

Figure 5.1 Main forms of communication skills.

(Riemer 2007), project presentations, event meetings, and communication competitions.

In education, academic institutions should not depend only on communication courses. Both written and oral communication should be a major part of the curriculum, especially in project-based courses. The engineering education system should also recognize the importance of complementary courses in nurturing communication skills such as history, philosophy, psychology, and management.

5.3   Communication skills for professional effectiveness

The art of communication is the language of leadership.

James Humes

The term "communication skills" has outgrown the vague notion in layman's terms and has felicitously taken shape as an integrated concept with each of its constituent elements: verbal, nonverbal, and interpersonal (Atre et al. 2013). Communication is a key interpersonal skill. It is speaking, listening, or writing that is precise, thorough, and clear to its audience; it tells the truth about a case directly and clearly. Therefore, communication must be effective in addition to being professional.

5.3.1   Communicating ethically

Communication is the use of various resources to express information, to move, to inspire, to persuade, and to connect in an integrally ethical undertaking. Ethics are the preset morals and values that reflect someone's identity, education, or dignity. Regardless of context, communication involves choice, reflects values, and has consequences. These three key elements of communication form the basis of its ethical makeup (Makau 2018). Ethical communication is fundamental to thoughtful decision-making and responsible thinking. Historically, responsible and ethical communication has fostered devoted connection, compassion, and understanding (Mayhew 2018).

Ethical communication is extending the medium and even the language of delivering messages. Today, communication technology, which refers to texting, email, video chat platforms, social media platforms, websites, or other types of online services, has become an integral part of everyday life, where technology has been transforming the delivery and dissemination of information and how people and organizations interact with each other. With growing technology evolving at the rate of the thought, the efficiency can be taken care of only if the object in charge, the professionalism, is effective enough. As these technologies quickly evolve and embed themselves in everyday lives, these topics are worthy of further exploration. However, ethics should always be upheld. After the heavy usage of social media, ethics of communication have started to change, and society is experiencing a paradigm shift.

Ethical communication has several principles including communicating fact-based messages honestly and accurately, acting with sensitivity, acting with curiosity, acting with openness, and acting responsibly. It values freedom of expression, diversity of perspective, and tolerance of dissent. But while ethical communication should be honest and straightforward, it should never offend or provoke listeners (Mayhew 2018). The content of the message is extremely important, as is the delivery of the message. With so many different modes of communication, it is essential to know what type of information is ethical to send electronically versus information that should be communicated face-to-face.

Communication ethics are the rules driven by an individual's or group's preset morals that create some effects in that particular communication. Morals depend on the mindset of that communicator. Usually it is seen that when a person communicates with another person, mostly the individual tries to communicate with good morals. These types of communications include interpersonal, group, and mass communications (Mukherjee 2017). Communication ethics has impact not only on individual or group communication, but also on organization communications.

5.3.2   Communicating real-world skills versus academic skills

Real-world skills are not like academic skills but include competencies and interpersonal skills that help people make educated decisions, solve problems, think critically and creatively, communicate and network effectively, leverage relationships, always see the big picture, and set realistic expectations for professional growth and development.

Professionals like engineers and computing specialists use communication for many different purposes, for example, pitching ideas, describing solutions, reporting results, discussing work with collaborators, customers, etc. Therefore, graduating students need to acquire the necessary communication skills and become familiar with a broad selection of styles during their education (ABET 2013). It is a well-known complaint from real-world organizations that the recent graduates they hire are ill-prepared for acting and, especially, professionally communicating in the workplace. Yet as part of their curriculum, students do a lot of formal writing and, sometimes, speaking. However, most student communication, such as papers, reports, and exams, encourages the development of communication skills that are at odds with those useful in the real world. Specific writing and speaking courses can help, of course, but are too often disconnected from the materials students must learn in other courses. Yet appropriate learning activities in these other courses can help students develop effective real-world communication skills (Doumont 2002). The above observation is one of the reasons why the accreditation board has shifted its focus from the documentation of required courses (or learning input) to that of learning outcomes. In other words, it does not matter how many papers students write; what matters is whether they acquire useful writing skills.

Designing activities that foster real-world communication skills may well be uncomfortably straightforward, once the desired purpose is recognized. While engineering and computing classes are known for group projects, professors must deal with group members to develop original communication tasks in addition to design and implementation tasks. The challenge is to make students write for and speak to other students, not teachers, usually on topics that that are related to the content of projects using real-world skills. This integration is vital for realizing and transforming knowledge and skills related to the project content and principles effectively as well as for transition to future career's workplaces.

5.3.3   Communicating professionally and effectively

In a profession, eventually everything stands to serve the purpose of bringing efficiency and effectiveness (Atre et al. 2013). Planning and preparing are part of the objectivity and formality of professional communication. To be effective, the topic should be revealed to audiences early in the communication process. Professionalism in communication depends on choosing the best way in which to express a subject, understanding the mindset of others, and then following basic guidelines for conveying the message to the recipient. Effectiveness, traditionally the focus of the professional world, has been on the so-called hard skills, the technical skills necessary to effectively perform within the organization. Figure 5.2 shows three phases that integrate professionalism and effectiveness in communication.

Apparently there are many ways of communication, though they tend to fall into four categories: speaking, listening, writing, and non-verbal. Each of these types can be formal or informal. The level of formality and familiarity are determined by the recipients of communication, the audience. Another important consideration is gender neutrality. Using gender neutral language avoids preference and bias.

The most common professional communication barriers are non-attentive listening, interrupting others, inappropriate reactions, jumping to conclusions, failure to recognize body language synchronicity, and gender differences. The first four barriers are self-explanatory: not listening, acting disproportionately to a situation or information, and making a judgment before having all the information. Most people are aware these are negative actions in the workplace. However, the last two are more understated (Richason 2018).

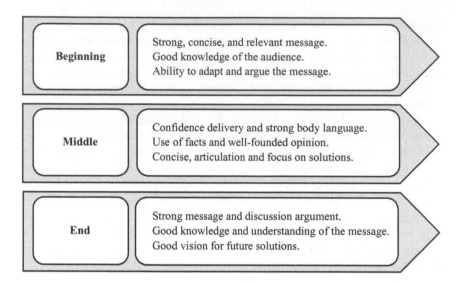

Beginning

Strong, concise, and relevant message.
Good knowledge of the audience.
Ability to adapt and argue the message.

Middle

Confidence delivery and strong body language.
Use of facts and well-founded opinion.
Concise, articulation and focus on solutions.

End

Strong message and discussion argument.
Good knowledge and understanding of the message.
Good vision for future solutions.

Figure 5.2 Phases of integrating professionalism and effectiveness in communication.

5.4   *EQ to communicate and lead*

> *Emotional awareness is necessary so you can properly convey your thoughts and feelings to the other person.*
>
> **Jason Goldberg**
> *[from Communication Skills for Success (2014)]*

EQ includes the ability to observe, perceive, distinguish, reason about, and recognize emotions, and to employ emotions to lead actions, solve problems, develop thought, and stimulate growth. EQ was first defined in 1990 by Salovey and Meyer (Salovey and Meyer 1998). It may generally be defined as a set of non-cognitive competencies that are linked to interpersonal effectiveness at work. Communication is a core leadership skill, and there is a deep connection between one's ability to successfully communicate and one's ability to successfully lead. It is about being able to listen well, to motivate and inspire others, to control your reactions, and to build strong relationships (Franchetti 2016). Figure 5.3 shows the impact of EQ on communications and leadership skills.

EQ comprises five components: self-awareness, self-regulation, motivation, empathy, and social skill. These components have a direct relationship on a person's EQ that further drives a person's performance (Lakshmi 2016). Given that communication is ranked as one of the prime characteristics required by employers in the workplace, EQ has an important role to play in strengthening communication skills when certain EQ elements are enhanced. Similarly, it has been shown that incorporating a greater

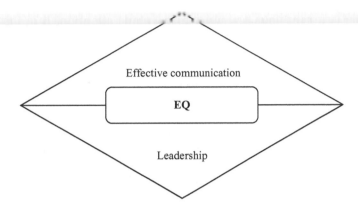

Figure 5.3 Impact of EQ on communication and leadership skills.

emphasis on communication activities serves to enhance EQ aspects, including more active participation, greater self-control and awareness, heightened motivation, and a better understanding of duties and assignments (Upchurch and Sims-Knight 1999).

EQ directly impacts on communication competences by targeting particular elements that improve and enhance the process of communication. In the US, the biggest complaint of workers is poor communication with management, sometimes even preventing employees from doing their best work. Further, the key to empathy is listening well. Being in control of personal emotions also makes the worker more accessible to other people, both inside and outside the workplace (Goleman 1998).

In the workplace, to improve management, teams, and individual effectiveness, significant effective communication skills are required which rely heavily on EQ. Students' skills in communication and EQ, which reinforce these competences, should be initiated and taught at the initial stages of learning. Also, EQ skills improve team-working skills, especially with regards to communication between team members (Riemer 2007). Furthermore, the context for the receiver of the communication (whether it be written, non-verbal or oral), is taken into account through empathy and self-awareness, whether the context is cultural, educational, professional, social, or otherwise.

5.5 *Learn to listen*

> *The word "listen" contains the same letters as the word "silent".*
>
> **Alfred Brendel**

Listening is a conscious activity which entails attention. It is the most important component of interpersonal communication and is a significant part of communication skills. Good listening is critical for building strong communication relationships.

Aristotle classified listeners into those who would be using a speech to make decisions about past events, those who would make decisions affecting the future, and those who would evaluate the speaker's skills (Wrench et al. 2011). Watson et al. (2012) classified listeners into four styles. First, people-oriented listeners, who are interested in the speaker and how the speaker thinks. They are more attentive to the speaker than to the message. Second, action-oriented listeners, who are primarily interested in finding out what the speaker wants. Third, content-oriented listeners, who are interested in the message itself, whether it makes sense, what it means, and whether it is accurate. Fourth, time-oriented listeners, who prefer a message that gets to the point quickly. This kind of listener may be receptive for only short periods of time and may become rude if the speaker takes a longer time. They convey their impatience through eye rolling, shifting about in their seats, checking their phones, and other unsuitable behaviors.

5.5.1   Active listening

Active listening is an advanced communication skill based on the work of psychologist Carl Rogers, which involves giving free and undivided attention to the speaker (Robertson 2005). Active listening skills are an extension of broad communication skills and involve both verbal and nonverbal communication (Silverman et al. 1998). Active listening means being deeply engaged in and concentrating on what the speaker is saying. It requires far more listening than talking, including intense concentration and attention to everything the person is conveying. It is a process of attending carefully to what is being said. It also involves the listener observing the speaker's behavior and body language by remaining neutral and non-judgmental.

Active listening involves a meaningful understanding of what the speaker said and sending it back to them. One way to demonstrate this neutral attention is for the listener to show understanding by paraphrasing what the speaker is saying. Paraphrasing may confirm the accuracy of the listener's understanding or identify the need for explanation. To be an active listener means to fully understand and positively respond to what the audience is communicating.

Active listening is a significant skill that requires both time and practice to acquire. |It requires patience, because listeners need time to explore their own thoughts and feelings. This requires avoiding the urge to jump with questions or comments every time the speaker pauses.

Active listening is a vital element of constructive discussions because it allows for the considerate exchange of ideas. It is mainly valuable in situations of disagreement or misunderstanding where an atmosphere of cooperation should be created to increase the possibility of clarifying the disagreement.

5.5.2 Reflective listening

Reflective listening is a special type of listening that involves paying deep attention to the content and feeling of the speaker. It is a process in which a conscious decision is made to listen to and understand the message of the speaker. It focuses on personal elements of the communication rather than the abstract ideas (Katz and McNulty 1994). Reflective listening involves two key steps: seeking to understand the speaker's idea, and offering the idea back to the speaker, to confirm that it has been understood correctly. The process involves responding to others to check out the listeners' understanding of the communication. The process should be feeling-oriented and responsive. The listener should show empathy and concern for the person communicating.

Reflective listening has many objectives. It may help one understand what the speaker is saying. It also allows the speaker to feel understood and achieve outcomes. Listening may help the speaker clarify thoughts, decide on a course of action, or explore feelings to a certain extent. It is useful for both the speaker and the listener. Being able to understand and communicate the meaning of the words helps receivers better interpret the received information. In general, reflective listening is effective during demanding conversations. A reflective listener focuses on the discussion at hand while allowing the speaker to communicate the message. Verbal reaction is essential for reflective listening. Listeners should make statements that summarize what is said, clarify what appears to be understood, and reflect the feeling from the speaker.

5.5.3 Critical listening

Critical listening is a demanding form of listening that involves analysis, critical thinking, and judgment. It is a process that requires reflective, reasonable, rational thinking to assemble, understand, and evaluate information in order to develop a judgment. The main idea is to try to understand others before evaluating them. When listeners are not critical of the messages they are attending to, they are more likely to be influenced by unreasonable arguments based on opinions but not actual facts. Critical listening encompasses all aspects of professionalism, especially in technical training. It entails the mode of thinking about any subject, content, or problem in which the thinker improves the quality of judgment by capably analyzing and assessing it. However, education sometimes may discourage critical thinking by presenting the student with only well-structured theories and best practices during the student's learning, not requiring a critical attitude from the students, an opportunity to reflect a high level of professionalism.

Critical listening can be improved by employing one or more strategies to help the listener analyze the message: recognize the difference between facts and opinions, uncover assumptions given by the speaker, be open to new ideas, use both reason and common sense when analyzing messages, relate new ideas to old ones, and take useful notes (Wrench et al. 2011).

5.5.4   Ethical listening

Ethical listening depends heavily on authentic intentions. Coopman and Lull (2008) emphasize the creation of a climate of caring and mutual understanding, observing that "respecting others' perspectives is one hallmark of the effective listener. Respect, or unconditional positive regard for others, means treating others with consideration and decency whether agreeing with them or not".

Ethical listeners should not interrupt a speech, should not give advice, should not do something else while listening, and should not convey distraction through nervous mannerisms (Wrench et al. 2011). Polite listening can be used when it is not required to either agree or disagree with the speaker. In general, people learn ethical communication by listening, by being courteous and polite, and by maintaining a free and open expression of ideas.

5.6   Prepare to speak

> *Think before you speak. Read before you think.*

> **Fran Lebowitz**
> *[from The Fran Lebowitz Reader (1994)]*

Speaking is the process and act of giving a speech, lecture, or talk in a structured, thoughtful manner intended to inform or influence a listening audience. Knowing the value of the speech and how to conduct oneself as a confident, good speaker might mean the difference in getting a job or moving throughout the ladder of profession for a leadership position.

5.6.1   Ethical speaking

Ethical speaking is a responsible process that begins with brainstorming the topic of speech with honesty and openness. Elspeth Tilley, a public

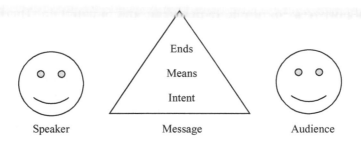

Figure 5.4 Conceptual model of speaking incorporating the ethical pyramid.

communication ethics expert from Massey University, proposes a structured approach to thinking about ethics (Tilley 2005). Her ethics pyramid involves three basic concepts: intent, means, and ends. Figure 5.4 shows a conceptual model of speaking incorporating the "ethical pyramid".

The ethical pyramid is an illustrative way of understanding the three fundamental parts: intent, means, and ends. The first major consideration to be aware of when examining the ethicality of something is the issue of intent. To be an ethical speaker or listener, it is important to begin with ethical intentions. This means that ethical speakers will prepare their remarks with the intention of telling the truth to their audiences. The "means" incorporate communication with others as the second level of the ethics pyramid. McCroskey et al. (2003) describe this part as the tools or behaviors employed to achieve a desired outcome. It should be realized that there are a range of possible behavioral choices for any situation and that some choices are good, some are bad, and some fall in-between. Whereas the means are the behavioral choices to make, the ends are the results of those choices. Eventually, understanding ethics is a matter of weighing all three parts of the ethical pyramid: intent, means, and ends.

5.6.2   Public speaking

Without a speaker, there cannot be an oral message. Without an audience, the message cannot be public. Without an organized message, the speech is not likely to be effective. Public speaking is the process and act of speaking or giving a lecture to a group of people in a structured manner intended to inform or influence a listening audience. It is an art form nearly as old as humanity itself (SSBA 2018).

Effective public speaking involves understanding audience and speaking goals, choosing elements for the speech that will engage the audience with the topic, and delivering the message skillfully. Modern public speaking scholars typically use a classification system of three general purposes: to inform, to persuade, and to entertain. The first is about helping audience members acquire information that they do not already possess. The primary purpose of informative presentations is to share one's knowledge of a subject with an audience. To persuade means to get listeners to embrace a point of view or to adopt a behavior that they would not have done otherwise. Entertaining speaking involves an array of speaking occasions including social, political, educational, etc. An entertaining speech can be either informative or persuasive at its root, but the context or theme of the speech requires speakers to think about the speech primarily in terms of audience enjoyment (Wrench et al. 2011).

The interchange between the verbal and nonverbal components of speech can either bring the message intensely to life or confuse the audience. Therefore, it is best that the speaker neither overdramatize the speech delivery behaviors nor downplay them. This is a balance achieved through practice, trial and error, and experience.

Experiencing some nervousness about public speaking is normal. The energy created by this physiological response can be functional if you harness it as a resource for more effective public speaking. Anxiety typically peaks at the anticipatory stage. This level of anxiety is called communication apprehension. This can cause a variety of involuntary responses, such as heart pounding, stomach butterflies, mouth drying, shaking hands and legs, nausea, sweating, and forgetting the information, among other things (McCroskey and Beatty 1986). Communication apprehension is a psychological response to evaluation. This psychological response, however, quickly becomes physical as the body responds to the threat the mind perceives. It is connected to the idea of judgment from the audience (Wrench et al. 2012). Speakers are likely to be most anxious right before they get up to speak. As a speech progresses, the level of anxiety is likely to decline. Planning the speech to incorporate techniques for managing nervousness at different times will help decrease the overall level of stress experienced.

5.6.3   Learn to debate

Debate is about decision-making for everyday life. The skills that can be sharpened by debating are critical thinking, listening, research, information processing, creative thinking, communication, and persuasion (NAUDL 2007). Debate is the presentation of ideas in conflict. It brings diversity, fun, and motivation. It is the method through which decisions are made in any organization. Debate is essential in life; the only alternatives are passive acceptance of decisions or the violent overthrow of the decision-makers. The rules of debate vary from place to place; however,

Table 5.1 Possible examples of students' debates

Debate 1	Can the current laws keep up with development on Internet technology?
Debate 2	Is development on AI a threat to humanity?
Debate 3	Will robotics reduce human employment?
Debate 4	Is nuclear energy too dangerous and expensive, or it is an important future power source?
Debate 5	Is it a benefit or downfall to engage technology in education?

the general basis of debating remains unchanged: each participant is given equal time and is expected to clarify the benefits of their own point of view and to show the weaknesses in the opponent's point of view.

In education, Bloom's taxonomy identifies roleplay and debates in the "affective goals domain" because they require that the students' values, attitudes, or interests be affected in the class (Anderson et al. 2001). Debate in its easiest form requires a question, statement, or idea with at least two opposing positions, each of which is defended against the others by an advocate, often with an impartial moderator ensuring that the discussion remains focused. In the end, students acquire an enhanced grasp of the knowledge content and skills simply because they are an active participant in the learning process. Table 5.1 shows several examples of debate ideas that can be performed in the class.

5.6.4 Prepare for interviews

Planning for an interview is an important stage in the hiring process; accordingly, it is important to understand what approach to take and to develop appropriate answers for anticipated questions. Planning can also increase awareness of potential drawbacks and areas where one may need to show more sensitivity.

Most interviews have some degree of planning involved, as can be seen in job interviews, in which questions are targeted to assess role-relevant skills. In general, interviews can be either fully-structured, where all questions are delivered to each respondent consistently, regardless of their responses; semi-structured, where there are some set questions that are delivered to all respondents; and unstructured, like an exploratory interview with few or no set questions. Clearly more planning is needed in structured interviews than unstructured interviews, which enable more consistency (McDaniel et al. 1994). Interviewing reveals information about the person's experience and also provides the chance to observe communication skills firsthand. Table 5.2 outlines several possible interview questions that cover a wide range of interpersonal skills.

Table 5.2 Several possible interview questions

Motivation	What are your reasons for applying for this position?
Experience/Skill	What do you consider to be the most significant work accomplishment of your career?
Intelligence	Describe a position which you have held that required you to analyze the facts and prepare a final product.
Judgment	If you were given several important tasks to accomplish, how would you go about prioritizing them?
Responsibility	Describe a project or assignment which you were required to complete from start to finish.
Relationship	Talk about a coworker you like working with the best and the least.
Leadership	How do you handle crisis situations?
Habits	What do you view as the characteristics of a person best suited for this position?

5.7   Viewing and representing

> We are drowning in information but starved for knowledge.
>
> **John Naisbitt**
> *[from Megatrends: Ten New Directions*
> *Transforming Our Lives (1988)]*

Professionals today require sound viewing and representing skills, as is conceptualized in Figure 5.5. In a world that is full of media images on television, on the Internet, on billboards, in newspapers, and in magazines, people need to understand the impact of such images on learners.

5.7.1   Digital literacy

Media is a powerful force in everyone's life. Music, TV, video games, magazines, and other components of the media have a strong influence on how people see the world, an influence that often begins in infancy (CDML 2018). Globally, the International Society for Technology in Education (ISTE) frames its benchmarks for digital literacy around six standards: creativity and innovation; communication and collaboration; research and information fluency; critical thinking, problem-solving and decision-making; digital citizenship; and technology operations and concepts.

Media education is the process through which individuals become media literate. In education, media in general and digital media in

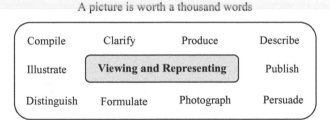

Figure 5.5 The process of viewing and presenting.

particular has a place in nearly every course and subject. It embodies and furthers current pedagogy, which emphasizes student-centered learning, recognition of multiple intelligences, and analysis and management rather than just the simple storing and reciting of information.

Unlike traditional media, there is no one-way connection in digital media. In traditional media, content only flows one way: producers create it, then it will be sold or licensed to distributors, who then bring it to customers. On the other hand, digital literacy is an important part of this skillset, alongside communication, problem-solving, critical thinking, teamwork, and other skills that are complementary to technology (BCC 2016). It is the ability to understand, use, and interact with technology, media, and digital resources in real-world situations. In digital media, by contrast, users are no longer the final link in a distribution chain but a node in the middle of an infinite network. Collaboration and dialogue are the norm, rather than solitary creation and broadcasting (Jenkins et al. 2006).

5.7.2   *Knowledge transformation*

Digital literacy is more than technological know-how: it includes a wide variety of ethical, social, and reflective practices that are embedded in work, learning, leisure, and daily life (Jenkins et al. 2006). Figure 5.6 shows a model that illustrates the many interrelated elements that come under the digital literacy umbrella, including knowledge acquisition, possession, and creation. These range from basic access, awareness, and training to inform user confidence to advanced and more complex creative and critical literacies and outcomes. There is a logical progression from the more basic skills towards the higher, more transformative levels.

Knowledge acquisition represents data, information, and technical fluency that is needed to engage with computers and the Internet. Technical fluency includes basic knowledge of computer components; understanding of software programs; coding skills, which are the ability

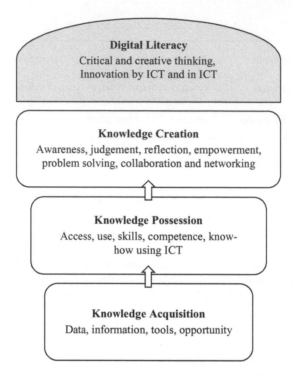

Figure 5.6 Digital literacy model for knowledge creation through transformation.

to apply computational thinking skills in a specific coding language to solve problems and create solutions; computational thinking skills, including problem-solving skills and different approaches based on the context or environment of the problem; and understanding the capabilities of digital presentation tools to create presentations that help prepare for the expectations of the users.

Knowledge possession helps users use, understand, comprehend, contextualize, and critically evaluate knowledge and ICT-related digital skills. The future careers of students depend on their ability to understand and harness digital tools. Skills and competencies include understanding the basis of how digital information is created and how digital tools operate, and even how to create digital tools.

Knowledge creation is the ability to produce knowledge content and professionally communicate through a variety of digital media tools. Creation with digital media includes being able to adjust to various contexts and receivers. This means using multimedia such as images, sound, and video and to effectively and responsibly engage with Web 2.0 user-generated content through the design of social processes that engage blogs and forums, video and photo sharing, and other forms of social media.

5.8   Non-verbal communication (NvC)

The human body is the best picture of the human soul.

Ludwig Wittgenstein
[from Philosophical Investigations (1953)]

NvC is a process of communication through exchanging wordless messages. It may be communicated in many ways including, for example, facial expression and eye contact, body movement or posture, gestures, and touch.

5.8.1   Facial expressions

The expressions used to convey emotions like fear, anger, sadness, and happiness are similar throughout the world. The human face, for example, is very expressive, able to show numerous emotions without a need to say a word. The ability to understand facial expressions is a significant aspect of NvC. Unlike some forms of NvC, facial expressions are universal. The facial expressions for happiness, sadness, anger, wonder, fear, and hatred are all similar across cultures. The value in understanding facial expressions is to collect information about how the other person is feeling and guide mutual interaction accordingly (Cuncic 2018). Not all facial expressions remain for a long time. Those that pass fast are called micro-expressions and are nearly invisible to the casual observer.

5.8.2   Eye contact

The eyes may indicate understood processes or cognitive function. Eyes can also perform monitoring functions. Eye contact means when two people in conversation are looking at each other's eyes at the same time. It is a non-verbal ability to communicate and makes conversations flow smoothly. Eye contact is used to acknowledge or avoid the presence of others and may tell information about attitudes, emotion, and influence in social relationships. It is often equal to ability to verbally express a thought.

Since the visual sense is dominant for most people, eye contact is thought to have a big influence on social behavior. In many Asian cultures, avoiding eye contact is seen as a sign of respect. However, those in Latin and North America consider eye contact important for conveying equality among individuals (Drucker 2017).

Eye contact is also essential in maintaining the flow of conversation and for guessing the other person's response. The eyes are frequently referred to as the "windows to the soul" since they are capable of revealing a great deal about what a person is feeling or thinking. By engaging in conversation with others, taking note of eye movements is a natural and important part of the communication process (Cherry 2018).

5.8.3 Body movements and posture

Posture refers to the position of the body, limbs, and muscular tone. The positioning of the body is often regarded as NvC. The way the body moves communicates a lot of information. Posture may reveal a great deal about emotional status. Posture could be closed when positioning the arms so that they are folded across the body and/or crossing the legs. It could be open posture when positioning the arms so they are not folded across the body and not crossing the legs. A key aspect of showing confidence is the maintenance of a relaxed and open posture.

5.8.4 Gestures

Gestures are also known as kinesics. They are movements that communicate information, intentionally or not (McNeill 2008). Gestures refer to the study of arm movement, hand movement, body movement, and face movement. They may be used when speech is not reaching the message (for example, a language barrier) or insufficient (for example, complex content in the message). However, gestures may vary across cultures and regions, so it is important to be careful to avoid misinterpretation.

Mostly hand and arm gestures are used in NvC. They are usually separated into the following categories: emblems, illustrators, and adaptors. Emblems are gestures that convey meaning by themselves and are assumed to be deliberately performed by the speaker. They are conventionalized symbols and are strongly culture-dependent (Kendon 1983). Illustrators are gestures that accompany the speech such as simple, repetitive, rhythmic movements that bear no obvious relation to the semantic content of the accompanying speech. Adaptors are not communicatively intended or perceived to be meaningfully related to the speech, such as scratching one's head, stroking the chin, hand-to-hand movement, and lip licking (Ekman and Friesen 1967). The importance of understanding NvC using hand gestures and its implications on information sharing may make communication more effective.

5.8.5 Touch

Touch, or haptic communication, is a form of NvC in which information is conveyed by physical contact between people. Touch, like any other communication message, may elicit negative and positive reactions depending on the configuration of people and the circumstances (Knapp 1972;

Knapp and Hall 2002). It describes how people communicate with each other through the use of touch.

There are great cultural differences in the amount of touch allowed between individuals. In the US, for example, using a handshake is considered proper to greet a person or a business professional (Drucker 2017). There are also various cultural viewpoints on the right rules regarding physical contact between both similar and opposite genders.

5.8.6   Personal space

Most interactions between engineers and clients require face-to-face communication. A position and space express the nature of interest, acceptance, and trust between the two sides. Personal space is the distance maintained between a person and other people in everyday life. The distance differs depending on the situation. Everyone has a personal space that provides that individual with a sense of security and a kind of control. Personal space is based on several factors including gender, cultural norms, and sensitivity due to personal differences. Figure 5.7 shows the typical personal distances of individuals.

5.8.7   Voice

Voice is not just what people say, it is how they say it. When people speak, other people read their voices in addition to listening to their words. Things they pay attention to include timing and pace, how loudly they speak, tone and inflection, and sounds that convey understanding, such as "ahh" and "uh-huh". Think about how tone of voice, for example, can show irony, anger, care, or confidence.

5.9   Write to learn: learn to write

> *How can I know what I think until I see what I say.*
>
> **E.M. Forster**
> *[from Aspects of the Novel (1927)]*

Writing to learn is based on the observation that an individual's thoughts and understanding can grow and be clarified through the process of

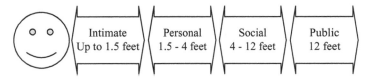

Figure 5.7 Typical personal distances.

writing. These can be short, unrehearsed, or otherwise informal writing tasks that help one think through key concepts or ideas.

5.9.1   Writing to learn

Language is any formal system of gestures, signs, sounds, and symbols used or conceived as a means of communicating thought. In today's world, effective use of language helps in interpersonal relationships at home and at work (Wrench et al. 2012).

Many authors from diverse disciplines have discussed the merits and techniques of using writing to solicit deeper learning at all levels of education. For example, Wheeler and McDonald (2000) highlight that writing helps students learn because it makes them establish and shape their thoughts, ideas, and facts; allows them to develop and enrich those ideas to a deeper level of understanding; and causes students to engage in the material directly and personally. Writing drives students to exercise their reason and to think more comprehensively and more broadly about the problems at hand.

Writing promotes learning better than activities that involve only studying or reading. It enables students to experiment every day with written language and increase their fluency and mastery of written conventions. Writing to learn involves much more than just writing down passages from a text or copying what the instructor is writing on the board. It involves a variety of recursively operating sub-processes (for example, planning, monitoring, drafting, revising, and editing) rather than a linear sequence (Applebee 1984). Therefore, instructors should incorporate writing in their courses in various ways, from research papers to short writing assignments to describe a concept, process, or device.

The writing to learn strategies are examples of some of the many ways instructors may help students engage in what they are learning by summarizing information, visualizing, and in other ways continuing to build and apply comprehension skills.

- **Journals.** Student journals are a remarkable forum for writing that may be implemented with any subject matter. While there are various forms of journals, in content-area classrooms most teachers use content-focused journals.
- **Think and write.** This strategy allows students as they read a text, listen to a lecture, observe a demonstration, or watch a video a chance to evaluate their understanding of the topic, to make a connection to something they have learned previously or experienced outside of school, to make a prediction, and to question anything that they might not fully understand. Asking students to think and

write about what they are learning promotes remembering and comprehension.

- **Structured note taking.** This helps students actively process the material they are learning. Creating an outline or graphic organizer for students' note taking provides a framework of support as students write their thoughts and questions.

5.9.2 Journaling

Journaling is defined as expressive personal writing about ideas that the writer perceives as important. Journaling can aid the various thought processes including, in particular, summarizing, observing, classifying, critiquing, interpreting, collecting and organizing data, and hypothesizing (Zacharias 1991). Journals can be an effective tool to enhance student learning and simultaneously provide the instructor with unique insight into students' thinking processes. However, students require significant guidance in journaling (Sobek 2002).

Journals may take on numerous forms, such as the reflective journal (Kerka 1969). Students are asked to reflect upon a certain concept or idea and create a written response that discusses, elaborates upon, or applies that idea. Reflection journals are chronicled entries of the learner that examine the process of learning and the acquiring of knowledge in a course or across courses. Beyond the training of newcomers to a discipline, they can be used in the professional development process or in continuous professional development (Steele 2013). The journal should be a reflective document that provides personal, thoughtful analysis of an individual's participation and progress on a task or group project, and an assessment of the group interactions that may have occurred during a period of time such as a week, for example.

A second journal form is the dialog journal, where students write entries which the instructor collects, reads, provides written responses to, and returns to the students. A third form is the literary journal, where students generate written responses to assigned readings (Burrows et al. 2001).

Journaling may work very well with student group projects. In considering student interactions with classmates as they proceed with a group project, the journal may address the following:

- What did the student learn during the interaction?
- What did the student contribute to their project tasks?
- What did the other members of the project group contribute?
- What are the group's plans for the next task?
- What is the student assessment of how the group is functioning so far?

- What happened when students tried something new? Why did they succeed or fail?
- Did the students consider a different perspective? Why or why not?
- Did the students have a theory background about tasks?

Also, it is needed to add few other issues, including:

- Literature review and/or readings that have been done to support investigating the project tasks
- New technological skills needed to plan and develop the task
- An individual feeling and opinion about the project
- The progress on achieving the course's learning outcomes
- Planning for the next task

5.9.3   Technical reports

Reports may be written for many reasons, for example they may intend to inform, recommend, motivate, play a part in debate, persuade, impress, record, reinforce, build on existing situations or beliefs, instruct, etc. If a report is to be well-received, then it must meet certain expectations of its readers. Overall, what gives people the feeling, both at first glance and as they get further into it, that a report is not to be avoided on principle? Readers in general like if a document is: brief, precise, simple, and descriptive. All these characteristics have in common that they can act to make reading easier and clearer (Forsyth 2010). A well-written report allows the reader to quickly understand what has been included. The report also provides sufficient detail to make the reader recreate the results, although the level of details provided depends heavily on the report's readers and any proprietary nature of the work.

The goal of a technical report is to completely and clearly explain technical work, why it was done, results obtained, and the implications of those results. The formal technical report contains a comprehensive, concise, and well-organized description of the work accomplished and the results obtained. All reports have certain aspects in common regardless of expected usage. Typical report sections are presented first, and all possible sections potentially included in the report are discussed subsequently.

A technical report typically follows the pattern described by the acronym IMRaD: introduction, methods, results, and discussion; see Figure 5.8. Usually, this format can be adjusted to certain needs, but it is helpful to commit the format to memory (Johnson-Sheehan 2018). An abstract must not be longer than half a page and must not contain figures or make reference to them. The results may be summarized in the abstract, but qualitatively, not quantitatively. The introduction section should provide the reader with an overview of why the work is performed, how the

Title page
Short, concise, and refers to a leading project activity

Abstract
Concise description, purpose and most important results

Introduction
Subject; purpose; main points; significance; background,
organization information

Theory; analysis; materials; methods
Description of methods; materials; steps, techniques, methodology

Results
Overview; data

Discussion
Purpose and importance; future work

Conclusions and recommendations
Project purpose; main points

How a reader peruses a technical report?
The reader will first read the title page and abstract. It should
encourage the reader into looking further into the report. The
conclusion is often the next section to be read. If the conclusion,
relative to the title page, sounds interesting the reader will continue
reading the other sections to learn more.

Figure 5.8 Basic structure of a technical report.

work is presented, and the most interesting results. This can usually be
accomplished with ease if the work has clearly stated the objectives. The
theory section may be divided into subsections if appropriate. Discussion
should be kept brief and refer the reader to outside sources of information where appropriate. Design details should be provided. If there is no
design but strictly analysis, then important details of all the analysis and
procedures performed should be provided. The results of the work should
be presented using neatly organized and completely labeled tables and/
or graphs whenever possible. When comparative data is available, data in
a way that facilitates the comparison should be facilitated with meaningful discussion. In the final section of the body of the report, the author

should briefly bring everything together. Conclusion is similar to the abstract except that the results are concluded upon in a quantitative way. Therefore, the conclusion should be a concise description of the report, including its purpose and the most important results, providing specific quantitative information (Akins and Akins 2009). Finally, all works should be cited in the report, including all the important bibliographical information. An appendix section may not always be present. Materials included in an appendix may include lab sheets, parts list, diagrams, extensive calculations, and probably lengthy computer programs, if required.

5.9.4   Project proposals and grants

A project proposal is a persuasive detailed description of a series of activities aimed at solving certain problems. Its objectives are to identify what work is to be done; to explain why this work needs to be done; to persuade the reader and/or the funder that the proposers are qualified for the work; to have a plausible management plan and technical approach; and to have the resources needed to complete the task within the specified time and cost constraints.

What makes an effective proposal? One major quality is artistic appearance. A robust proposal should have an attractive, professional, and inviting appearance. In addition, its information should be easy to understand. A second quality is substance, where a convincing proposal should include a well-organized plan of action. An effective proposal should have technical details, because technical depth is needed to promote the project and qualify it for funding.

Once the groundwork has been completed, proposal writing can commence. The key decision to be made at this stage is the structure of the project proposal (including the content and length). The structure is determined by the nature of the project as well as by the funding agency's requirements, including formats, application forms, project design outlines, and grant application guidelines (Nebiu 1990). The project proposal should explain the approach chosen for solving the problem and precisely how it will lead to improvement. It should be a detailed and directed manifestation of the project design. It is a way of presenting the project to the outside world in a format that is immediately recognized and accepted. It is helpful to include a table of contents at the end of the document. The contents page enables readers to quickly find relevant sections of the document.

The implementation plan should describe activities and resource allocation in as much detail as possible. It is exceptionally important to provide a good overview of who is going to implement the project's activities, as well as when and where. The implementation plan may be divided into two key elements: the activity plan and the resource plan. A simple table with columns could be prepared for activities, sub activities, tasks, timing, and responsibility.

In simple terms, a budget is an itemized summary of an organization's expected income and expenses over a specified period of time. Budgeting forms and financial planning procedures vary widely.

At the end, a brief description of the project personnel, the individual roles each one has assumed, and the communication mechanisms that exist between them should be given. All the additional information (such as CVs) should be attached to the annexes. Any specific jobs or course experiences that are relevant to the project should be highlighted. Figure 5.9 shows a basic structure that may be followed while writing a grant proposal.

5.10   Learn to present

> *Your slides should be a billboard not a document.*
>
> **Lee Jackson**
> *[from PowerPoint Surgery: How to Create Presentation*
> *Slides that Make Your Message Stick (2013)]*

An effective oral presentation is much more than just presenting ideas or delivering a speech. It is about skillful communication and relating to the audience, whether it is just a few people or a large gathering. It is one that matches the message to the audience, matches the content and delivery to the purpose, and it is delivered in a clear and engaging manner.

5.10.1   Preparing

Oral presentations are one of the most common tasks in the education system and various professions. Students, scholars, and professionals in all fields desire to propagate the new knowledge they produce, and this is often achieved by delivering oral presentations in class, at conferences, in public lectures, or in organization meetings. Therefore, learning to deliver effective presentations is a necessary skill to master both for education and further endeavors.

Robust presentations have one key component in common: they tell a story. Storytelling engages the audience, supports in understanding, and increases retention. Effective presentations require a good deal of researching, planning, and preparation. It is estimated that the majority of all mistakes in an oral presentation actually occur in the planning stage. The task may start with research by conducting a general review of the topic. The goal at this step is to find general information from books, journals, and the Internet that may help guide a presentation in the right direction.

Proposal title
Short, concise, and refers to a leading proposal activity

Introduction
Subject; purpose; main points; significance; background information

Statement of problem: the "why"
Statement; causes and effects; solving techniques

Implementation plan: the "what" and "how"
Objectives; plan; approaches; deliverables

Conclusion
Purpose and importance; cost and benefits; future work

Qualification
Personnel biographies; history of organization; prior experience

Budget plan

Proposal evaluation

Project proposal is largely evaluated based on the existence of clear innovative elements across the phases of the project. A clear comprehensive review of the current, relevant literature to both the problem statement and the proposed innovation should be presented. Action plan should be insightfully outlined in light of several relevant educational research and best practice elements. Ideas should be organized to fully address the problem statement and desired outcomes of the project. Relevant information should be richly described from data collection process. Recommendations should be clear, reasonable and can be backed by the results of the project.

Figure 5.9 Basic structure of a proposal.

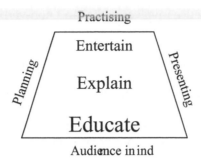

Figure 5.10 Key principles of effective presentations.

In general, effective presentations involve the three major "E" principles as well as the following three major steps: planning, practicing, and presenting, as shown in Figure 5.10.

While planning for the presentation, the following issues should be taken into consideration:

- Know the audience; this is an important factor in deciding what material to prepare and share.
- With the audience in mind, select the topic, identify the topic, outline the presentation to clarify key messages, and establish a logical sequence.
- Use the introduction to establish credibility by demonstrating familiarity with the topic; create an effective opening that will interest the audience; then a question may be posed to present a fact or tell a short story.
- Maintain a smooth flow from one topic to the next and establish logical sequence to tell the audience the "what, why, and how".
- Fix the number of key points as a checklist to convey the content.
- Reduce the amount of text; use presentation aids like photos or graphics to illustrate key points.
- Use visualization to boost the appeal and analogies and stories to explain complicated ideas and to build repetition.
- Briefly summarize the outcomes and refer to future action, if needed.

5.10.2   *Practicing*

Effective communication requires practice to get it right. Practicing is an important part of preparing to deliver an effective oral presentation. To practice, the following actions may be helpful.

- Remember, practice involves verbal and non-verbal delivery.
- Rehearse the presentations, do it either alone or with a team, or videotape oneself and review the performance after.
- Consider using different colored highlighters as a reminder to pause, to emphasize on a particular point, to have a slide change, etc.
- Plan ahead by anticipating the types of questions that will be asked and practice answers.
- The more you practice, the more comfortable you will be with the ideas, and you will look more professional.

5.10.3　Presenting

During a presentation, open with an attention-getting introduction. It is always the presenter's job to make the audience feel comfortable and engaged. The following steps may assist in the process:

- Dress appropriately.
- Arrive early and test the equipment. Check the visuals for various locations within the room.
- Make contact before the presentation by breaking the imaginary barrier with the audience.
- Act as natural and relaxed as possible.
- Smile and maintain eye contact with people. Only look at notes or slides very briefly.
- Be enthusiastic about the presentation topic.
- Read the audience's body language in order to modify the pace of delivery to keep as many people engaged as possible.
- To reduce misunderstanding, use presentation aids to clarify or to emphasize.
- Effective presentations can be set to a quick pace, a calm pace, or a combination.
- To engage the audience, it is better to move around in the available space rather than remain behind a podium.
- Do not underestimate the challenge of running a successful question and answer session. Always acknowledge the questions.

5.11　Learn to meet

> *In meetings philosophy might work, on the field practicality works.*
>
> **Amit Kalantri**

Meetings are essential in any form of human venture. They bring people together to discuss a scheduled topic. Today, meetings are so common

that turning the resources they tie up into sustained results is a priority in high-performance organizations (Serrat 2010). They are necessary to
coordinate individual efforts, collaborate on joint projects, sell ideas, solve
problems collectively, and make consensus-based decisions.

5.11.1   Effective meetings

Knowing how to plan and facilitate an effective meeting is a highly
effective skill. A successful meeting begins with good preparation and a
structured agenda through writing. They are crucial to ensure that teams
stay on schedule. The more productive the meeting, the less chance the
team is unfocused. This is important because the meeting time is a valuable setting to discuss points of view and gain agreement on a general
course of action. Each team member has an opportunity and obligation to provide feedback and share concerns if the best results are to be
accomplished.

Attention to meeting preparation, facilitation, participation, and
evaluation processes is the recommended approach for ensuring effective outcomes. Therefore, the most effective way to have a good meeting
is to follow guidelines. This systematic approach ensures that everyone's
point of view is noted for discussion and follow-up. Meetings become an
opportunity for team members to come together and focus their ideas in
a single direction (Pigeon 2018).

5.11.2   Meeting procedures

Meeting procedures may vary according to the level of formality required
to meet the requirements of the agenda efficiently. It is useful to use the
first meeting to determine and agree upon procedures for meeting conduct. At the meeting, a facilitator acts as a "content-neutral" person who
leads the group through the agenda but does not contribute to the substance of the discussion and has no decision-making authority.

There are three different types of group behaviors. First is task-oriented behavior, where the focus concentrates on the task at hand. Second,
relationship-oriented behaviors, which focus on relationships involved.
Third is self-directed behavior, which is destructive, since it focuses on
self-serving objectives. Effective meetings should have a combination of
both task-oriented and relationship-oriented behaviors, with the individual participants showing positive self-oriented behaviors. These are
the behaviors that a team leader wants individuals to display during the
meeting and should be encouraged.

Productive meetings usually follow a standard format; an example is
shown in Figure 5.11. Initially, the agenda is an important part of the meeting. It should be sent out and reviewed by the team members before the

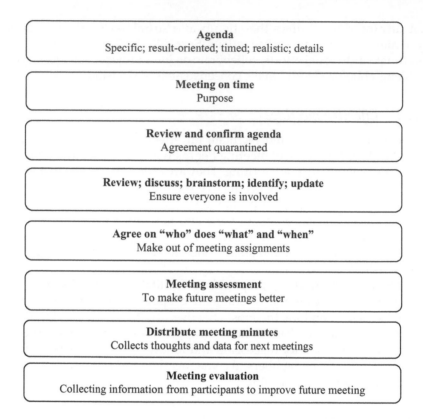

Agenda
Specific; result-oriented; timed; realistic; details

Meeting on time
Purpose

Review and confirm agenda
Agreement quarantined

Review; discuss; brainstorm; identify; update
Ensure everyone is involved

Agree on "who" does "what" and "when"
Make out of meeting assignments

Meeting assessment
To make future meetings better

Distribute meeting minutes
Collects thoughts and data for next meetings

Meeting evaluation
Collecting information from participants to improve future meeting

Figure 5.11 Basic structure of a meeting plan.

meeting so that all members are prepared for the agenda work. During the first part of the meeting, rules are assigned. This helps the team stay on the assigned task. Several general dominant rules for a meeting are: participate, get focus, maintain momentum, and reach closure.

One of the most challenging tasks is time management. Time limits are an essential part of well-run meetings. Usually participants appreciate and expect starting and ending on time. The biggest challenge is mapping out time limitations for each activity of the meeting agenda and sustaining momentum to keep the process moving. It is important to leave some time at the end of the meeting to evaluate the outcomes. It is necessary to review actions and assignments, and set the time for the next meeting and ask members if they can make it or not, meaning to get their commitment.

Finally, the minutes of the meeting should be distributed to the team members after a short period of time, probably a day or two. The minutes of a meeting act as the record for all the interactions throughout the meeting.

5.12 Intercultural competence in practice

Everybody believes that their reality is the real reality.

Paul Watzlawick

Increasingly, the ability to work with people of different cultures is becoming the order of the day. It has its benefits and its disadvantages. Intercultural competence represents knowledge, skills, and attitudes that encompass a person's ability to get along with, work, and learn with people from different cultures. It is the ability to discriminate and experience relevant cultural differences. It can be conceptualized as an individual's ability to develop a positive emotion towards understanding and appreciating cultural differences that promotes an appropriate and effective behavior within intercultural communication. This definition shows that intercultural sensitivity is a dynamic concept. It reveals that interculturally sensitive persons must have a desire to motivate them to understand, appreciate, and accept differences among cultures and to produce a positive outcome from intercultural interactions (Erasmus 2015).

Intercultural competence is the ability to think and act in interculturally appropriate ways. Openness, flexibility, and adaptation to diverse social and cultural situations are notable intercultural traits. Through practice, people become flexible by observing and reacting to others' behaviors. Therefore, flexible behavior leads to adaptability so that people perceive themselves as competent in other cultures (Gudykunst 2004).

Today, the importance of intercultural competence in both global and domestic contexts is well-recognized. New communication technologies such as the Internet, the increasing speed and reduced costs of international transport, migration flows, and the internationalization of business have resulted in an ever-increasing number of people, including engineers, engaged in intercultural communication, such as when dealing with foreign professionals or working in a foreign nation (Riemer 2007). The advantage of working in a cross-cultural situation is that you often gain insights on work and life that you never would have before.

Developing intercultural competence involves gaining more understanding of how one engages cultural diversity. Culture has incredible impacts on the way people think, perceive, communicate, learn, teach, and live. It is cited here as an aspect of a country or community, not in relation to organizational culture, and may be defined as a social organization, way of life, attitudes, customs, and beliefs held by a particular country or group. Communication styles are affected by the culture of those engaged in communication (Hofstede 2007). Culture is socialized in individuals and often reinforced in the education process. Various cultural dimensions impact on communication, with many appearing to be somewhat

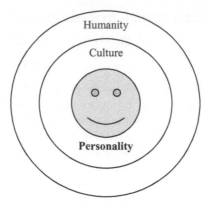

Figure 5.12 Layers of humanity, culture, and personality.

interlinked. Importantly, these dimensions are relative and not absolute, so variations can be expected; in effect (Hofstede and Hofstede 2005), Figure 5.12 shows the intercultural layers that have impact on personality.

5.13   *Knowledge acquisition*

Attempting to answer the following questions involves acquisition of knowledge from this book and other books, documents, and the Internet.

- What is effective professional communication?
- Why are communication skills important to engineering and computing students?
- Explain how the levels of the ethics pyramid might be used in evaluating the ethical choices of a public speaker or listener.
- What are some of the consequences of poor listening?
- Is it more important to be a good listener or a good speaker?
- Describe why the understanding of nonverbal communication is important in engineering.
- Why is digital literacy important?
- What level of digital skills should university students develop upon entering the workforce?
- What do you think gestures are, in terms of non-verbal communication?
- Differentiate among the three types of public speaking purposes.
- What is communication apprehension?
- What makes a good grant proposal?
- How is a project proposal assessed?
- What is the primary purpose of meeting minutes?

- How do students apply their intercultural skills in the classroom?
- Why are presentation aids important in public speaking?
- What is the role of culture in communication?

5.14   Knowledge creation

Collaborate with peers on learning or work with others outside the class to narrow down the objectives of each activity. You may access class and online resources and analyze data and information to create new ideas and balanced solutions. High-level digital tools may be used to develop multimedia presentations, simulations or animations, videos and visual displays, digital portfolios, reflective practice (online publishing and blogging), or well-researched and up-to-date reports.

5.14.1   Assessing communication skills

Good communication is central to working with people. It is important to be able to communicate both on a one-to-one basis and in a group context. Communication is not just about the words used but also about the manner of speaking, body language, and, above all, the effectiveness of listening. To reflect all of the above, you may produce an e-poster that displays the characteristics of good listening in an artistic way.

5.14.2   Creating a funding proposal

Imagine you have been assigned the task of writing a proposal for funding of a start-up company in one of the contemporary areas of digital technologies. For this task, write a 500-word essay to convince investors to join this new venture. Also, present your proposal to the class and note to what degree communication skills play a role in the tasks you have prepared.

5.14.3   Debate to foster real-world communication

In groups of six, students debate a philosophical question such as "Do machines think?" Each student defends a point of view except one student who plays the moderator. Besides being moderated by a student, this asynchronous conversation is also monitored and steered by a teacher. Each student (not just one per group) must dig into a potentially vast and complex philosophical view on the question. The other students have no knowledge of this view, but, interestingly, defend a different view on the same question. The moderator should be neutral in the discussion.

5.14.4   Why are image-making skills important to engineering and computing students?

Engineering is a multidisciplinary profession. A single project may involve teamwork with specialists from other disciplines. The ability to collaborate and communicate effectively with a diverse team, as well as convey complex concepts to a non-technical audience, is an asset. For this task, a group of students may think of a transdisciplinary project that requires, in addition to science and technology, involvement of arts and digital media. The group may produce an e-Portfolio of five to eight pages that reflects the importance of images in conveying the message of the project.

5.15.5   Can AI master interpersonal skills?

Interpersonal skills are what make us different from machines, these are things they cannot do, the things that make us human. Interpersonal and non-verbal communication skills are probably the skills that we need to nurture in order to thrive in a future driven by AI. For this task, two teams of three students each may investigate and debate this subject. The two groups may debate in front of the class, reflecting two opposing opinions about the subject.

References

ABET. 2013. Computing accreditation commission. Criteria for Accrediting Engineering Technology Programs, 2013–2014. http://www.abet.orglDispl ayTemplateslDocsHandbook.aspx?id=3. 150.

Akins, M. A., and J. H. Akins. 2009. Technical report writing guidelines. Poughkeepsie, New York: Dutchess Community College. http://www8.sun ydutchess.edu/faculty/akins/documents/TechnicalReportWritingGuide lines.pdf.

Anderson, W. L., D. Krathwohl, W. P. Airasian, A. K. Cruikshank, E. R. Mayer, R. P. Pintrich, J. Raths, and C. M. Wittroch. 2001. *A Taxonomy for Learning, Teaching, and Assessing: A Revision of Bloom's Taxonomy of Educational Objectives.* Second Edition. New York, NY: Longman.

Applebee, A. N. 1984. Writing and reasoning. *Review of Educational Research* 54(4): 577–596.

Atre, S., S. Jain, and V. Sharma. 2013. Impact of communication skills on professional effectiveness at the top level of hierarchy. *Global Journal of Management and Business Studies* 3(7): 751–756.

BCC. 2016. Developing Canada's future workforce: A survey of large private-sector employers. Business Council of Canada. http://thebusinesscouncil.ca/ wp-content/uploads/2016/03/Developing-CanadasFuture-Workforce.pdf.

Burrows, V. A., B. McNeill, N. F. Hubble, and L. Bellamy. 2001. Statistical evidence for enhanced learning of content through reflective journal writing. *Journal of Engineering Education* 90(4): 661–668.

CDML. 2018. Media literacy fundamentals. Canada's Centre for Digital and Media Literacy. http://mediasmarts.ca/digital-media-literacy/general-information/digital-media-literacy-fundamentals/media-literacy-fundamentals.

Cherry, K. 2018. Understanding body language and facial expressions. https://www.verywellmind.com/understand-body-language-and-facial-expressions-4147228.

Coopman, S. J., and J. Lull. 2008. *Public Speaking: The Evolving Art*. Stamford, CT: Cengage Learning.

Cuncic, A. 2018. 5 Tips to better understand facial expressions. https://www.verywellmind.com/understanding-emotions-through-facial-expressions-3024851.

Doumont, J.-I. 2002. Developing real-world communication skills in non-communication classrooms. https://ieeexplore.ieee.org/stamp/stamp.jsp?tp=&arnumber=1049098.

Drucker, P. K. 2017. 7 Cultural differences in nonverbal communication. https://online.pointpark.edu/business/cultural-differences-in-nonverbal-communication/.

Ekman, P., and W. V. Friesen. 1967. Head and body cues in the judgment of emotion: A reformulation. *Perceptual and Motor Skills* 24(3): 711–724.

Erasmus. 2015. Intercultural sensitivity. http://www.europskiput.com/index.html.

ESF. 2008. *Handbook for effective, professional communication*. Faculty of Forest and Natural Resources Management Undergraduate Education Committee, Syracuse, SUNY ESF. https://www.esf.edu/fnrm/documents/FNRM_Communications_Handbook2008.pdf.

Forsyth, P. 2010. *How to Write Reports and Proposals?* Revised Second Edition. London, UK: Kogan Page.

Franchetti, S. 2016. Emotional intelligence and its impact on communication in the workplace. https://franchetti.com/emotional-intelligence-impact-communication-workplace/.

Goleman, D. 1998. *Working with Emotional Intelligence*. London, UK: Bloomsbury Publishing.

Gudykunst, W. B. 2004. *Bridging Differences: Effective Intergroup Communication*. Fourth Edition. Thousand Oaks, CA: Sage.

Hofstede, G. A. 2007. European in Asia. *Asian Journal of Social Psychology* 10(1): 16–21.

Hofstede, G., and G. J. Hofstede. 2005. *Cultures and Organizations: Software of the Mind*. New York, NY: McGraw-Hill.

Jenkins, H., K. Clinton, R. Purushotma, A. J. Robison, and M. Weigel. 2006. Confronting the challenges of participatory culture: Media education for the 21st century. An Occasional Paper on Digital Media and Learning. https://www.macfound.org/media/article_pdfs/JENKINS_WHITE_PAPER.PDF.

Johnson-Sheehan, R. 2018. Planning and organizing proposals and technical reports. https://owl.english.purdue.edu/media/pdf/20080628094326_727.pdf.

Katz, N., and K. McNulty. 1994. Reflective listening. https://www.maxwell.syr.edu/uploadedFiles/parcc/cmc/Reflective%20Listening%20NK.pdf.

Kendon, A. 1983. Gesture and speech: How they interact. In Weimann, J. M., and R. E. Harrison (eds.). *Sage Annual Reviews of Communication Research: Nonverbal Interaction*, Vol. 11. Beverly Hills, CA: Sage, pp. 13–45.

Kerka, S. 1969. Journal writing and adult learning. EPIC Digest No. EDO-CE-96–174.

Knapp, M. L. 1972. *Nonverbal Communication in Human Interaction*. New York, NY: Holt, Rinehart and Winston.

Knapp, M. L., and J. A. Hall. 2002. *Nonverbal Communication in Human Interaction*. Crawfordsville, IN: Thomson Learning.

Lakshmi, N. 2016. Influence of emotional intelligence on communication skills: A survey and selective analysis. *Journal of English Language and Literature* 3(2): 97–102.

Leathers, D. G. 1992. *Successful Nonverbal Communication: Principles and Applications*. New York, NY: Macmillan.

Makau, J. M. 2018. Chapter 48: Ethical and unethical communication. In Eadie, W. F. (ed.). *21st Century Communication: A Reference Handbook*. San Diego State University. https://danielciurel.files.wordpress.com/2011/10/21stcentury communication2.pdf.

Mayhew, R. 2018. What are key principles of ethical communication? https://bi zfluent.com/info-8406730-key-principles-ethical-communication.html.

McCroskey, J., and M. Beatty. 1986. *Shyness: Perspectives on Research and Treatment*. New York, NY: Plenum Press.

McCroskey, J. C., J. S. Wrench, and V. P. Richmond. 2003. *Principles of Public Speaking*. Indianapolis, IN: The College Network.

McDaniel, M. A., D. L. Whetzel, F. L. Schmidt, and S. D. Maurer. 1994. The validity of employment interviews: A comprehensive review and meta-analysis. *Journal of Applied Psychology* 79: 599–616.

McNeill, D. 2008. *Gesture and Thought*. Chicago, IL: University of Chicago Press.

Mukherjee, K. 2017. Comparison between communication ethics and social media communication ethics: A paradigm shift. *Global Media Journal-Indian Edition* 7(2): 1–10.

NAUDL. 2007. Learning to debate: An introduction for first-year debaters. http:// chicagodebateleague.org/wp-content/uploads/2010/10/Learning-to-Debat e.pdf.

Nebiu, B. 1990. Project proposal writing. The Regional Environmental Center for Central and Eastern Europe, Szentendre, Hungary. http://documents.rec .org/publications/ProposalWriting.pdf.

Pigeon, Y. 2018. Leadership lesson: Tools for effective team meetings: How I learned to stop worrying and love my team. https://www.aamc.org/memb ers/gfa/faculty_vitae/148582/team_meetings.html.

Richason, O. E. 2018. What is effective workplace communication? http://sma llbusiness.chron.com/effective-workplace-communication-822.html.

Riemer, M. J. 2007. Intercultural communication considerations in engineering education. *Global Journal of Engineering Education* 11(2): 197–206.

Robertson, K. 2005. Active listening: More than just paying attention. *Australian Family Physician* 34(12): 1053–1055.

Salovey, P., and J. M. Meyer. 1998. Emotional intelligence. In Jenkins, J. M., Oatley, K., and Stein, N. L. (eds.). *Human Emotions: A Reader*. Malden, MA: Blackwell.

Serrat, O. 2010. Conducting effective meetings. Cornell University ILR School. https://digitalcommons.ilr.cornell.edu/cgi/viewcontent.cgi?referer=htt ps://www.google.ca/&httpsredir=1&article=1127&context=intl.

Silverman, J., S. Kurtz, and J. Draper. 1998. *Skills for Communicating with Patients*. Oxford, UK: Radcliffe Medical Press.

Cobel,, D. K. 2002. Use of journals to evaluate student design processes. Proceedings of the American Society for Engineering Education Annual Conference and Exposition, Montreal, Canada, June 16–19.

SSBA. 2018. Effective public speaking for boards of education: Module 13. Saskatchewan School Boards Associations. https://saskschoolboards.ca/wp-content/uploads/2015/08/Module_13_Public_Speaking.pdf.

Steele, A. L. 2013. Use of a reflection journal in a third year engineering project course. Proceeding 2013 Canadian Engineering Education Association (CEEA13) Conference, Montreal, QC, June 17–20.

Tilley, E. 2005. The ethics pyramid: Making ethics unavoidable in the public relations process. *Journal of Mass Media Ethics* 20: 305–320.

Upchurch, R. L., and J. E. Sims-Knight. 1999. Reflective essays in software engineering. Proceedings of 29th ASEE/IEEE Frontiers in Education Conference, San Juan, Puerto Rico.

Watson, K. W., L. L. Barker, and J. B. Weaver. 2012. The listening styles profile (LSP-16): Development and validation of an instrument to assess four listening styles. *International Journal of Listening* 9(1): 1–13.

Wheeler, E., and R. L. McDonald. 2000. Writing in engineering courses. *Journal of Engineering Education* 89(4): 481–486.

Wrench, J. S., A. Goding, D. I. Johnson, and B. A. Attias. 2011. Stand up, speak out: The practice and ethics of public speaking. https://catalog.flatworldknowl edge.com/catalog/editions/wrench-stand-up-speak-out-the-practice-and-ethics-of-public-speaking-1-0.

Wrench, J. S., A. Goding, and D. I. Johnson. 2012. Public speaking: Practice and ethics. https://2012books.lardbucket.org/books/public-speaking-practice-and-ethics/.

Zacharias, M. E. 1991. The Relationship between journal writing in education and thinking processes: What educators say about it. *Education* 112(2): 265–270.

module six

Professional practice in reflection

6.1 Knowledge and understanding

Having successfully completed this module, you should be able to demonstrate knowledge and understanding of:

- Reflection as a pedagogically and theoretically contentious concept
- Critical reflection as a process of questioning feelings, beliefs, values, and behaviors
- The three reflection processes: reflection "in", "on", and "for" action as central to the view of experiential learning
- The way reflection improves understanding of professional practice and actions taken as a result of reflective thinking
- Reflective practice and its models, including common sense, ERA, the what, experiential learning, and iterative cycle
- Conditions, situations, or circumstances that prompt engagement in the reflective process
- Categories of reflection for learning, including listening, speaking, reading, and writing
- Structured reflection on design, including education and practice
- Reflection tools in engineering learning, including journaling, portfolios, studios, and case studies

6.2 Reflection

> *By three methods we may learn wisdom: First, by reflection, which is noblest; second, by imitation, which is easiest; and third, by experience, which is the bitterest.*

Confucius

Reflection in the sense described in the quotation above is not effortless or just about looking back on past actions and events but is an influential concept for professionals who embrace lifelong learning experiences that resonate with the head as well as the heart. Many professional experiences are challenging in many ways, such that it may be difficult to thoroughly and systemically think through them and pay attention (Figure 6.1).

Reflection

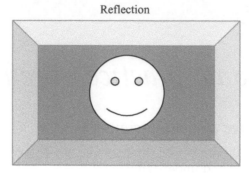

Figure 6.1 Think through and pay attention.

Reflection is a necessary bridge in the learning process that connects how we would like to practice and what we actually do (Driscoll 1994). It links experience and knowledge by providing an opportunity to explore areas of concern in a critical way and to make adjustments based on these reflections.

Aristotle emphasized the importance of reflecting in the real world and developing experience in it. He emphasized the requirement of paying attention to emotions and imagination in order to develop our perception of the world so that emotion and imagination are not relegated to unwanted self-indulgent urges or corrupting influences that get in the way of good rational thinking, but rather are a responsive and elective part of our thinking. In this way, Aristotle believed it was possible to develop real practical insight, responsiveness, and understanding (Nussbaum 1990).

The educationalist and philosopher John Dewey has been extremely influential in contemporary discussion about the concept of reflection. Dewey (1933) developed his ideas on thinking and learning and focused on the concept of thinking reflectively. Dewey saw reflective thinking as thinking with a purpose and focused strongly on the need to test out and challenge true beliefs by applying the scientific method through deductive reasoning and experimentation. Dewey suggests that when confronted with a problem, a reflective thinker reflects on theories to find a solution. These theories are based on past experience and prior knowledge.

The philosopher Donald Schön has been a huge influence on the development of reflection in professional education. Importantly, Schön (1983, 1987) believed that practice should be central to professional curricula; consequently, he saw "learning by doing" becoming the core of programs rather than an add-on, with students investing in practice and time in order to learn from it.

Reflection is a way of approaching an understanding of one's life and actions, as exemplified by Socrates' notion of reflection as "the examined life" for ethical and compassionate engagement with the world and its moral dilemmas (Nussbaum 1997). It is an important human activity in which people recapture their experience, think about it, and mull over and evaluate it. It is this working with experience that is important in learning (Boud et al. 1985).

Reflection is a pedagogically and theoretically contentious concept in higher education. It is a form of mental process – thinking about what has been done, learned, and experienced – which is used to fulfill a purpose or to achieve some anticipated outcome (Moon 1999). Reflection is at the heart of the learning process. It has an important role in solidifying an experience in the learner's memory, which raises the potential for further learning. It is an active process of witnessing one's own experience in order to take a closer look at it, sometimes to direct attention to it briefly, but often to explore it in greater depth.

In fact, all forms of education can encourage reflection. Lecture-based teaching, for example, albeit a mode that's "primarily one-way", can still offer opportunities for reflection, especially if the educator makes the lecture interactive or if the lecture is accompanied by practical lab sessions. Project-based courses further encourage reflection: group-based projects, in particular, offer many opportunities for reflection (Bull and Whittle 2014).

Figure 6.2 shows the reflection model. The model simply indicates that reflection and realization are intertwined and that it is up to the designer to choose which one is applicable or realistic for the purpose.

6.3   Reflection "on", "in", and "for" action

> *Learning without reflection is a waste. Reflection without learning is dangerous.*
>
> **Confucius**

Reflection in, on, and for actions are central to Donald Schön's view of experiential learning. There have been times when one gains new insight

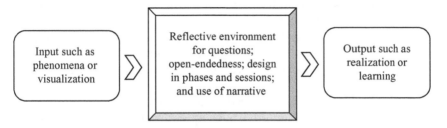

Figure 6.2 Reflection in three phases.

by approaching a problem from a different perspective. This is what Donald Schön refers to as reflection during the problem-solving process.

6.3.1 Reflection-on-action

Reflection-on-action refers to the retrospective contemplation of practice undertaken in order to uncover the knowledge used in practical situations by analyzing and interpreting the information recalled (Fitzgerald 1994). This is the process of thinking about a past experience after it is finished. It is perhaps the most common form of reflection. It is defined as reflection that comes after an experience. Donald Schön defined reflection-on-action (or reflecting back on past experience) as reflecting on how practice can be developed, changed, or improved after the event has occurred. The aim is to develop more effective ways of acting in the future. It is perhaps the most common form of reflection. It involves carefully re-running in one's mind events that have occurred in the past. Once the problem was solved, it might be worthy to consider what could have been done differently or what one would do differently next time.

Questions that may arise when reflecting on action could be: What went well and what did not go as well? What is needed to change/what is learned as a result of that experience? What was achieved, and did you really achieve it? How successful was it? Could the deal with the situation be different (Hamilton 1994)?

6.3.2 Reflection-in-action

Reflection-in-action refers to active evaluation of thoughts, actions, and practices during action as an incident happens. It is a conscious attempt to make professional actions more reasoned and purposeful (Schön 1987). It is described as reflecting on the situation while changes can still be made to affect the outcome, rather than waiting until a later time to reflect on how things could be different in the future.

For workers, it may also be described as "thinking on one's feet", which means exercising self-awareness and learners do consciously and subconsciously throughout each working day to overcome various issues (Dyba 2000). Reflection-in-action concerns thinking about something whilst engaging in doing it, having a feeling about something and practicing according to that feeling. This model celebrates the intuitive and artistic approaches that can be brought to uncertain situations (Schön 1983).

Reflection-in-action is triggered in situations of doubt, when unexpected situations are encountered. Subsequently, after the action has been completed, it is possible to think about what happened and how the action was undertaken in the previous evaluative process, reflection-on-action.

6.3.3 Reflection-for-action

Reflection-for-action is a proactive way of thinking about future experiences (Schön 1987). This is the process of thinking about what is needed in preparation for an activity, for example a procedure or teaching session (Hamilton 1994). It may be triggered by past experiences but might also involve thinking about future events and how an educator or service might respond. This might include being responsive to shifts in the community, considering different approaches, and refining inclusive practices and communication strategies to develop and maintain relationships with others.

Reflection-for-action is thinking about the future with the intention of improving or changing a practice. In learning, this type of reflection requires that teachers anticipate what will occur during a lesson as well as reflect on their past experiences before a lesson occurs (Farrell 2013).

6.4 Critical reflection (CR)

> *Critical reflection on practice is a requirement of the relationship between theory and practice.*
>
> **Paulo Freire**
> *[from Pedagogy of Freedom: Ethics, Democracy, and Civic Courage (1998)]*

Frequently, "reflection" and "CR" are used interchangeably in the literature. However, CR denotes another level of reflection beyond what might or might not be covered in other forms of reflection, including diaries and journals (Eraut 1994). This is why a CR framework may be better suited, as it requires reflection in relation to past and future action.

6.4.1 Definition and domain

CR is defined in two main ways. The first involves the ability to unearth, examine, and change very deeply-held or fundamental assumptions (Mezirow 1991). Brookfield (1995), however, emphasizes a second meaning, which is that what makes reflection critical is the focus on power. Critical in both these senses, is about the ability to be transformative, to involve and lead to some fundamental change in perspective. CR is therefore not mutually exclusive but can be based on similar assumptions and processes of thinking.

CR, when used specifically to improve professional practice, is reflection that focuses on the power dimensions of assumptive thinking and therefore on how practice might change in order to bring about change in the social situations in which professionals work. In order to be able to critically reflect, obviously one must be able to reflect first. However, not all reflection will lead to CR, that is, to fundamental changes (Fook 2007).

CR is a process of questioning feelings, beliefs, values, and behaviors in order to justify actions and describe why things are done the way they are, and what other differing views or behaviors there might be. This process would help practitioners to develop a rationale for their practices and to make informed decisions in these contexts. Such reflective action, based on critical assessment of assumptions underlying their beliefs and behaviors, becomes an integral element in decision-making (Mezirow 1990).

6.4.2   Traditions of thinking

A central goal of contemporary education is to improve the thinking skills of students; the notions of critical thinking and of creative thinking provide focuses for this effort. Critical thinking is seen as analytic. It is the means for arriving at judgments within a given framework. Creative thinking, on the other hand, is seen as imaginative, constructive, and generative (Bailin 1987).

In order to understand the idea of CR and the processes involved, it is helpful to explore the main traditions of thinking from which it arises, including: reflexivity, postmodernism, critical social theory, and deliberate reflection. These traditions are not mutually exclusive and, of course, share many commonalities. It is helpful to understand some of the basic tenets of each of these traditions in order to build up a more complex understanding of the theoretical underpinnings of CR. In addition, a better understanding of some of this thinking will enable learners to make more substantial connections between assumptions and social and cultural contexts (Fook 2007).

In the sociology of knowledge, reflexivity means a bidirectional relationship between cause and effect. It is the ability to look both inwards and outwards to recognize the connections with social and cultural understandings. Reflexivity is an important practice skill and central to working ethically in uncertain contexts and unpredictable situations, as opposed to instrumental accountability by following rules and procedures. It can be conceptualized as a learning tool and as a process for creating rules to guide practice and enhance practice wisdom. Participants alluded to the idea that reflexivity can be used to sort out "what works" in a particular situation, without having to "reinvent the wheel" (D'Cruz et al. 2007). In order to be reflexive, it is necessary to be aware of the many and varied ways in which people might create, or at least influence, the type of knowledge they use.

The influence of postmodern thinking brings with it particular ways of thinking, which to some degree transcend yet complement those associated with reflexivity (Fook 1999). It represents a questioning of the idea that knowledge must be arrived at in a progressive way and that it is non-conflictual.

Critical social theory points to how a CR process might help forge bridges between one's own experience and that of others to bring about desired social changes. It provides a broader framework for understanding what CR can and should help achieve (Fook 2007). Critical theory is a social theory oriented toward critiquing and changing society as a whole, in contrast to conventional theory oriented only to understanding it.

In the following section, the fourth tradition, "RP", will be discussed for its importance to the core objectives of this module.

6.5   Reflection practice (RP)

Reflection practice is a dialogue of thinking and doing through which I become more skillful.

Donald A. Schön
[from Educating the Reflective Practitioner (1987)]

The term "RP" is a popular concept in teaching and learning domains. It involves an ongoing scrutiny of practice based on identifying the assumptions underlying it. RP has developed and expanded its domain in various professional disciplines and contexts, each with their own differences and distinctions. RP carries multiple meanings that range from the idea of professionals engaging in solitary introspection to that of engaging in critical dialogue with others (Oluwatoyin 2015). According to Schön (1983, 1987), RP is centered on the three common processes: knowledge-in-action, reflection-in-action, and reflection-on-action. Knowledge-in-action is a type of knowledge that is not derived from any intellectual operation and is embedded within the action itself. According to Schön, the focus is on professional practice, for example, the ways in which professionals act in real situations and how they can be helped to develop their reflective processes through action (da Costa et al. 2009).

RP can be seen as a process of researching practice theory by developing it directly from concrete practice. The role of the emotions is also often emphasized (Fook 1999). A reflective practitioner is characterized by the ability and willingness to question routine ways of thinking and acting, either after having acted (reflection-on-action) or in the midst of acting (reflection-in-action). The latter makes it possible to alter one's current course of action by framing the problem in a new way or by improvising on new ways of solving the problem at hand (Prudhomme et al. 2003).

The teaching and application of RP have generated a range of ethical concerns. These relate to confidentiality, rights to privacy, informed consent, and professional relationships. Practitioners who are engaging in RP need to aware of the risks and also of the potential for conflicts of interest.

RP does not have a limit. It is as long a process as it needs to be to critique the practice situation. RP can be flexible; it can happen before, during, and after lessons; and it can focus on different aspects of learning. There is a range of RP models that can be used, as discussed in the following subsections.

6.5.1   Common sense model

Moon (1999) defines a "common sense" reflection as a form of mental processing with a purpose and/or anticipated outcome that is applied to relatively complex or unstructured ideas for which there is not an obvious solution. In this regard, five stages of learning, called the "map of learning", have been identified. To see that learning has occurred, it is important to "notice". It can be successful by getting to know the material as coherent "making sense" and the meaningness to develop a holistic view "making meaning" which can be done by creating relationships of new material with other ideas "working with meaning". To ensure that the new learning has been transformed, it is necessary to "transform learning".

6.5.2   ERA cycle

This simple cycle summarizes the three main components of RP: experience, reflection, and action (ERA), as shown in Figure 6.3. Experience means what happened, reflection is the process which helps us think through the experience, and action is what is done as a result of reflection.

6.5.3   The "What?" model

This model for reflection comes from the work of Driscoll (1994), called the "What?" model. Driscoll provides trigger questions that can help thinking

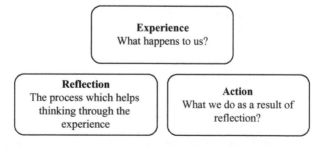

Figure 6.3 ERA RP model.

| **What?** Describe the whole experience. For example, description about who, what, why, when, where. | **So What?** Describe the consequences, meaning, and significance. This is the sense-making phase. | **Now What?** Describe the action taken. This phase makes connections from the experience to further actions. |

Figure 6.4 RP worksheet for the "What" model.

about an experience and develop a plan for improved practice. Driscoll's model applies well to situations of reflecting -on or -for practice. Figure 6.4 highlights the "What?" model.

6.5.4 Experiential learning model

The EL model is popular in professional programs like engineering, computing, business, medical, and education. It is an important part of making connections between theory and practice. Reflection upon experience in a placement not only describes the experience but evaluates it based on ideas from participants by assessing a theory or approach based on observations and practice, and evaluates one's own knowledge and skills within the professional field.

The model (Kolb 1984) illustrates an iterative cycle of four stages: concrete experience; reflection; abstract conceptualization; and active experimentation, as shown in Figure 6.5. According to this model, learning occurs between active and reflective modes, emphasizing the significance of reflecting upon the experience for learning to happen.

The model is used as a context for realizing learning from experience. Its four components (doing, reflecting, learning, applying) work together to make learning from experience possible. From the experiential reflection, it is better to discuss experiences in a work placement or practicum within the context of personal or organizational goals; doing so provides important insights and perspective for one's own growth in the profession.

6.5.5 Iterative model

Learning through repetition model (Gibbs 1988) provides some key points in development, especially description, evaluation, analysis, and action. Gibbs' popular model was developed from the earlier theoretical model of David Kolb's four-stage EL cycle (Kolb 1984). It requires practitioners to provide a clear description of the situation, an analysis of feelings, evaluation of the experience, analysis to make sense of the experience, a conclusion where other options are considered, and reflection upon the

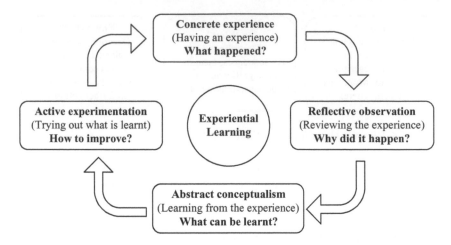

Figure 6.5 Experiential learning cycle model.

experience to examine what to do if the situation arose again. This model encourages the use of CR in converting new learning and knowledge into action and change.

The work of Gibbs (1988, 1998) allows the reflective practitioner to analyze and evaluate the practice and make necessary improvements into their practice. Gibbs (1988) introduces an experimental reflective cycle comprising six elements of reflection, which shows a clear "description" of the situation, analysis of the "feeling", "evaluation" of the experience, "analysis" to make sense of the experience, "conclusion", and reflection upon the experience to examine what to do if the situation occurred again or "action plan". Figure 6.6 shows the iteration model.

6.6   Reflection categories in learning

> *We do not learn from experience … we learn from reflecting on experience.*
>
> **John Dewey**
> *[from How We Think (1933)]*

Professional education in general should develop in students their own conceptions and theories of the profession, which allow them to generate best practices. To achieve this aim, professional education should involve not only developing students' competencies in content knowledge and professional attitudes, but also provide opportunities for students to reflect on their experience and practice. Figure 6.7 outlines a path for reflection based on three theme questions to choose from: "What, How, Whom".

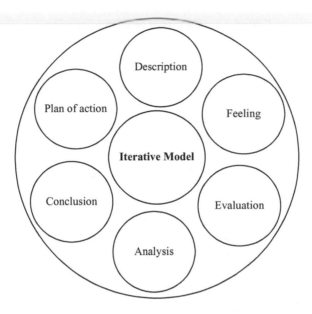

Figure 6.6 Iterative RP model.

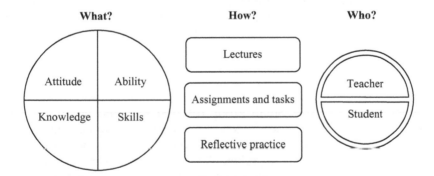

Figure 6.7 Path for reflection based on three theme questions to choose from.

6.6.1 *Reflective listening*

Reflective listening, also called mirroring, is a special type of listening that involves paying respectful attention to the content and feeling expressed in another persons' communication. It is hearing and understanding, and then letting the other know that he or she is being heard and understood. Reflective listening is one of the key building blocks of effective communication and one of the most difficult skills to learn and practice. It can help with understanding what the speaker is saying. It

Table 6.1 Categories of reflective listening

Reflective content	This process involves placing the content of the speaker's message into the listener's words and then verbally restating. This helps the speaker to know that the listener understands the subject matter.
Reflective feelings	This requires more work for the reflective listener than merely reflecting content because it requires the listener to listen for feelings behind the speaker's content.
Reflective meaning	This is listening accurately to someone and reflecting both the content and feeling of their message in a single response.
Reflective skills	These include the checking out process.

also allows the speaker to feel heard. It can help the speaker achieve the outcomes of the speech. It is useful for both speaker and listener. In general, there are several categories of reflective listening; the major ones are outlined in Table 6.1.

6.6.2 Reflective speaking

Reflective speaking is the other side of the coin of reflective listening. Speakers can reflect in a simple, literal way (sometimes called parroting) via a more complicated way (summarizing, paraphrasing) to achieve more reflective understanding by reflecting feelings, needs, essence, or meaning.

Structured reflection sessions may be facilitated during discussion in the class. For example, it is helpful for students to hear stories of success from the teacher or others. Students can offer feedback and collaborate to identify other stories. Small group discussions could be an alternative to full-class reflection sessions when students need more time to talk individually. Two students or a student and a teacher may be matched to reflect upon an experience together. Class presentations or serving on a panel are other ways for students to share their learning experience with peers, communities, or interested groups.

6.6.3 Reflective reading

Reading reflections offer an opportunity to recognize and perhaps break down assumptions which may be challenged by the texts. In education, many interdisciplinary courses may ask students to submit a reading reflection. Often instructors should indicate to students what they expect of a reflection, but the general purpose is to produce informed opinions about ideas presented in the text and to consider how they affect interpretation.

A main challenge for teachers is the need for students to have a frame of practice to appreciate the theory they learn. In engineering science classes like physics, chemistry, and other basic courses, getting students to read the textbook and other course materials and not focus specially on problem-solving may be a challenging task. In order to help students learn the material, the teacher may allocate one or several readings during the semester with a reflection assignment. The purpose of the assignment is to encourage students to process and identify important concepts from the given material. For each reading assignment, students may respond to a series of questions including: write a short summary of thoughts on the reading assignment; what parts seem to be the most difficult to understand, and what parts are comfortable for realization and application in real life?

6.6.4   Reflective writing

Writing reflectively involves critically analyzing an experience, recording its impact, and making a future plan. The means to reflective writing is to be analytical, not descriptive. Journals, logs, diaries, portfolios, research papers, essays, emails, and evaluations are containers for writing that is recorded over a period of time. They are increasingly used in higher education as means of enabling and/or assessing learning. Table 6.2 shows several types of reflective writing.

It is increasingly common to require learners to maintain reflective writings as a source of data and information to demonstrate achieved learning outcomes for a module or course. Table 6.3 lists reasons for keeping a reflective writing log.

For reflective writing, it is important to balance reporting or descriptive writing with CR and analysis. In such cases, it is good to consider the following questions:

- **Contextualize reflection:** What are the learning goals? What are the objectives of the organization? How do these goals fit with the themes or concepts from the experience?
- **Provide important information:** What is the name of the host organization? What is its mission? Who does it serve? What was your role?
- **Analytical reflection:** What is the learning experience?
- **Lessons from reflection:** Did the experience fit with the goals or concepts of the course or organization? Why or why not? What are the lessons learned for the future? What was successful? Why? How should one prepare for a future experience?

Table 6.2 Types of reflective writing

Journal	Participants should reflect on how they felt: excited, troubled, impressed, or unnerved about an experience.
Diary	It is similar to a journal but may require group participation. The diary then becomes a place to communicate in writing with others.
Log book	It is often used in disciplines based on experimental work, such as science or engineering. A log provides an accurate record of a process and helps in reflecting on past actions and making better decisions for future actions.
Note	A reflective note encourages students to think about personal reactions to an issue raised in an activity.
Peer review	It usually involves individuals showing their work to their peers for feedback.
Learning portfolio	Learning portfolios can be used in combination with the other types of reflections, like papers and individual journal reflections.
Essay	Reflective essays may focus on personal development, academic connections, or ideas.
Research paper	Through research work, participants may develop their research methodology and the skills they need for their research project.
Email	Through emails, individuals can create a dialogue with the facilitator and peers involved in a learning task.
Self- and peer evaluation	Participants may respond to a questionnaire with open-ended questions on a self-evaluation, peer evaluation, or program evaluation.
Publications	Individuals may share their thoughts about their learning tasks through writing newspaper and magazine articles.
Quotes	Using quotes is an effective way to initiate reflection. Quotes may be used to fit various learning tasks.

6.7   Structured reflection on design

Bad design is a smoke, while good design is a mirror.

Juan-Carlos Fernandez

The design process offers a variety of events to reflect on the visionary level of the practice. Structured reflection means reflection performed on a regular basis and is performed in a systematic way. To perform regular reflection, the structure of the design process must permit and stimulate regular reflection.

Table 6.3 Reasons for keeping reflective writing

Process Reason	Outcome
To record experience	By maintaining a journal and/or professional portfolio, as an initial step in reflective learning
To improve personal learning	By asking critical questions to develop an awareness of taken-for-granted assumptions
To engage in deep learning	By exploring the theory to understand personal situations
To foster creative interaction	By exploring options through organized group discussion in supervision
To increase self-awareness	By increasing personal insights into personal and professional behavior
To enhance creativity	By helping to connect with the inner intuitive elements of self
Outcome Reason	
To learn from experience	By analyzing critical incidents, possibly by using a model of reflection to question the concept
To enhance other forms of learning	By supporting the research processes through reflexivity
To understand personal learning processes	By becoming aware of the personal learning style and utilization of that approach
To boost problem-solving skills	By transferring skills in the problem-solving process
To develop professional practice	By developing awareness of disagreement between concepts and actions
To promote change	By helping to implement changes toward personal and professional development
To free up writing and learning	By overcoming personal impedance around writing ability
To enrich self-expression	By expressing self in different ways
To assess formal learning	By demonstrating the effectiveness of the learning outcomes

6.7.1 Reflection on design education

To develop reflections on learning, students may be invited to write an essay or any other form of reflection in which they explicate their personal vision of themselves as designers. The purpose of the essay is to go beyond the obvious. To transform superficial statements such as "I want to make this world a better place" and "I want to design products that fulfill people's real needs" into meaningful statements about what is a better world, and about what are real needs. Possible questions that may be addressed during the reflection are (Sonneveld and Hekkert 2008):

- What are values, goals, and dreams?
- What is a designer's role in society, and what are their responsibilities towards people?
- Do you have a method? Do you need one?
- What inspires you and how do you keep inspired?
- How are these ideas reflected in your design projects?

Based on the above, students reflect on the development of personal competences, such as creative thinking and mastering design tools, and articulate what they will do next to improve these competences. The reflection may be expressed in a variety of forms and structures, such as plain text, puzzles, shapes, or using digital media to produce design portfolios, posters, and videos.

6.7.2   Reflection on design practice

Continuous improvement of design processes is always essential. To achieve that goal, it is necessary to consider the design process as a sequence of design situations, changed by design activities and changes in the design context. A design situation at a certain moment is defined as the combination of the state of the design process, the product being designed, and the design context at that moment (Reymen and Hammer 2002).

A design process is usually structured as a series of design phases (defined by milestones), as shown in Figure 6.8. The concept of design sessions should be introduced within each phase of the design to help designers improve the design process and its flow performance with regular reflection on segments of the design process. A designer, when

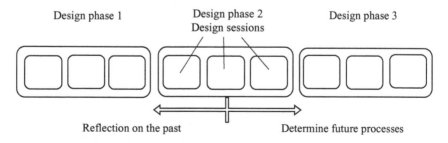

Figure 6.8 The concepts of design phases and design sessions.

designing, is inside a design process and is not always in the position to consider the process critically and logically. A designer that wants to be in control of the design process, by means of regular reflection on the design process, must step out of the "designerly way of thinking" every now and then (Cross 1994). Based on these observations, it seems important to reserve certain moments during the design process for reflection. Reflection only at the beginning and end of a whole design process is often too superficial; reflection must take place at many more moments during a design process.

Reflection on a design situation is divided into two parts. Reflection on the state of the design context is mainly done at the beginning of a design session; reflection on the state of the product being designed and the state of the design process is mainly done at the end of a design session. At the beginning of a design session, designers should also concentrate on the product being designed and the design process to know where the previous design session stopped. This can be done based on documents made at the end of the previous session. Reflection on a sequence of design activities is also split into two parts. Reflection on interactions with the design context and on transitions in the design context is mainly done at the beginning of a design session. Reflection on design activities about the product being designed and design activities about the design process is mainly done at the end of a design session (Reymen 2001).

Finally, reflection helps designers to learn from their experiences, to integrate and coordinate various aspects of a design situation, to judge the progress of the design process, to evaluate interactions with the design context, and to plan suitable future design activities. From reflection on the performed design activities one can, for example, learn which activities were not successful for reaching the design objectives (Reymen and Hammer 2002). In summary, reflection on a design process can influence a steeper learning curve of designers for a smoother design process and an enhanced product as an outcome.

6.8   Reflection tools in learning

> *What lies behind us and what lies before us are small compared to what lies within us.*

> **Ralph Waldo Emerson**

Reflection in engineering and computing is about "doing" rather than "telling"; it is about first-hand knowing through experience rather than second-hand knowing through reading textbooks; it is about subjectivity (you) rather than objectivity (the collective other); it is about the journey (process) rather than arriving (outcome).

6.8.1 Reflective journal

A reflective journal is usually a vehicle to facilitate the development of the process of reflective learning (Woodward 1998). It is a collection of notes, observations, thoughts, and other relevant materials built up over a period of time, a placement experience, or fieldwork. Possibilities of journal developing that come to mind are notebooks, written files, computers, blogs, recordings, and videos. In this context, the learning journal provides an opportunity for students to record their observations, reflections, and lessons learned from class lectures and activities, cases, and projects. This means that a learning journal should not be a purely descriptive account but an opportunity to communicate the thinking process.

Journals are extensively used in professional education and development, including engineering and computing. They are usually aimed towards the development of practitioners who are willing to reflect on events, theory, design projects, and other experiences. In addition, journals are used in many disciplines and fields (Steele 2013). Table 6.4 supplements a rubric that illustrates the type of entries of any typical learning journal.

6.8.2 Learning portfolio

The creation of portfolios as a form of learning and professional preparation is becoming more common in education. Learning portfolios can

Table 6.4 A reflection journal rubric

Reflection	Unsatisfactory	Satisfactory	Excellent
Ability to reflect experiences and critically assess work and outcomes.	Limited or no reflection. Straightforward description provided.	Evidence of correct analysis. Shortage of extended analysis and examination from diverse perspectives.	Strong critical thinking and creative solutions. Examination of issues from different perspectives.
Presentation			
Organization of ideas, opinions, and perspectives. Linguistic quality.	Mindless thinking. Confusing organization. Several linguistic mistakes.	Good ideas and arguments. Better arrangement for enhancement. Some linguistic mistakes.	Mindful thinking. High linguistic quality.

help students engage in meaningful goal-setting and develop a desire for achieving their goals. In general, a learning portfolio has two major elements: a narrative reflective log and a list of structured professional artifacts that demonstrate accumulated knowledge, skills, and practice about teaching that are reinforced by CR. It works to help students reflect throughout the learning experience on what they learn, how learning can be more meaningful, and what else they should be focusing their attention on.

The learning portfolios can also be used to monitor development and progress as a form of self-assessment or for institutional assessment. Their main outcome is the enhancement of the students' learning experience. The portfolios discuss the challenges and knowledge construction by responding to issues such as the content (what the students learned); context (how learning is connected to real life); and process (how learning can be accomplished effectively).

Portfolios can be written in electronic format (e-Portfolio), which is recognized as a high-impact practice that allows students to reflect on their experiences, uncover ways they are interconnected, and come to a deeper understanding of their learning progress. Rather than just using an e-Portfolio as a digital repository, it may be regarded as a space for students to declare their goals and pose their own questions. In general, the e-Portfolio takes significant effort and time by their creators, and need thorough learning by curriculum designers (Eynon and Gambino 2017).

The pedagogy of the e-Portfolio falls in the space between students' social realm of Facebook/Twitter and future professional persona on LinkedIn. Because of the increased access to digital media, students today may have practice posting, reflecting within social realms. However, they do not yet have as much practice in learning spaces to question, to admit to not-knowing, and to ask for guidance. An e-Portfolio provides a unique pedagogical space that is explicitly for posing questions or demonstrating "not knowing" and for recognizing that one knows enough to realize gaps in knowledge.

6.8.3   Reflection in studio

Studio education originates from disciplines such as architecture, design, and art (Bull and Whittle 2014). A studio is a room for supporting collaborative and individual learning that is very practical and often project-based, employs coaching (as well as formal and informal critiques), and usually acts as the student's second home (Schön 1983).

The aspect of studio education that is most important to its success is the culture that the students and staff foster. Elements of this culture include sharing ethics, being social, treating the space like a second home, maintaining good work ethics, and utilizing peer learning. Common examples of reflective activities from studios include constant question-ing, open-ended complex problems, rapid iterations of design, a culture of critique, teamwork, collaborative learning, interactive problem-solving, student presentations, peer review, and coaching (Bull et al. 2013). Studio culture is important to RP because it provides many opportunities that allow for a valuable element of being reflective: constant questioning (Tomayko 1991).

Given that design projects are crucial ingredients in graduate and undergraduate engineering design education for providing concrete experiences, it is not sufficient to have a good knowledge of engineering theory; it is also important to be able to design a product that solves an open-ended complex problem, ideally in an interdisciplinary team envi-ronment. Such experiences are fundamental components in Kolb's model of experiential learning (Kolb 1984).

Creative design inherently requires reflection (Schön 1983). Design is also an inherently complex activity. Design professionals deal often with uncertainty, uniqueness, and conflict, so bite-sized or limited-scope activ-ities wouldn't make sense in courses with a focus on software design. The ability to design is learnable, but some claim that it can't be taught via traditional classroom methods (Schön 1987). RP are of particular nec-essary when addressing typical complex and ill-structured problems in engineering design. In the design disciplines, it is a commonly held belief that designers "learn how to design largely by doing it". It seems almost impossible to learn design without actually doing it. This gives credibility to why it is important to practice engineering(Lawson 2012).

Experience alone, however, is not helpful for students unless they learn something in the process, as noted in Dixon's survey of engineering education (Dixon 1991). The learning process involves metacognition (the monitoring of one's own learning), and while this is a natural process, it often needs reinforcement and improvement through practice (Bransford et al. 1999). As reflective activities, learning journals are intended to help students enhance their own learning processes.

6.8.4   Reflection on case study

Case studies are a significant approach to learning because long-term process analysis is required that is sensitive to technical and professional development. This involves initiating, tracking, and realizing the context information and process of change. Case studies are usually presented in class, and students discuss the situation and identify how they would solve the problem.

Ethical case studies are an example that gives students the opportu-nity to analyze a situation and gain practice in ethical decision-making as they choose a course of action. This reflection strategy may foster the exploration and clarification of values. In this regard, students write or discuss a case study of an ethical dilemma they have confronted, including a description of the context, the individuals involved, and the controversy or event that created an ethical dilemma.

Technical case studies expose students to the breadth of technical and nontechnical issues in practice, including software development. The students extract and effectively communicate the key information in a fixed time frame, apply concepts of domain and application of engineering, and identify the business case for product design and development.

For effective reflection experience in the class, students should be given time to present their cases. The time limit should be strictly enforced. Students may explore one or two topics in some depth and reflection instead of covering many aspects of the case. During the presentations, feedback sheets may be handed out, and it should be expected that every student is able to recognize some key lessons and is able to ask one question. During presentations, the case should be communicated to the entire class, and presenters should listen to other presentations and provide feedback to presenters.

6.9   Knowledge acquisition

Attempting to answer the following questions involves acquisition of knowledge from this book and other books, documents, and the Internet.

- What is reflection? Who needs to reflect?
- How is reflection different from critical reflection?
- Can reflection and critical thinking be taught?
- What is reflective learning? What benefits are related to students reflecting?
- What is your purpose for keeping a reflective journal?
- How do student and instructor orientations to e-Portfolios change over the course of a semester?
- What is RP? Why is it important to engage in RP?
- What is a learning journal? What are the purposes for learning journals in an academic setting?
- Can you think of an event that had a major impact on you? Pause for a while and then write down what happened and how you feel you changed as a result.
- Do you have any experiences of keeping a journal or diary? When have you used them and how useful have they been?
- Identify some examples of reflective activities in the studio environment.

6.10   Knowledge creation

Collaborate with peers on learning or work with others outside the class to narrow down the objectives of each activity. You may access class and online resources and analyze data and information to create new ideas and balanced solutions. High-level digital tools may be used to develop multimedia presentations, simulations or animations, videos and visual displays, digital portfolios, reflective practice (online publishing and blogging), or well-researched and up-to-date reports.

6.10.1   Reflection on reading

This activity involves reading a research paper, an article, or a group project. After reading, students may ask themselves the following questions, or other questions that require reflection on the reading (Allard 2013): What happened? What did we learn from the reading? How can we apply what we have learned? What would we like to learn more about, related to the reading? What would we do otherwise if we were to do the reading again? Students may simply record the answers to the questions in writing and think about them. This task will enable the students to track learning over time, and they will have the option to keep reflection via a personal learning journal or to share learning via a reflection blog.

6.10.2   Reflection on a course

To help students understand the process of reflection via a journal, consider Table 6.5, which can be used as a supplemental rubric to illustrate the type of entries that could be used in this task. Consider a professional practice or any other related course designed to give engineering and computing students the knowledge and experience of various topics, in addition to a possible group project or paper assignment that reflects from a series of modules that range from profession, ethics, design, entrepreneurship, project management, AI, and career development. Table 6.5 may be considered a guideline to reflect on the content and learning experience of the course.

Table 6.5 Supplemental rubric

Description of modules encountered in the course.
Reflect on the teacher experience.
Reflect on an interesting module or topic of your choice.
Reflect on the style of project presentations.
Makes an explicit link between everyday life and the module(s).
You may add more.

6.10.3   Reflection guiding questions

Think about what you learned from a lecture on professional practice course or any other course of interest. This task will enable you to track learning over time, and you will have the option to keep reflection via a personal learning journal or to share your learning with the instructor or via a reflection blog. Try in writing to answer the following questions.

Guiding questions: How has this changed your way of thinking? What will you do with this information? What surprised you the most about your experience from this lecture? What disappointed you the most about your experience from this lecture? If you had a chance to make a change (task-related), what would that change be? What might some obstacles be? What do you plan to investigate further (task-related) (Moussa-Inaty 2015)?

6.10.4   Reflection on change about engineering and computing learning

Learning is an active process that is required to be meaningful and relevant to the learner; it is a social process that is enhanced by interaction between learners. For this task, try to design a blog or a website to incorporate the principles of effective learning and reflect knowledge of the change process in your design.

Guiding questions: What is your vision for engineering and computing teaching, learning, and practice? What is your vision for teachers' learning? What does professional development, in which your new vision of teaching and learning will be playing out, look like? What is the knowledge and beliefs that inform your professional development plan? How does your design reflect the knowledge and beliefs? What are the goals or desired outcomes of your plan?

6.10.5   Designing a reflective classroom activity

Classroom-based EL may take different forms, including role-playing, games, case studies, simulations, presentations, and various types of group work. For this task, students may design a reflective classroom activity for one of their academic courses. Students should decide which parts of the course can be instructed more effectively with the EL model. They should think about how any potential activities match the course learning objectives; how the potential activity complements the overall course of study; grading criteria; and evaluation methods that would match the proposed activity.

References

Allard, E. 2013. Reflection. McMaster University. http://avenue.mcmaster.ca/help /docs/reflection_student_handout.pdf.

Bailin, S. 1987. Critical and creative thinking. *Informal Logic* IX(1): 23–30.

Boud, D., R. Keogh, and D. Walker. 1985. *Reflection: Turning Experience into Learning.* London, UK: Kogan Page.

Bransford, J. D., A. Brown, and R. R. Cocking. 1999. *How People Learn: Brain, Mind, Experience, and School.* Washington, DC: National Academy Press.

Brookfield, S. 1995. *Becoming a Critically Reflective Teacher.* San Francisco, CA: Jossey-Bass.

Bull, C. N., and J. Whittle. 2014. Supporting reflective practice in software engineering education through a studio-based approach. *IEEE Software* 31(4): 44–50.

Bull, C. N., J. Whittle, and L. Cruickshank. 2013. Studios in software engineering education: Towards an evaluable model. Proceedings of 35th International Conference on Software Engineering (ICSE 13), pp. 1063–1072.

Cross, N. 1994. *Engineering Design Methods: Strategies for Product Design.* Second Edition. Chichester, UK: John Wiley and Sons.

D'Cruz, H., P. Gillingham, and S. Melendez. 2007. Reflexivity: A concept and its meanings for practitioners working with children and families. *Critical Social Work* 8(1): 1–18.

Da Costa, C., L. D. Ribas, and J. Ueta. 2009. Reflective processes and competencies involved in teaching practice at university: A case study. *Interface (Botucatu)* 13(31): 409–422.

Dewey, J. 1933. *How We Think: A Restatement of the Relation of Reflective Thinking to the Educative Process.* Boston, MA: DC Heath and Company.

Dixon, J. R. 1991. New goals for engineering education. *Mechanical Engineering. Engineering Design Science* 113(3): 56–62.

Driscoll, J. 1994. Reflective practice for practice: A framework of structured reflection for clinical areas. *Senior Nurse* 14(1): 47–50.

Dyba, T. 2000. Improvisation in small software organizations. *IEEE Software* 17(5): 82–87.

Eraut, M. 1994. *Developing Professional Knowledge and Competence.* London, UK: Routledge.

Eynon, B., and L. M. Gambino. 2017. *High-Impact e-Portfolio Practice: A Catalyst for Student, Faculty and Institutional Learning.* Sterling, VA: Stylus.

Farrell, T. S. 2013. Reflecting on ESL teacher expertise: A case study. *System* 41(4): 1070–1082.

Fitzgerald, M. 1994. *Theories of Reflection for Learning.* Oxford, UK: Blackwell Scientific.

Fook, J. 1999. Critical reflectivity in education and practice. In Pease, B., and J. Fook (eds.). *Transforming Social Work Practice: Postmodern Critical Perspectives.* Sydney, Australia: Allen and Unwin.

Fook, J. 2007. Chapter 26: Reflective practice and critical reflection. In Lishman, J. (ed.). *Handbook for Practice Learning in Social Work and Social Care: Knowledge and Theory.* London, UK: Jessica Kingsley, pp. 363–375.

Gibbs, G. 1988. *Learning by Doing: A Guide to Teaching and Learning Methods. Further Education Unit.* Oxford, UK: Oxford Polytechnic.

Hamilton, J. 1994. The power of reflection. https://www.manitobaphysio. com/wp-content/uploads/The-Power-of-Reflection-by-Joanne-Hamilt on-2017.pdf.

Kolb, D. A. 1984. *Experiential Learning: Experience as the Source of Learning and Development*. Englewood Cliffs, NJ: Prentice Hall.

Lawson, B. 2012. *How Designers Think*. Fourth Edition. London, UK: Routledge.

Mezirow, J. 1990. How critical reflection triggers transformative learning. International Journal of Mezirow (ed.). *Fostering Critical Reflection in Adulthood*. San Francisco, CA: Jossey-Bass, pp. 1–20.

Mezirow, J. 1991. How critical reflection triggers learning. In Mezirow, J. (ed.). *Fostering Critical Reflection in Adulthood*. San Francisco, CA: Jossey-Bass.

Moon, J. 1999. *Reflection in Learning and Professional Development*. London, UK: Kogan Page.

Moussa-Inaty, J. 2015. Reflective writing through the use of guiding questions. *International Journal of Teaching and Learning in Higher Education* 27(1): 104–113.

Nussbaum, M. 1997. *Cultivating Humanity: A Classical Defence of Reform in Liberal Education*. Cambridge, MA: Harvard University Press.

Nussbaum, M. C. 1990. *Love's Knowledge: Essays on Philosophy and Literature*. Oxford, UK: University Press.

Oluwatoyin, F. E. 2015. Reflective practice: implication for nurses. *IOSR Journal of Nursing and Health Science* 4(4): 28–33.

Prudhomme, G., J. F. Boujut, and D. Brissaud. 2003. Toward reflective practice in engineering design education. *International Journal of Engineering Education* 19(2): 328–337.

Reymen, I. M. M. J. 2001. Improving design processes through structured reflection: A domain-independent approach. PhD Thesis, University of Technology, Eindhoven, the Netherlands.

Reymen, I. M. M. J., and D. K. Hammer. 2002. Structured reflection for improving design processes. International Design Conference, Dubrovnik, May 14–17.

Scholz, K., C. Tse, and K. Lithgow. 2017. Unifying experiences: Learner and instructor approaches and reactions to e-Portfolio usage in higher education. *International Journal of ePortfolio* 7(2): 139–150.

Schön, D. 1983. *The Reflective Practitioner*. London, UK: Temple Smith.

Schön, D. A. 1987. *Educating the Reflective Practitioner*. San Francisco, CA: Jossey-Bass.

Sonneveld, M. H., and P. Hekkert. 2008. Reflecting on being a designer. International Conference on Engineering and Product Design Education, Universitat Politecnica De Catalunya, Barcelona, Spain, September 4–5.

Steele, A. L. 2013. Use of a reflection journal in a third year engineering project course. Proceedings of the Canadian Engineering Education Association (CEEA13) Conference.

Tomayko, J. E. 1991. Teaching software development in a studio environment. *ACM SIGCSE Bulletin* 23(1): 300–303.

Woodward, H. 1998. Reflective journals and portfolios: Learning through assessment. *Assessment and Evaluation in Higher Education* 23(4): 415–423.

part three

Practices of innovation, entrepreneurship, safety and sustainability in design

module seven

Innovation and entrepreneurship practice

7.1   Knowledge and understanding

Having successfully completed this module, you should be able to demonstrate knowledge and understanding of:

- The notions of creativity as a habit and attitude, critical thinking, and creative thinking
- The difference between invention and innovation
- Incremental and radical innovations; disruptive and sustaining innovations
- Paradigms of innovation, including product, process, and management
- The practice of innovation, including closed innovation and open innovation, technological innovation, and social innovation
- Habits of mind as essential traits for enhancing entrepreneurial mindset
- Entrepreneurial skills that are necessary for innovations in either business, service institutions, or new ventures
- Key characteristics and skills often associated with successful entrepreneurs
- The power of intrapreneurship in driving innovation
- The distinct phases of the entrepreneurship process including identification and evaluation, development of a business plan, and determination of resources
- Marketing concepts and principles that could be applied in the field of entrepreneurship
- The interface between ethics and entrepreneurship

7.2   Creativity

> *Creativity is a habit, and the best creativity is the result of good work habits.*
>
> **Twyla Tharp**
> *[from The Creative Habit: Learn It and Use It for Life (2006)]*

Creativity, in the sense perceived in the quotation above, is not just a personality trait, it is a behavior, habit, and attitude. Habits are the fabric of creative lives and creative careers. With routine and repetition, habits evolve into skills, and skills open up the pathway to opportunity (Rao 2017). Attitude is the ability to believe in change, a readiness to play with ideas and potentials, and the habit of appreciating the noble. The earlier an opportunity is created, the sooner it can be converted into innovation.

Creativity is marked by the ability to bring into existence something new, to invent into a new form, and to produce through imaginative skill. It is characterized by an extensive and systematic search for solutions, especially innovative ones. Creativity basically contains four stages: preparation, generation, incubation, and verification (Baillie 2002), as outlined in Figure 7.1. One approach says that creativity, at least in the technological sense, is the ability to recognize a problem in multiple dimensions (Habash 2017). According to Taylor (1996), creativity is perceived as a hierarchy from a low to a progressively higher level, as outlined in Table 7.1.

Creativity starts with an idea, but the truth is that ideas do not arise in an intellectual vacuum. The brain requires preparation in advance,

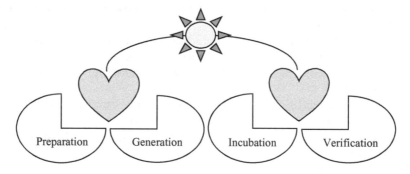

Figure 7.1 Main stages of creativity.

Table 7.1 Hierarchy of creativity

Expressive	The ability to develop a unique idea with no concern about its quality
Technical	The proficiency to create products with consummate skills but with little expressive freedom
Inventive	The skill to develop a new use of old parts and new ways of seeing old things in an ingenious manner
Innovative	The ability to penetrate foundational principles or establish a school of thought and formulate innovative ventures
Emergent	The ability to incorporate the most abstract ideational principles or assumptions causing a body of knowledge

including feeding materials to work with in order to generate creative ideas. The ideas need to stay in one's mind for a while (the insight step) in order to realize, evaluate, elaborate, and verify their feasibility. The above process is iterative as well as recursive. It involves lots of conversations, including about goals and actions, and conversations with co-creators and colleagues. The collaborators' experiences and values have an impact on the conversations.

Critical thinking and creative thinking may very well be different sides of creativity; however, they are not identical when it comes to their inner meanings. Critical thinking is the art of thinking *about* thinking, in such a way as to identify its strengths and weaknesses and recast it in an improved form (where necessary). The first characteristic requires the thinker to be skilled in analytic and evaluative thinking. The second requires the thinker to be skilled in creative thinking. Thus, critical thinking has three dimensions: the analytic, the evaluative, and the creative (Paul and Elder 2016). On the other hand, creative thinking may be defined as the art of generating solutions to problems by the force of imagination and reasoning. Every idea is a product of thinking, and every product is the manifestation of a naked idea in a thinker's mind (Okpara 2007). Critical thinking is convergent, but creative thinking is divergent, where the mind is free to stray. Creative thinkers are people who see problems as opportunities to improve something or make something new, whether a thought or idea, a product or a process. In the context of education, creative thinking is about applying imagination to finding a solution to learning tasks.

7.3   Innovation

> *Innovation is the act that endows resources with a new capacity to create wealth.*
>
> **Peter Drucker**
> *[from Innovation and Entrepreneurship (2006)]*

Innovation involves creativity but is not the same as creativity. It involves acting on creative ideas to make some specific and substantial difference in the domain in which the innovation occurs.

7.3.1   Invention and innovation

An invention is a novel idea that proves workable in theory and has been transformed into reality for the first time and given a physical form. It is the discovery or development of a product or process by applying previous knowledge in new ways.

Invention comprises the process of discovery, from basic science through R&D. In general, it requires scientific skills. It may also include the repurposing of existing knowledge of technologies for new applications. The key distinguishing feature of invention is discovery and the creation of new knowledge that is made tangible and reproducible (Anadon et al. 2013). Inventions can be patented, as this provides security to the inventor for IP rights.

Invention is vital. It is the creation of something new, but it is not innovation. Invention covers all efforts aimed at creating new ideas and making them work. For example, Thomas Edison began to work on inventing the incandescent lamp powered by electricity in 1878. The moment at which the electric light became available on the market was the moment the invention became an innovation (Taylor 1996).

Innovation involves the application of basic discoveries or inventions to produce a useful product or process for a specific application. Product innovation is the development of new and improved products or services, while process innovation refers to new or improved methods of production or distribution. Innovations cannot be patented, even though often times the distinction between inventions and innovations is blurry (Gaynor 2014).

Innovation is really what drives economic growth. Joseph Schumpeter (Schumpeter 1934), who was a professor at Harvard University and is considered one of the twentieth century's major economists, said that innovation was the product of new combinations, and he proposed five combination patterns: (1) the production of a new good; (2) the introduction of a new method of production; (3) the development of a new market; (4) the acquisition of a new source of supply of raw materials; and (5) the emergence of a new organization of any industry.

7.3.2   Incremental or radical

Innovation may be classified according to the object of innovation, for example innovation of sociocultural systems, of ecosystems, of business models, of products, of services, etc. Most innovations are incremental, meaning that they are of an evolutionary nature. Incremental innovation involves slightly upgrading a pre-existing product. Examples include making a phone slightly thinner or a computer slightly faster. Incremental innovation involves doing things in a different way. It refers to the small changes in a product that help improve performance, lower costs, and enhance appeal, or simply to announce a new model release.

Radical innovations, on the other hand, are revolutionary and imply major changes in the way a product or service works. Successful radical innovation occurs rarely within any particular area, perhaps once every 10 years. Radical innovations are considered to be associated with high levels of uncertainty. They seldom live up to their potential when initially introduced. At first, they are often challenging to use, expensive, and limited in capability. Incremental innovation is necessary to renovate the radical idea into a form that is acceptable to those beyond early adopters (Norman and Verganti 2012). Without radical innovation, incremental innovation reaches a limit. Without incremental innovation, the potential enabled by radical change is not realized.

7.3.3   Disruptive and sustaining

The term disruptive innovation has been widely used as a synonym of disruptive technology, but the first is now more popular, because market disruption has been found to be a function usually not of technology itself but rather of its changing application. Sustaining innovations are typically innovations in technology, whereas disruptive innovations change entire markets (Habash 2017). Sustaining innovations allows organizations to advance markets the same way, such as the development of a more efficient car.

Historically, disruptive technological innovations have transformed society through the ages, from the horse-drawn carriage to the first steam engine, to the car and airplane, to the PC and the mobile phone. Today, the increase in competitive pressure coming from globalization in combination with disruptive technologies means that innovation has become an essential principle of economic existence.

The theory of disruption goes that a smaller company with fewer resources can unseat an established, successful business by targeting segments of the market that have been neglected by the incumbent, typically because it is focusing on more profitable areas. Disruption happens when the incumbent's mainstream customers start taking up the start-up's products or services in volume. Take Uber, for example, a company that is often referred to as a beacon of disruptive innovation because of its seismic impact on the taxicab industry (Hutt 2016). Another example of disruptive innovation is Apple's iPhone disruption of the mobile phone market.

In addition, sustainability is another driver for disruption, because the world needs to deal with environmental and social issues such as air and water pollution, climate change, a growing and aging population, and the needs of an emerging wealthy middle class.

7.4   Paradigms of innovation

There is an innovator inside of all of us.

Rowan Gibson

Innovation may take several paradigms, primarily including process, product, and management, as shown in Figure 7.2.

7.4.1 Process innovation

Innovation in processes includes changes and improvements to techniques. These contribute to increases in productivity, which lowers cost and helps to increase demand. It is the adoption of new or significantly improved production methods. These methods may involve changes in equipment or production organization or both. The methods may be intended to produce new or improved products, which cannot be produced using conventional plants or production methods, or essentially to increase the production efficiency of existing products (Reguia 2014). Process innovations often have a big impact on the economics of production. It can slow down competitors by granting firms benefits from the production perspective, such as cost efficiency, production speed, and quality reliability. However, process innovation can be a costly and difficult practice if knowledge and experience are not available.

7.4.2 Product/service innovation

The continuance and the persistence of any company depend on its capacities to maintain its spot in the marketplace and face the competition, which spreads rapidly and aggressively with the globalization and expansion of new technologies. While a product reflects the producer's image, its whole success depends also on the product success through realizing consumer desires and needs and developing new products (Reguia 2014).

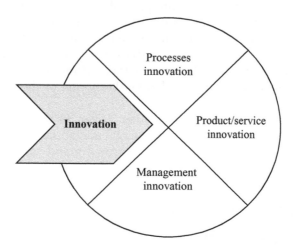

Figure 7.2 Paradigms of innovation.

Product innovation contributes in reducing production costs and time of the production process. It usually emerges largely in the public imagination. From a commercial perspective, the value of product innovations is that the innovation of a new product will encourage consumers to make a purchase. Examples of product innovation may include new products or service inventions, technical specification and quantity improvement, or the inclusion of new features. These lead to increases in effective demand, which fosters increases in investment and employment. Sustaining products and services is also the kind of innovation companies often need to develop just to stay in the business and involves opening up new markets. It contributes also to improving products' quality and making products more competitive in markets.

Product innovation includes many processes, including development of the old products; innovating new products to realize the market's needs; and using new techniques in the production process.

7.4.3 Management innovation

Management innovation can be defined as a marked departure from traditional management principles, processes, and practices or a departure from customary organizational forms that significantly alters the way the work of management is performed (Hamel 2006). It involves the introduction of novelty in an established organization, and as such it represents a particular form of organizational change (Hamel and Mol 2008).

Management innovation implements new management practices to enhance human and material resources together with the capacity to anticipate techniques. It simply changes how managers do what they do. This innovation is based on new principles that challenge management convention; it should be systemic, encompassing a range of processes and methods; and part of an ongoing program of invention, where progress mounts over time. McDonald's, as a business entity, did not invent anything. Its final product was what any decent American restaurant had produced years ago. But it applied management concepts and management techniques (what is the value to the customer?), standardized the product, designed processes and tools, and based training on the analysis of the work to be done and then set the standards it required. Accordingly, McDonald's drastically upgraded the yield from resources and created a new market (Drucker 1986).

Management processes include setting goals and laying out plans; acquiring knowledge and discipline through the chaotic process of scientific discovery; project and brand management that challenges management orthodoxy; budgeting, hiring, and promotion; employee assessment, executive development, and identifying and developing talent; and other areas that focus management principles into strategic practices.

7.5   Innovation practice

> *Innovation is the specific instrument of entrepreneurship*
> *... the act that endows resources with a new capacity to*
> *create wealth.*

Peter Drucker
[from Innovation and Entrepreneurship (2006)]

Innovation is an exclusive tool of entrepreneurs, the means by which they use change as an opportunity. It can be learned and practiced. For innovation to occur, something more than a creative idea or insight is required. The idea must go into action to make a real difference, resulting in new business processes or changes to existing products or services.

7.5.1   Closed innovation and open innovation

The difference between open innovation and closed innovation is determined by the way in which innovation is created. Closed innovation is developed in a self-contained company environment. The aim is to discover and develop the best technologies and be the first to introduce them to the market.

Open innovation is a practice that encourages opening up the innovation process beyond company boundaries in order to increase its own innovation potential through active strategic use of the environment (Zapel 2018). It is the opening up of innovation processes to allow ideas, new technologies, or feedback from external partners to flow into the firm. Open innovation helps integration of customers, partners, and other stakeholders in the innovation process. This is helped by a mindset change specifically related to R&D. In open innovation, a firm commercializes both its own ideas as well as innovations from other firms and seeks ways to bring its in-house ideas to market by deploying pathways outside its current businesses (Bitterly 2015). In this approach, a firm should not restrict the source nor the use of ideas and technologies.

One of the biggest reasons for the possibility of transition from closed to open innovation is the increasing connectivity provided by the Internet, social media, and other forms of communication. Small businesses and individuals have also gained the benefits of open innovation. Crowdfunding platforms like Kickstarter and Indiegogo allow backers to contribute money in exchange for rewards.

Open innovation offers a variety of opportunities for any type of business and innovation project. By the advance of the Internet and Web 2.0, the practice of crowdsourcing experienced its rise, and many new opportunities evolved. Through Internet platforms, it is possible to involve a large number of customers, users, inventors, and innovators around the world in the innovation process (Hengsberger 2018). Examples of current platforms include innocentive.com; atizo.com; and quirky.com. The trendiest activity in open innovation is collaboration with start-ups. This is mainly important for companies that have high potential through digital transformation.

7.5.2   Technological innovation

Following Schumpeter (1934), innovations were increasingly reduced to technological innovations relating to products and processes. In general, technological innovations involve three types of technological change: platform, component, and design. Platform innovation is the emergence of an entirely new technology based on scientific principles distinctly different from those of the existing technologies. For example, the incandescent lamp used a new technology, electric resistance, to provide light, where the prior technology used combustion.

Technologies co-evolve with societies (Saviotti 2005). Technological developments influence society, and vice versa. The question about who makes decisions about the development and direction of new technologies have seldom been asked and even less often answered. In academic circles during the 1960s and 1970s, questions were increasingly voiced about wanted and unwanted consequences, both foreseen and unforeseen, and the direction and steering of new technologies.

Component innovation is one that uses new parts or materials within the same technological platform. For example, various types of halogen lamps, like tungsten quartz, parabolic aluminized reflectors, and dichroic reflector lamps, all rely on the incandescent principle but use different gases and parts.

Design innovation is a reconfiguration of the linkages and layout of components within the same technological platform. For example, compact fluorescent lamps and circular fluorescent lamps are also design innovations based on the same principles of fluorescents (Sood and Tellis 2005).

7.5.3   Social innovation

Since Schumpeter (1934), the concept of innovation has focused predominantly on economic and technical developments. Meanwhile, the importance of social innovation successfully addressing social, economic, political, and environmental challenges of the twenty-first century has been recognized just recently, and technology might be a great catalyst of such change.

Social innovation is any initiative or business that works in meeting social goals, including a product, process, program, or platform. In time, the initiative develops and deploys effective solutions to challenging and often systemic social and environmental issues in support of social progress. Under this perspective, social innovation is a new combination of social practices in certain areas of action or social contexts prompted by certain actors in an intentional targeted manner with the goal of better satisfying needs and problems (Howaldt et al. 2016).

Historically, the most important social innovator from the eighteenth century was possibly Robert Owen, born in 1771 at the dawn of the Industrial Revolution. By the turn of the century he had bought four textile factories in New Lanark and was determined to use them not just to make money but to remake the world. Under Owen's management, the cotton mills and village of New Lanark became a model community. Owen stopped employing children under 10 and sent young children to newly built nursery and infant schools, while older children combined work and secondary school. In addition to schools, New Lanark set up a crèche for working mothers, free medical care, and comprehensive education, including evening classes (Mulgan 2007).

Social innovation might not only be about products but putting innovative new systems in place so businesses may ascend to demanding social and environmental challenges in a more ethical way. It involves turning today's prevailing business model of maximizing short-term profits for shareholders on its head and returning to the way companies operated a few decades ago, when they were more rooted in the physical communities in which they operated and there was greater accountability (Slavin 2013).

7.6   Entrepreneurship

> *The entrepreneur always searches for change, responds to it, and exploits it as an opportunity.*
>
> **Peter F. Drucker**
> *[from Innovation and Entrepreneurship (2006)]*

The word "entrepreneur" comes from the French, where it literally means "undertaker". The word was a loanword into English in the mid-nineteenth century, perhaps the golden age of the entrepreneur, when the number of new economic niches was exploding.

Innovation is the specific instrument of entrepreneurship. Entrepreneurship is neither a science nor an art; it is a practice (Drucker 1986). It has a knowledge and mindset base, which this module attempts to present. But, as in all practices, like engineering and computing for example, knowledge and mindset in entrepreneurship are a means to an end.

7.6.1   Mindset and habits of mind

A mindset is defined as a mental attitude or inclination. While mindset can be influenced by an intentional consciousness, it can also largely be guided by experiences. In this sense, a mindset is a habit that requires practice. Mindset depends largely on habits of mind (HoM), which means one's character toward behaving logically when challenged with problems the answers to which are not immediately known. HoM are traits or ways of thinking that affect how a person looks at the world or reacts to a challenge. These six HoM (Figure 7.3) are so encouraged, even rewarded by engineering experiences that, over time, they become part of an engineer's everyday thinking. These ways of thinking are not exclusive to engineering. There are HoM of math, science, engineering, and art; however, we are discussing engineering HoM (EHoM) in this module. EHoM allow engineers to routinely come up with solutions to problems or improvements to current technologies or ways of doing things. When engineers develop EHoM, they are not just learning how to pass a test; they are learning to make meaning out of the world around them (Katehi et al. 2009). Figure 7.4 shows the 16 EHoM.

7.6.2   The entrepreneurial mindset

The entrepreneurial mindset is the tendency to discover, evaluate, and exploit opportunities. It is also about how an entrepreneur perceives needs, problems, and challenges as opportunities. It is about coming up with innovative ways to deal with challenges and problems and creating business value. People with an entrepreneurial mindset are drawn to opportunities and innovation; are effective at taking calculated risks; are capable of accepting the realities of change and uncertainty; and may take a step back to see the larger picture.

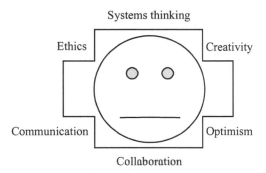

Figure 7.3 The six HoM.

1. Persisting
2. Managing impulsivity
3. Listening with understanding and empathy
4. Thinking flexibly
5. Thinking about thinking
6. Striving for accuracy
7. Questioning and posing problems
8. Applying past knowledge to new situations
9. Thinking and communicating with clarity and precision
10. Gathering data through all senses
11. Creating, imagining, innovating
12. Responding with wonderment and awe
13. Taking responsible risks
14. Finding humor
15. Thinking interdependently
16. Remaining open to continuous learning

Figure 7.4 The 16 EHoM.

Entrepreneurial mindset means a combination of technical, management, and personal skills. As such, there is no established, simple definition of the entrepreneurial skillset. However, the Organization for Economic Cooperation and Development (OECD) has identified three main groups of skills required by entrepreneurs (EU 2015):

- Technical, including communication (listening, reading, writing, speaking, viewing, and representing), environment monitoring and awareness, problem-solving, technology implementation and use, interpersonal, and organizational skills
- Business management, including planning and goal-setting, decision-making, human resources management, marketing, finance, accounting, customer relations, quality control, negotiation, business launch, growth management, and compliance with regulations skills
- Personal entrepreneurial, including self-control and discipline, risk management, innovation, persistence, leadership, change management, network building, and strategic thinking

This blend of skills, competencies, and attributes is required by commercial managers and creative workers. In addition, entrepreneurs require knowledge of the sectors in which they operate.

7.6.3 Personality characteristics of successful entrepreneurs

The possession of certain personality characteristics predisposes an individual toward entrepreneurial behavior (Westhead et al. 2011). An entrepreneurial personality is an important aspect in the context of business venture performance. The success of a business venture is the outcome of many different factors; personality characteristics are only one of them. Entrepreneurial characteristics are defined as the individual competences including attitude and behavior, which allow the entrepreneur to achieve business success, as shown in Figure 7.5. In particular, entrepreneurial competencies include aptitude, vision, risk tolerance, attitude, confidence, creativity, initiative, perseverance, passion, and many more.

Most people have a wide range of the above characteristics, starting with aptitudes including natural talents, tendencies, or capacities. Entrepreneurs apply their aptitudes to their career and business ventures. Entrepreneurs can envision their end results or goals. They have a vision of their success, and they constantly work toward making it real. Another pillar of entrepreneurial characteristics may include risk tolerance, which is the degree to which they can comfortably accept taking chances. Entrepreneurs need to have a pretty high tolerance of risks. Calculated risk-taking is a significant feature of entrepreneurship, however, entrepreneurs cannot be generalized as universal risk-takers in any circumstances. Therefore, the concept of innovation and newness is an integral part of entrepreneurship in this aspect. Perseverance is the determination that pushes the entrepreneur to keep going and keep trying. Initiative is the readiness and willingness to start a new enterprise. Entrepreneurs are usually self-motivated and quite willing to take on this leadership role

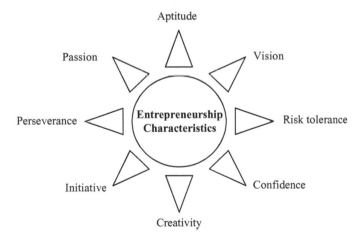

Figure 7.5 Main personality characteristics of successful entrepreneurs.

and make themselves personally responsible for the success or failure of a venture. Finally, entrepreneurs are passionate about their ideas, their company, and their vision.

7.7   Intrapreneurship

Of the top 10 sources of innovation, employees are the only resource that you can control and access that your competitors cannot. Employees are the one asset you have that can actually be a sustainable competitive advantage.

Kaihan Krippendorff

The term intrapreneurship (entrepreneurship within an existing business structure; also termed corporate entrepreneurship or corporate venturing) is derived from a combination of "intra", or internal, and "entrepreneurship". Intrapreneurship is defined as a collection of formal and informal activities within an organization leading to the implementation of innovative ideas and behaviors (Toftoy and Chatterjee 2005).

Intrapreneurship has become part of the business lexicon for the last 30 years. *TIME* and *Newsweek* articles about intrapreneurship were both published in 1985. But three years earlier, Howard Edward Haller's completed formal academic case study and master's thesis documented the terms intrapreneurship and corporate entrepreneurship.

The word intrapreneur is iconic for many millennials. They use it as shorthand for the freedom to pursue their own ideas and the chance to make a meaningful difference early in their careers. This is what millennials are demanding. As millennials spread the word, companies are implementing intrapreneuring to recruit and retain the best and the brightest (Pinchot 2016).

At the level of an individual intrapreneur, the trigger for innovation could arise from the aspiration to challenge oneself beyond the obvious. Intrapreneurs seeking to reinvent a company in order to increase efficiency may do so by removing unproductive layers of bureaucratic hierarchy, harnessing the power of technology, proper delegation of authority and power, or finding other ways to improve efficiency and effectiveness (Seshadri and Tripathy 2006).

Figure 7.6 outlines several insights of intrapreneurship.

7.8   The entrepreneurial practice

An entrepreneur must deal with more uncertainty than a professional with a well-defined role.

Peter Thiel

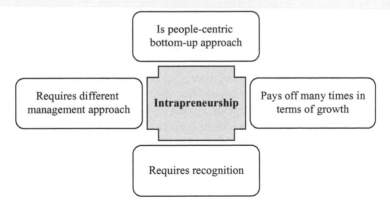

Figure 7.6 Insights of intrapreneurship.

The process of developing a new venture is expressed in the entrepreneurial practice, which entails multiple phases starting with an opportunity and ending with managing the resulting enterprise. There are four major stages of the entrepreneurial process, which are innovation, a triggering event, implementation, and growth (Figure 7.7). This model is supported by Hisrich et al. (2010), who presented the four-stage entrepreneurial process.

7.8.1 Innovation: Identifying and evaluating the opportunity

Innovation means creating the business idea, searching for the market opportunity, creating the concept, identifying the value, and evaluating the opportunity. Most good business opportunities do not suddenly emerge but rather result from an entrepreneur's readiness to exploit possibilities or, in some cases, the establishment of mechanisms that identify

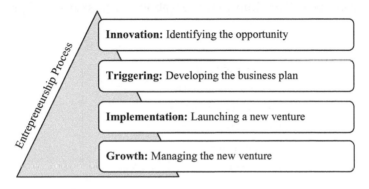

Figure 7.7 The four distinct phases of entrepreneurship process.

potential opportunities. Opportunities do not appear quickly but are results of the entrepreneur's devotion to these opportunities.

Inspiration for opportunities generally comes from monitoring the market environment and its factors, such as demand for certain products and export possibilities. The idea may also come from a new discovery of an important commodity's sources, the discovery of new products and technologies. Ideas and inspiration may also be taken from life situations and surroundings. There are many sources for new ideas and venture opportunities for individuals. Ideas for business may come from one's own skills, hobbies, and interests; another's successful ideas; separation from the parent company; inefficiency in the market; and ability to correct that inefficiency (Habash 2017).

Examination or filtering product ideas is the initial stage of evaluation. Business opportunity evaluation means that the resources should be allocated on further enhancement and elaboration. This evaluation is perhaps the most critical element of the entrepreneurial process, as it allows the entrepreneur to assess whether the specific product or service has the returns needed compared to the resources required.

The following step is to carry out what is called "customer analysis" for market identification and to realize the existence of the marketplace. This may be accomplished by conducting surveys or simply by trying to answer a series of questions like: who will buy the product; does a market exist for the innovation; and what price is the customer willing to pay? Figure 7.8 reflects the components of identification and evaluation of the opportunity process.

7.8.2 Triggering: Developing the business plan

Triggering includes the motivation to start a business, developing a business plan, assessing the risk, resource acquisition, and the determination to proceed. The business plan is a written statement intended to crystallize business objectives, inform readers about the business, and provide a

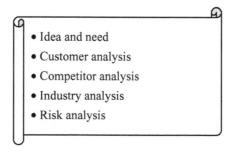

- Idea and need
- Customer analysis
- Competitor analysis
- Industry analysis
- Risk analysis

Figure 7.8 Identification and evaluation components of the opportunity process.

guidebook for managing the company. Importantly, preparing a business plan requires entrepreneurs to split excitement and emotion from the new idea and verbalize the concept, mission, and feasibility of the new business (Habash 2017).

A good business plan must be developed in order to exploit the defined opportunity. This is a very time-consuming phase of the entrepreneurial process. Most potential investors will want to see a business plan before they consider funding your business. A business plan is regarded as a filter, cleaning and screening ideas with the absence of potential for developing a successful entrepreneurship. In particular, it should cover strategies for improving your existing sales and processes to achieve the desired growth. Figure 7.9 describes what a business plan needs to include. The marketing objectives entail, for example, how many new customers to gain and the anticipated size of the customer base at the end of the period; better understanding the characteristics and preferences of customers; identifying opportunities to increase sales and grow business; and monitoring the level of competition in the market.

The business plan should evolve in much the same way as technology. At first simple and brief, then more detailed and complex as the marketplace evolves. Despite its inevitably greater complexity, the plan must remain framed in plain, simple, declarative sentences that tell what you want to achieve and how you plan to achieve it. Above all, the plan must always reflect you and your objectives (OEERE 2000). Any basic plan will contain the components shown in Figure 7.10 and will prove an invaluable tool for making decisions about your commercialization strategy.

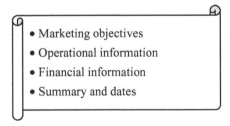

- Marketing objectives
- Operational information
- Financial information
- Summary and dates

Figure 7.9 Elements of a business plan.

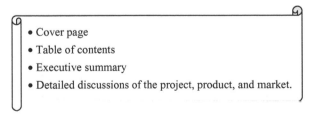

- Cover page
- Table of contents
- Executive summary
- Detailed discussions of the project, product, and market.

Figure 7.10 Basic components of a business plan.

The cover page should include the contact information: the name of the business, the address, phone numbers, principals, and the date of the plan. A very brief synopsis on the company purpose or any other appropriate information about the company and plan may be added. The table of contents should be about one page. It is an essential part of a good business plan. It should be specific enough to let readers get to the sections they want to find them quickly. The executive summary should be brief; one page should be enough.

The discussion part should be written in simple technical language where the story is told, remembering that non-technical people like potential investors and prospective licensees need to understand the plan. The description should be reduced to the simplest terms that will convey a full understanding of the technology as given in Figure 7.11.

The size and nature of the market should be demonstrated to convince the reader that the project is a good bet. This is how the validity and business potential of product definition is documented.

To produce and/or sell the invention, a business plan is a must. An effective, polished commercialization plan can serve as a strong foundation; however, a business plan demands a significant step upward in the sophistication of information and presentation. Thus, if the intention is to venture the invention, some sections should be added to a commercialization plan, as given in Figure 7.12.

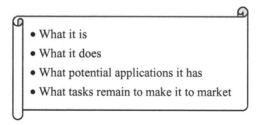

Figure 7.11 Understanding of the technology.

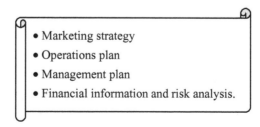

Figure 7.12 Commercialization plan.

7.8.3   Implementation: Launching a new venture

Implementation includes setting up and launching a new venture, running a business, managing a venture, deploying resources, and incorporation. Leadership is required to organize resources toward the goal while simultaneously preserving and encouraging a strategic vision. To successfully execute a business plan, in order to translate the business concept into an action, entrepreneurs have to surround themselves with the right mix of resources, which includes people, capital, and partners (Habash 2017). The entrepreneur should also assess the downside risks associated with insufficient or inappropriate resources. As the business develops, more funds will probably be needed to finance the growth of the venture. Figure 7.13 outlines the required resources.

7.8.4   Growth: Managing the new venture

Growth means maximizing profit, getting rewards, and continually growing the venture to include other opportunities. After resources are acquired, the entrepreneur must use them to implement the business plan. The management part of any planning remains the most important factor in the success of a new business and effective partnering. Understanding how to run the day-to-day operations of a business is essential to long-term planning strategies and success. The operational problems of the growing enterprise must also be examined. This involves implementing a management style and structure, as well as determining the key variables for success. A control system must be established so that any problem areas can be quickly identified and resolved. Some entrepreneurs have difficulty managing and growing the venture they created (Habash 2017). The significant task an entrepreneur may do is to distinguish those tasks that can be performed well from those that should be delegated.

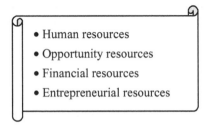

- Human resources
- Opportunity resources
- Financial resources
- Entrepreneurial resources

Figure 7.13 Required resources for the entrepreneurship process.

7.9   *Entrepreneurial marketing*

> *Word-of-mouth marketing has always been important. Today, it's more important than ever because of the power of the Internet.*
>
> **Joe Pulizzi and Newt Barrett**
> *[from Pulizzi's Get Content Get Customers: Turn Prospects Into Buyers with Content Marketing (2008)]*

Marketing is not only about selling. Relatively, that is right, because that is the eventual goal of marketing; however, it is more than just selling. It is about approaches in attracting the attention of target customers. One common characteristic between entrepreneurship and marketing is the study of approaches through which marketing concepts and principles could be applied in the field of entrepreneurship.

Entrepreneurial marketing is a concept that was developed at the interface between two sciences, marketing and entrepreneurship. It came out in 1982 at a conference at the University of Illinois, Chicago (Hills et al. 2010). Marketing is of crucial importance for the success or failure of an enterprise, as its success is eventually decided in the market, competing for the target customers. In funding, venture capitalists will usually look at the way enterprise plans to enter the market, target groups to be addressed, and the approach by which the firm's product or service offered will be communicated and distributed to potential customers. Entrepreneurial marketing is difficult to calculate and is rather based on the entrepreneur's visionary and creative marketing ideas (Volkmann and Berg 2011). Such marketing is made up of six components, given as the "6Ps," as shown in Table 7.2.

Entrepreneurial marketing is difficult to calculate and is rather based on the entrepreneur's visionary and creative marketing ideas. Marketing activities of small companies with limited access to resources should be

Table 7.2 The 6Ps of marketing variables

Product	Product enhancement: What is the real product? What should or should not be offered?
People	Customer focus: Who uses the product? What do they care about?
Price	Market focus: Can customers afford the product or service? How do they value it?
Place	Product distribution: How do customers get to the product? Where is it distributed? How is it delivered?
Production	Unique proposition: Is it possible to meet the market needs? Is production flexible enough to meet changing market needs?
Promotion	Innovative marketing: How do people know about the producer? How well does promotion work?

creative and simple (for example, budget or guerrilla marketing). Guerrilla marketing is an unconventional way to advertise a product or a service. This strategy is more focused on helping small companies and entrepreneurs to advertise their products and services without spending a large amount of money. It involves word-of-mouth advertising and addressing consumers in their everyday work situation, for example via email, messages, stickers, and poster campaigns (Volkmann and Berg 2011).

Viral marketing is another customer-based approach for entrepreneurial marketing, which uses social networks like Twitter, Facebook, etc. to gain brand awareness. The term was coined in 1997 (Phelps et al. 2004). However, the more widespread use of social media has recently pushed this idea to a whole new level. The standard viral-marketing model is based on an analogy with the spread of infectious disease. Information about the product passes virally from human to human at a low-cost marketing method, which is very efficient. It assumes that one starts with a seed of people who send a message by infecting their friends, where the anticipated number of new infectious people generated by each existing one is called the "reproduction rate".

7.10   Ethical practice in entrepreneurship

> *As an entrepreneur building a business, you need to respect yourself and surround yourself with people you can respect ... Do not lie, steal, or cheat. Make your word your bond and always stand by your word. When you are wrong, own up to it and make good on the deal. Treat others as you'd want to be treated.*
>
> **Jana Matthews**

Ethics, whether applied to business, engineering, law, medicine, or any other professional practice, is derived from a set of universal values (Starcher 1997). It deals with the distinction between what is right and wrong. Ethics has a significant role to play in practices, as it gives a guideline as to which entrepreneurial practices are morally acceptable and which are not.

7.10.1   Interface between ethics and entrepreneurship

Entrepreneurship is more than being innovative or creative in coming up with new ideas for products or services. Entrepreneurs must also either create an organization or work through an organization (intrapreneurs) to develop the new opportunities and values they envision. This involves not only risks of various sorts, but also obstacles and barriers that may stand in the way of the entrepreneur's efforts (Brenkert 2009). Importantly, morals and ethics are among these obstacles and barriers.

The interface between ethics and entrepreneurship involves two main related issues. The first concerns the entrepreneurial framework for ethics, while the second involves the ethical framework for entrepreneurship. Basically, what many consider to be entrepreneurial behavior is a set of actions fraught with ethical dilemmas. Entrepreneurs are often admired for the creative ways in which they overcome significant limitations, obstacles, and sources of resistance to their new venture ideas (Fisscher et al. 2005). Practices such as bending or breaking rules, putting other people's resources at risk, creatively interpreting the facts, exaggerating one's position, and promising more than one is currently able to deliver are presented by some as clever manifestations of the entrepreneurial spirit. To the extent that these practices are entrepreneurial, and that the more a person engages in them the more entrepreneurial that person is, the ability to reconcile "entrepreneurial" and "ethical" can therefore become problematic (Tanwar 2013). It is through awareness of ethics that entrepreneurs abstain from engaging in lawless practices that lead to the harm of humans, compromise the environment, or bring about gain at the partial expense of other businesses, employees, consumers, etc.

Entrepreneurs face complex ethical problems related to basic fairness, personnel, and customer relationships; honesty in communications; distribution dilemmas; and other challenges. At the same time, entrepreneurs face difficulties of survival due to lack of brand recognition and sales and cash flow in order to survive, which may lead to unethical decision-making (Tanwar 2013). A compromise between entrepreneurial ambition and moral values surrounds businesses, especially at the early stages. Figure 7.14 shows the two faces of this challenge.

7.10.2   Approaches to ethical entrepreneurship

There are fundamental reasons to take the ethics of entrepreneurship more seriously than other topics. First, entrepreneurship has emerged as a distinctive area of academic inquiry, with unique problems and questions that can be productively studied in their own right. Second, entrepreneurship is an inescapably ethical activity: whether one views it from the societal, the organizational, or the individual level, entrepreneurial action has powerful ethical dimensions and implications (Dunham 2005).

In these different contexts, entrepreneurs sometimes break rules or do something that is morally wrong, and yet from a broader, ethical perspective, their actions may be viewed as acceptable or even, in some cases, admirable. Sometimes, it seems, doing something wrong may be preferable to aiming for moral perfection. This more complex vision of morality

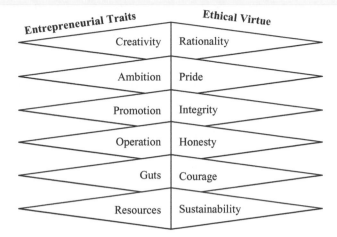

Figure 7.14 Entrepreneurial traits and corresponding ethical virtues.

and ethics is the context within which an ethics of entrepreneurship and the breaking of rules needs to be understood (Brenkert 2009).

One major approach to ethics is through virtue. Virtues are action-guiding character traits that aim at good results. The ethics literature is populated with many competing accounts of what the good results should be and, consequently, with competing accounts of what virtues we should uphold. Some virtue ethicists make the claim that a character has priority in ethical evaluation over rules or principles, actions, and consequences. Setting aside the issue of whether virtue has priority, my concern here is to connect entrepreneurial success traits to virtues (Hicks 2009).

The unique ethical challenges found in entrepreneurial ventures can be traced to the newness and smallness of these firms. Compared with larger, more established businesses, entrepreneurial firms are more vulnerable to environmental forces, especially given the limited cash reserves and debt capacity of such organizations, their frequent over-dependence on a limited product/service line, and their tendency to rely on a niche customer base. Moreover, there is a liability of newness, especially at the early stages of the venture, when entrepreneurs are unfamiliar with their roles and the roles of the firm and are apt to commit a variety of errors and blunders (Morris et al. 2002).

The virtues and values listed in the right column of Table 6.8 together constitute an entrepreneurial code for business ethics. That set of virtues is an abstraction of a description of entrepreneurial activity. The thoughts and actions of entrepreneurs are particulars of a general set of success traits. Those success traits of entrepreneurs are particulars of a general set of virtues (Hicks 2009).

7.11   *Knowledge acquisition*

Attempting to answer the following questions involves acquisition of knowledge from this book and other books, documents, and the Internet.

- What is the difference between creative thinking and critical thinking?
- Compare invention to innovation.
- How do innovative technologies evolve?
- Should firms make or buy innovations?
- What does social innovation look like?
- What is the difference between closed innovation and open innovation?
- What are the characteristics of management innovation?
- What is the difference between groundfunding and groundsourcing?
- What is the entrepreneurial mindset?
- What contributes to the development of a successful entrepreneur?
- What is the relationship between design, innovation, and entrepreneurship?
- Describe the benefits and drawbacks of entrepreneurship.
- What are major strategic constraints and challenges confronted by entrepreneurs today?
- What excites you about being an entrepreneur? What are your major concerns?
- How do engineers view entrepreneurship?
- What is the difference between entrepreneurship and intrapreneurship?
- How does technology entrepreneurship differentiate from other types of entrepreneurship?
- What are the personal characteristics required to be a successful entrepreneur?
- What is a project? What is a business plan?
- What is opportunity analysis?
- What is a market survey?
- What is venture capital?
- Do serial entrepreneurs succeed more than first-time entrepreneurs?
- Where do most entrepreneurs obtain their ideas from?
- Explain the forces that drive the growing of entrepreneurship.
- What is the role of ethics in technology entrepreneurship?
- How do entrepreneurs differ from non-entrepreneurs with respect to ethics?

7.12   Knowledge creation

Collaborate with peers on learning or work with others outside the class to narrow down the objectives of each activity. You may access class and online resources and analyze data and information to create new ideas and balanced solutions. High-level digital tools may be used to develop multimedia presentations, simulations or animations, videos and visual displays, digital portfolios, reflective practice (online publishing and blogging), or well-researched and up-to-date reports.

7.12.1   Entrepreneurial mindset

Think about something you dislike in your everyday life and try to find, as an entrepreneur, an innovative way to fix it. For this task, prepare an e-Poster to outline the above based on the following three principles and possibly more, if any: need, opportunity, and resources.

7.12.2   Entrepreneurial struggle

Imagine yourself in the position of an entrepreneur struggling to turn an idea into a successful business. Select a famous entrepreneur. Identify and record how many of the entrepreneurial characteristics from your checklist the entrepreneur has. How did the entrepreneur create value? How did the entrepreneur use the resources to satisfy their needs or solve problems? Present the outcome to the class in a five-minute presentation.

7.12.3   Marketing a new technology venture

Digital tools and technology continue to disrupt the world of marketing. Engagement on new platforms, such as messaging services and social media, is reshaping the future of marketing. This pattern shift represents the next opportunity to change the way consumers and brands engage with one another.

Key Point: There is a well-known story of two shoe entrepreneurs who go to China to do market research. They find, to their surprise, that no one in China wears shoes. One entrepreneur comes home and laments that there is no market of shoe-wearers to sell to. The other entrepreneur returns with a smile on his face, knowing that if he can access it, the market is enormous (Felser 2011). Be optimistic!

For this task, propose an approach for marketing a new technology venture, which combines viral-marketing tools with old-fashioned mass media in a way that yields far more predictable results than "purely" viral approaches like word-of-mouth marketing. You may use metaphors and symbols as long as those are clearly communicated or explained in supplementary materials.

7.12.4 *Supporting employee intrapreneurs*

Intrapreneurs are a real channel to generate and execute new thinking approaches within a corporate environment. For this task, form a team and work together in a collaborative environment to formulate a combined message through a three-minute video to encourage intrapreneurial efforts within an organization to create cultural change of accepting new ideas and thinking; engage existing employees; and attract new and high-potential individuals into the organization. Try to explore a wide range of approaches and models for organizations to support and improve the effectiveness of intrapreneurs. This may include incentives, training, and various types of support.

7.12.5 *Case of ethics on entrepreneurship*

X, as a computer science student, had an entrepreneurial idea that was developed due to support from the university. Upon graduation, X took a career, but at the same time took the entrepreneurial initiative and started her own venture, which was developed successfully. After a few years later, X sold the business for a large amount of money. X is now living the good life of building a dream home, raising family, managing a great portfolio of assets, and travel. Discuss the moral status of this case.

References

Anadon, L. D., G. Chan, E. Kempster, L. Vinsel, J. Stephens, K. Araujo, and P. Guardabassi. 2013. Background paper for the project on innovation and access to technologies for sustainable development. Harvard Kennedy School of Business. https://www.hks.harvard.edu/content/download/68197/1245598/version/1/file/2013–03.pdf.

Baillie, C. 2002. Enhancing creativity in engineering students. *Engineering Science and Education Journal* 11: 185–192.

Bitterly, P. 2015. Don't you know the difference between closed and open innovation? Implementing open innovation. https://www.linkedin.com/pulse/dont-you-know-difference-between-closed-open-ch1-pascal-bitterly.

Brenkert, G. C. 2009. Innovation, rule breaking and the ethics of entrepreneurship. *Journal of Business Venturing* 24: 448–464.

Drucker, P. F. 1986. *Innovation and Entrepreneurship: Practice and Principles*. New York, NY: Harper and Row Publishers Inc.

Dunham, L. 2005. Entrepreneurship and ethics. University of St. Thomas, St Paul, MN. http://www.stthomas.edu/news/entrepreneurship-and-ethics/.

EU. 2015. Analytical highlights: Focus on entrepreneurial skills. http://skillspa norama.cedefop.europa.eu/sites/default/files/EUSP_AH_Entrepreneur ial_0.pdf.

Felser, J. 2011. An Engineer's guide to applying appropriate technology. 2011 AHS Capstone Projects. Paper 21. http://digitalcommons.olin.edu/ahs_capstone_ 2011/21.

Fisscher, O. D. Frenkel, Y. Lurie, and A. Nijhof. 2005. Stretching the frontiers: Exploring the relationships between entrepreneurship and ethics. *Journal of Business Ethics* 60: 207–209.

Gaynor, G. H. 2014. Innovation: Transition from bottom-up to top-down innova-tion. *IEEE Engineering Management Review* 42(1): 5–7.

Habash, R. 2017. *Green Engineering: Innovation, Entrepreneurship, and Design*. Boca Raton, FL: CRC Taylor and Francis.

Hamel, G. 2006. The why, what, and how of management innovation. https:// hbr.org/2006/02/the-why-what-and-how-of-management-innovation.

Hamel, G., and M. J. Mol. 2008. Management innovation. *Academy of Management Review* 33(4): 825–845.

Hengsberger, A. 2018. Best practice open innovation – this is how the best are doing it. https://www.lead-innovation.com/english-blog/best-practice-o pen-innovation.

Hicks, S. R. C. 2009. What business ethics can learn from entrepreneurship. *The Journal of Private Enterprise* 24(2): 49–57.

Hills, G. E., C. M. Hultman, S. Kraus, and R. Schulte. 2010. History, theory and evidence of entrepreneurial marketing: An overview. *International Journal of Entrepreneurship and Innovation Management* 11(1): 3–18.

Hisrich, R. D., M. P. Peter, and D. A. Shepherd. 2010. *Entrepreneurship: Starting, Developing, and Managing a New Enterprise*. Eighth Edition. Irwin, NY: McGraw-Hill.

Howaldt, J., D. Domanski, and C. Kaletka. 2016. Social innovation: Toward a new innovation paradigm. http://www.scielo.br/scielo.php?script=sci_arttext &pid=S1678-69712016000600020.

Hutt, R. 2016. What is disruptive innovation? https://www.weforum.org/agenda /2016/06/what-is-disruptive-innovation/.

Katehi, L., G. Pearson, and M. Feder. 2009. *Engineering in K–12 Education: Understanding the Status and Improving the Prospects*. Committee on K–12 Engineering Education, National Academy of Engineering and NRC. Washington, DC: National Academies Press.

Morris, M. H., M. Schindehutte, J. Walton, and J. Allen. 2002. The ethical context of entrepreneurship: Proposing and testing a developmental framework. *Journal of Business ethics* 40(4): 331–361.

Mulgan, G. 2007: Social innovation: What it is, why it matters, and how it can be accelerated. http://eureka.sbs.ox.ac.uk/761/1/Social_Innovation.pdf.

Norman, D. A., and R. Verganti. 2012. Incremental and radical innovation: Design research versus technology and meaning change. *Norman and Verganti Incremental and Radical Innovation* March: 1–19.

OEERE. 2000. From invention to innovation. Office of Energy Efficiency and Renewable Energy, US Department of Energy, Washington, DC.

Okpara, F. O. 2007. The value of creativity and innovation in entrepreneurship. *Journal of Asia Entrepreneurship and Sustainability* III(2): 1–14.

Paul, R., and L. Elder. 2016. *The Miniature Guide to Critical Thinking Concepts and Tools*. Seventh Edition. Dillon Beach, CA: Foundation for Critical Thinking Press.

Phelps, J. E., R. Lewis, L. Mobilio, D. Perry, and N. Raman. 2004. Viral marketing or electronic word-of-mouth advertising: Examining consumer responses and motivations to pass along e-mail. *Journal of Advertising Research* 44(4): 333–348.

Pinchot, P. 2016. Why intrapreneuring is suddenly happening again. http://www.pinchot.com/intrapreneuring/.

Rao, S. 2017. Creativity is not a trait. It's a habit. https://medium.com/the-mission/creativity-is-not-a-trait-its-a-habit-f3ed184e88c4.

Reguia, C. 2014. Product innovation and the competitive advantage. *European Scientific Journal* 1(June): 140–157.

Saviotti, P. P. 2005. On the co-evolution of technologies and institutions. In Weber, K., and J. Hemmelskamp (eds.). *Towards Environmental Innovation Systems*. Berlin, Germany: Springer, pp. 9–32.

Schumpeter, J. A. 1934. *The Theory of Economic Development*. Cambridge, MA: Harvard University Press.

Seshadri, D. V. R., and A. Tripathy. 2006. Innovation through intrapreneurship: The road less travelled. *Vikapala* 31(1): 17–29.

Slavin, T. 2013. Social innovation means business becoming a force for good. https://www.theguardian.com/sustainable-business/blog/social-innovation-business-force-for-good.

Sood, A., and G. J. Tellis. 2005. Understanding the seeds of growth: Technological evolution and product innovation. PhD Thesis, Marshall School of Business, University of Southern California, Los Angeles, CA.

Starcher, G. 1997. Ethics and entrepreneurship, an oxymoron: A transition to a free market economy in Eastern Europe. European Baha'i Business Forum, Paris, France. http://bahai-library.com/starcher_ethics_entrepreneurship.

Tanwar, R. 2013. Interplay of ethics and entrepreneurship at various stages of an organizational life cycle. *Global Journal of Management and Business Studies* 3(9): 1041–1050.

Taylor, E. 1996. *Innovation Design Environment and Strategy. Block 1: An Introduction to Innovation*. Milton Keynes, UK: The Open University.

Toftoy, C., and J. Chatterjee. 2005. The intrapreneurial revolution: Now is the time for action. http://sbaer.uca.edu/research/icsb/2005/paper192.pdf.

Volkmann, V., and H. Berg. 2011. Entrepreneurial marketing. Guest Lecture Kosice. http://www.ekf.tuke.sk/files/utorok.pdf.

Westhead, P., G. McElwee, and M. Wright. 2011. *Entrepreneurship: Perspectives and Cases*. Essex, UK: Pearson Education Ltd.

Zapel, D. 2018. Open innovation vs. closed innovation. https://www.lead-innovation.com/english-blog/open-innovation-vs.-closed-innovation.

module eight

Safety in design practice

8.1 Knowledge and understanding

Having successfully completed this module, you should be able to demonstrate knowledge and understanding of:

- Design, design knowledge, design problems, and design safety
- Engineering habits of mind which are essential for design, like systems thinking, creativity, optimism, collaboration, ethics, and society
- Design methodology and engineering design process
- Hazard, risk assessment, risk management, and risk communication
- Risk management as an area of knowledge with which all engineers should be familiar
- System safety as an application of engineering and management principles
- Functional safety, safety integrity, and safety instrumented system
- System safety analysis techniques, including failure modes and effects analyses, and fault tree analysis
- Safety factor and design margin
- Ergonomics principles as a practice of designing products, systems, or processes to take proper account of the interaction with the people who use or operate them
- Types of standards and codes in engineering design

8.2 Engineering design

> At the end of the day, the goals are simple: safety and security.
>
> **Jodi Rell**

Safety in design, in the sense perceived in the quotation above, is not a physical object, but a status in which danger is absent; it's not just about designing for simpler, easier use and long-term economic benefits through reduced production and maintenance costs, but for health and safety-engaging standards and guidelines, change, remediation, and risk analysis (Figure 8.1).

Professional engineering and computing are about problem structuring and solving; applying theoretical knowledge in the conception, design,

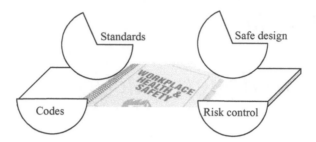

Figure 8.1 Design safety cycle.

implementation, and operation of new products, systems, processes, and services. Technical knowledge and skills are complemented by a sound appreciation of the process involved, along with an awareness of the ethical, safety, environmental, economic, and social considerations involved in practicing as a professional (HSE 2009).

The word "design" is ambiguous and may carry several meanings. In its noun form, it may be related to intellectual activities of sketching, drawing, planning, patterning, intention or purpose, the cognitive process of the designer, or the art of producing configurations, compositions, value, or purpose. In its verb form, it may involve representing an artifact, system, or society; fixing its look, function, or purpose; or all those things combined (Habash 2017). Artifacts are the end product of the design, which are supposed to meet the objectives for which they are built.

Design is now regarded as a new discipline of practical reasoning and augmentation (Buchanan 1992). It creates value for industries, users and, ultimately, for society. Practitioners are currently required to provide innovative solutions to complex problems, for example, corporate strategy, business management, product design, and manufacture. This requires the application of concepts and methods from other disciplines and speculates on broader social, cultural, and philosophic issues and subjects to explore design (Buchanan and Margolin 1995).

Design is the central creative process of engineering. It is, in fact, the "essence of engineering". The Canadian Academy of Engineering (CAE 1999) states: "Engineering is a profession concerned with the creation of new and improved systems, processes, and products to serve human needs. The central focus of engineering is design, an art entailing the exercise of ingenuity, imagination, knowledge, skill, discipline, and judgment based on experience".

Engineering design is a distinguished discipline since it (1) synthesizes new information for product realization, (2) establishes quality through defining functionality, materialization, and appearance of artifacts, and (3) influences the technological, economic, and marketing aspects of production (Horvath 2000).

The CEAB describes engineering design as integration of mathematics, basic sciences, engineering sciences, and complementary studies in developing elements, systems, and processes to meet specific needs. It is a creative, iterative, and often open-ended process subject to constraints that may be governed by standards or legislation to varying degrees, depending on the discipline. These constraints may relate to economic, health, safety, environmental, social, or other pertinent interdisciplinary factors. Obviously, successful engineering design requires a broad cross-section of knowledge, skills, and attitudes (CEAB 2004).

8.3 Design landscape

> *Design is the intermediary between information and understanding.*
>
> **Hans Hoffman**

The basic step of the design process is usually similar to the step used in a typical problem-solving process. Since design problems are usually defined more vaguely and have a variety of correct answers, the process may require backtracking and iteration. Solving a design problem is a liable process, and the solution is subject to unexpected complications and changes as it develops.

8.3.1 Design knowledge

Design knowledge links the three fields in the world of designing. All three have a relation with design knowledge; design practice applies and generates design knowledge, design education transfers this knowledge, and design research produces this knowledge (together with design practice). Ideal relation between the three fields is given in Figure 8.2.

Design research, sometimes called design science, includes the study of how designers work and think. It gets input from design education and practice and develops theories and support for future use in design education and practice. Design education uses the results of research, gets inputs from design practice, delivers good designers for practice, and gives feedback to design research. Design practice uses support developed in research and taught in education and gives input for design education and design research (Reymen 2001).

8.3.2 Design problems

The best way to design or build something is a problem, and how to create an artistic or innovative work may be a problem. Design problems are more than just story problems; they basically consist of three states: the

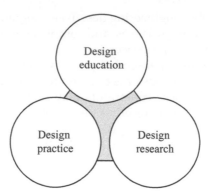

Figure 8.2 Interactions between the three components of design knowledge.

provided state, the goal state, and the problems that block the provided state from reaching the goal state. They are a mixture of all of the above three states, but tending towards the goal state, which has an absolute possibility of becoming an achievable result.

Design problems are usually more vaguely defined than analysis problems, which are well-defined. Unlike an analysis problem, a design problem often begins with an unclear, abstract idea in the mind of the designer. Creating a clear definition of a design problem is more difficult than defining an analysis (routine) problem, where a design problem evolves through a series of steps or processes as understanding of the problem is developed (Habash 2017). Design problems can be classified into three classes, as shown in Table 8.1.

8.3.3   *Engineering habits of mind (EHoM) in design*

EHoM allow engineers to routinely come up with solutions to problems or improvements to current technologies or ways of doing things. Modern engineering practice is dependent on the development of a mindset and

Table 8.1 Classes of design problems

Class 1	Open-ended, non-routine creative activities where the goals are ill-structured and there is no effective design plan specifying the sequence of actions to take in producing a design model.
Class 2	Existing, well-developed design and decomposition plans (for example, designing a new product).
Class 3	Routine where design and decomposition plans are known as well as customary actions taken to deal with failures (for example, writing a computer program).

Table 8.2 The six EHoM that are essential to design

EHoM	Impact on design
Systems thinking	It means seeing whole systems and parts and how they connect by examining the linkages and interactions, pattern-sniffing, and recognizing interdependencies.
Creativity	Creativity is an integral part of the engineering design process. It is the ability to use novel approaches for generating, investigating, and representing ideas.
Optimism	Engineers, as a general rule, believe that things can always be realized and improved
Collaboration	Collaboration involves both communication between and coordination among members of a design team.
Ethical criteria	Ethical considerations, reflections, and actions can make a difference in whether a particular innovation, design, or research finding will have a helpful or harmful impact on society.
Social criteria	Engineering is simply a social activity which relies more on social involvement, cooperation, and collaboration. Key to this understanding is that engineers generate technological solutions that are intended to add value to society but that may sometimes have negative consequences.

the skills necessary to transcend disciplinary limitations in solving problems. Table 8.2 shows the six EHoM that are essential to design.

8.4   Design methodology and design process

We design our world, while our world acts back on us and designs us.

Anne-Marie Willis
*[from Willis' paper, "Ontological designing
– laying the ground" (2006)]*

The combined use of tools, techniques, and methods, which are meant to support designers in their work, is a subject of design methodology and process as a concrete plan of action for the design of technical systems.

8.4.1   Phases of engineering design

Design methodology, which is strongly process-based, aims at the improvement of design processes particularly by exploiting scientific techniques. A methodology is a body of knowledge comprising the principles, guidelines, systematic analysis, practices, and processes. Design methodologies intend to structure the design process, to maintain planning of product development, and to provide support for related activities. There are a number of features that should be possessed by each and every design methodology. The features are noticeable elements characteristic of each and every successful engineering design endeavor. Therefore, methodology is a much broader concept than a process (Habash 2017).

Design process may be seen as a set of successive cycles of design information where the design problem cycle is gradually transformed into a solution cycle. The process should start with clear product requirements that determine the scope of the product. It should be flexible enough to meet the needs of both a particular organization and a particular project. While an effective design process provides a framework within which work is carried out, there is some need for innovation along the way when designing products (Habash 2017). Typically, engineering design involves three main phases; each entails several steps, as described in Figure 8.3.

8.4.2   Customer requirements and problem definitions

Engineering design ideas always occur in response to a human need. Before developing a definition statement for a design problem, it is necessary to recognize the need for a new product, system, or service. The initial source of ideas are customers, the motivating force in the design of products and services. Simply, a customer requirement is a statement that specifies what a product should do, but it does not define how it should do it. The customers may be people, institutions, or other companies. In some circumstances, the customer and designer may be one

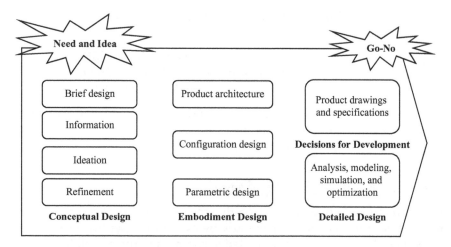

Figure 8.3 Phases of engineering design.

and the same person. The needs of customers are often many and difficult. However, establishing these needs is the most difficult aspect of market-led design, since customers do not always know what they want. Therefore, the customer requirements represent the system's actual requirements.

Once an idea is established for a product, it should be described by writing a problem statement. Often, the results of the activities in this design step determine how the design problem is decomposed into smaller and more manageable design tasks. Sometimes not enough information is known yet about the problem, and decomposition occurs later in the design process. At this phase, lots of time should be allocated and very little money should be spent. Critical thoughts and an in-depth review of literature should be the theme of this phase (OEERE 2000). All assumption should be challenged.

8.4.3   Engineering design process

Understanding the design process is important for the teaching of design, the improvement of products, and the efficiency of engineering-based companies; it is also the foundation on which a lot of design research is conducted. Design process is cyclic or iterative in nature, whereas analysis problem-solving is primarily sequential. There are several ways of describing the design process, of which the main phases have been identified in Figure 8.3. During each phase, the design engineer can focus on a portion of the problem, and the decisions taken are based on the accuracy of the forecasts made and the quality of criteria used.

Product conceptual design is the heart of product innovation and development, directly impacting detailed design in the latter phase of design. It is the very early phase of the product design process, in which drawings or prototypes are the dominant tools. It involves several activities, such as design briefs, information and background research, ideation, brainstorming, and concept evaluation.

The embodiment design phase takes the abstract conceptual path, chosen in the conceptual design phase, and molds it into a system that can actually be produced. When conceptual design is completed, a set of concepts are evaluated to produce a single concept or a small set of concepts for further development. The embodiment design involves three main activities, including product architecture, configuration design, and parametric design specifications, dimensions, and tolerances.

Detailed design is the last design activity before implementation begins. It is the phase wherein the necessary engineering done for every component of the product is identified and engineered. In this phase, the design is brought to a state where it has the complete engineering description of a tested and reproducible product. Engineers work closely with the product development team to ensure designs take full advantage of technological opportunities and observe all technical constraints (Habash 2017).

8.5   Hazard and risk

Risks must be taken because the greatest hazard in life is to risk nothing.

Leo Buscaglia

The assessment and management of risk are integral components of the daily activities of human beings in general and engineers in particular. Simply, the practice of engineering carries with it an instinctive level of risk that engineers must try to fully understand and manage.

8.5.1   Hazards

A hazard is any source of potential damage, harm, or adverse health effects on something or someone. It is the potential of a machine, equipment, process, material, or physical factor in the working environment to cause harm to people, the environment, assets, or production. Basically, a hazard is the potential for effects; for example, on people as health effects, on organizations as property or equipment losses, or on the environment.

Hazards may be grouped into five general categories: operational failure, organizational failure, human failure, economic failure, and natural failure (Apegga 2006). These groups are not mutually exclusive and are often compounding.

8.5.2   Risk

Risk is universal in technology, and safety has been a central concern of engineering. Risk arises from hazards. It is the chance or probability that a person will be harmed or experience an adverse health effect if exposed to a hazard. Risk relates to the combination of the likelihood of an accident occurring and to the severity of the outcomes of such accidents, where an accident is defined as an unintended event which results in loss. It is a measure of the probability that harm will occur under defined conditions of exposure to an agent (Amyotte and McCutcheon 2006; Renz 2009). There are two aspects to risk, probability and severity. The terms likelihood or frequency are sometimes used instead of probability. A hazard, therefore, is a main source of loss; risk is the chance of actually experiencing a loss of some degree of severity by virtue of coming into contact with a hazard.

$$Risk = Probability \times Damage$$

$$Risk = Probability \times Consequences$$

$$Risk = Hazard \times Vulnerability \times Exposure$$

In professional practice, the main risks may be characterized as occupational safety and health, environment and public health, legal and financial, and societal, depending on who or what is affected. Occupational health and safety risks include the health and safety of all workers present at a worksite and environmental impacts inside the organization property lines. If the consequences extend beyond the property line, there may be risks to the environment (air, surface water, groundwater, soil), quality and/or quantity, and to the public. Professional members and practices have significant legal obligations. Failing to diligently perform their tasks to the required standard of care can result in significant legal, economic, and other risks (Apegga 2006). Professionals including engineers can avoid these risks by knowing and complying with the standards of care as defined by contractual agreements, civil and tort law, and legislation and regulations.

8.5.3   Risk assessment (RA)

Effective collaboration between engineers, health and safety professionals, and workers themselves can lead to more effective risk control (IOSH 2013). RA is specifically valuable for detecting deficiencies in complex technical systems and in improving safety performance. The objectives of the RA process are to achieve a unified outcome from the following three main exercises:

- **Identify risk:** Identify hazards and risk factors that have the potential to cause harm (hazard identification). The risk (or event) identification process precedes RA and yields a comprehensive list of risks.
- **Analyze risk:** There are multiple tools available to help understand the risk components, probability, and consequences with risk analysis and assessment.
- **Assess risk:** Assessing risks consists of assigning values to each risk and opportunity using the defined criteria. The results of the RA process serve as the main input to risk responses whereby response options are examined.

RA may include model building to simplify the analysis. However, professional members must not rely on an over-simplified approach.

8.5.4   Risk management (RM)

RM is basically a closed-loop control process of identifying, analyzing, controlling, and reporting risk. It is a modern concept concerning the way to cope with natural and man-induced disturbances. It refers to coordinated activities to assess, direct, and control the risk posed by hazards to society. Its purpose is to reduce the risk. The management process is a systematic application of management policies, procedures, and practices. RM process is an integrated process, with RA and risk treatment (or mitigation) in constant communication and consultation, and under constant monitoring and review (Lacasse 2016). Figure 8.4 shows the possible options of risk mitigation.

In professional practice, the RM framework outlined in Figure 8.5 can be used to recognize and manage risks. Each step requires certain activities that are conducted in suitable formats. It begins with actively identifying possible hazards leading to the continuing management of the risks deemed to be acceptable. Risk reduction measures involve identifying mitigation strategies meant to reduce the likelihood that a hazard will result in an accident or reducing the severity of the possible accident.

If elimination of hazards is not possible, then the associated risks should be reduced to the lowest acceptable level within the constraints of cost, schedule, and performance by applying the design safety order of precedence as follows (Sojka 2018):

- Eliminate hazards through design selection.
- Reduce risk through design alteration.
- Incorporate engineered features or devices.

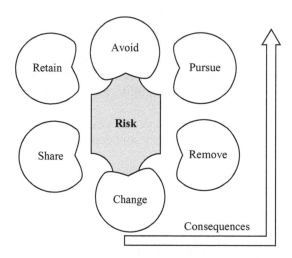

Figure 8.4 Possible options of risk mitigation.

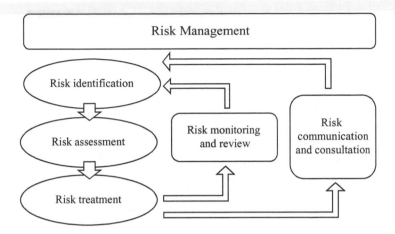

Figure 8.5 General RM framework.

- Provide warning devices.
- Incorporate signage, procedures, training, and personal protective equipment.

RA and RM must be part of every professional member's decisions. Many organizations develop a risk matrix describing what is a low-level risk (acceptable), a medium-level risk (acceptable with certain conditions), and a high-level risk (unacceptable). Such matrices clarify to employees what they must do and what is acceptable. The low-level risks are usually acceptable without any further mitigation. With respect to medium risk, management needs to be actively involved to ensure the risk is kept under control; it is worthwhile noting here that management's responsibilities come to the forefront as managers are assuming responsibility for accepting the risk (Amyotte and McCutcheon 2006; Renz 2009).

RM does not always require a formal and complex analysis. Often RM may be based on simple, common sense approaches. However, the identification of hazards, assessment of risk, RM, and rationale for decisions must be documented.

8.5.5   Risk communication (RC)

RC means the exchange of risk-related knowledge and information among stakeholders. It is an integral part of risk analysis and an inseparable element of the RM framework. RC is a prerequisite for effective RM and RA. It focuses on sharing timely, meaningful, relevant, and accurate information of risks to experts, responders, and the public. The key to RC success is anticipation, preparation, and practice in clear and understandable terms. The need for good RC skills is evident as engineers explain their risk studies not to other engineers but to regulators and the public in order to promote understanding of the process, so as to boost trust and confidence in the safety of the product.

8.5.6   Why RM for engineers?

The history of engineering has left a rich and varied collection of examples of mistakes and catastrophic failures. The challenge therefore is for engineers to learn through their own mistakes and those of others without endangering their own health and safety or that of others (HSE 2009). In general, engineers manage projects that naturally entail risk. Therefore, for a better understanding of health and safety, RM is needed at the conception stage of engineering projects and in all workplaces where problems can potentially be engineered-out (IOSH 2013). An engineer will either be a manager or will work for/with a manager. Also, engineers in management positions have different risk-related responsibilities than the workers they employ. Engineering decisions are increasingly being made on the basis of risk. It is therefore important for engineers to understand the process of RM (Amyotte and McCutcheon 2006). A number of RM models have been developed to describe risk complexity. These include among many, the 5M (Man, Machine, Medium, Mission, and Management) model, expanded by some to include (Method, Material, and Maintenance), and the SHEL (Software, Hardware, Environment, and Liveware) model.

Why RM for engineers? Not only is it the right thing to do, it is the professional thing to practice. Projects, products, and designs must be developed with the primary objective of maintaining the well-being of the public. This does not mean that engineering activities must be conducted with no risk, but it does mean that the risks inherent in these activities must be well-managed (CEAB 2005). Figure 8.6 shows how risk analysis is an integral part of the design process that is fit for product objectives.

8.6   Safe design

> *The minimum we should hope for with any display technology is that it should do no harm.*
>
> **Edward Tufte**
> *[from Envisioning Information (1990)]*

In codes of ethics, the engineer's responsibility for the safety of workers and the public is greatly emphasized. Safety practice starts by considering the possible hazards of the system, including states and conditions that may lead to an accident. It is concerned with ensuring that the system

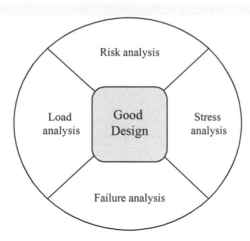

Figure 8.6 Risk analysis as an integral part of good design.

will not cause damage regardless of whether or not it conforms to its specification. Safety practice is devoted to the application of scientific and engineering principles and techniques to the elimination and control of hazards. This requires a great deal about many different engineering aspects, especially in recognition and control of hazards. Safety practice involves the recognition (and sometimes anticipation), evaluation, and control (engineering or administrative) of hazards and risk and management of these activities.

Safety in design means the integration of control measures early in the design process to eliminate or, if this is not reasonably practicable, minimize risks to health and safety throughout the life of the system being designed (Matthews 2015). Quality and safety in design should be fundamental practice concerns, not only because a tenet of the code of ethics is to ensure the well-being of the community, but also because it makes good common sense to develop products, processes, and systems that ensure the profession's continued existence and reputation. Engineers have a professional and legal duty of care to design products, processes, and systems that are as safe as is reasonably practicable (Australian Government 2006).

Safe design is concerned with eliminating hazards at the design stage or controlling risks to health and safety as early as possible in the planning and design of systems and items that comprise a workplace or are used or encountered at work. Safe design is also good practice in that if design flaws can be identified and corrected early in the life cycle, it is much less costly than trying to remedy them later, and essentially a more effective product exists for the entire life cycle (Australian Government 2006). Figure 8.7 shows a typical model for safety in design, while Table 8.3 outlines the key elements that impact achieving a safe design.

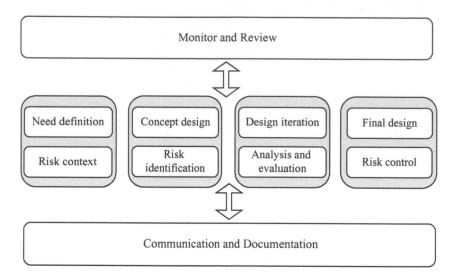

Figure 8.7 Model for safety in design.

Table 8.3 Key elements that impact achieving a safe design

Principle	Summary
Persons with control	Persons who make decisions that affect the design of products, facilities, or processes.
Product life cycle	Safe design applies to every stage in the life cycle from conception to disposal. It involves eliminating hazards or minimizing risks as early in the life cycle as possible.
Systematic risk management	The application of hazard identification, risk assessment, and risk control to achieve safe design.
Safe design knowledge and capability	Knowledge acquired by individuals with control over the design process.
Information transfer	Effective communication and documentation of design and risk control information between all individuals involved in the phases of the life cycle.

8.7   System safety

The safety of the people shall be the highest law.

Marcus Tullius Cicero

System safety is the application of engineering and management principles, criteria, and techniques to achieve acceptable risk within the constraints of operational effectiveness and suitability, time, and cost, throughout all phases of the system life cycle (Sojka 2018). The safety requirements of a system should be distinctly specified. These requirements should be based on an analysis of the possible hazards and risks.

8.7.1 Functional safety (FS)

Engineers use varieties of analytical methods to evaluate design safety, which lead to proper system functioning. FS is that part of overall safety that depends on whether a system or component operates accurately with the input signals that it receives. It is part of the overall safety that depends on the correct functioning of the electrical, electronic, or programmable electronic safety-related systems (SrSs) and other risk reduction measures. A SrS is an element that has the potential to contribute to the violation of or achievement of a safety goal (Sojka 2018), as shown in Figure 8.8.

FS must not be mistaken with electrical safety, which is concerned with protection against short circuit, electric shock, and fires caused by electricity. Examples of FS include an over-speed trip to prevent a grinding wheel from running too fast; fire alarms in a building; or seatbelts in a car. Such SrSs are used to reduce the identified risks to a tolerable level. Therefore, the safety of the whole system depends on the proper function of these systems.

SrSs are designed to implement safety functions in order to achieve or maintain safe states of equipment, systems, or installation in respect to specific hazardous events (Brissaud and Turcinovic 2015). In designing control and protection systems, FS solutions are implemented in various industrial sectors (IEC 2000). However, there are still methodological challenges concerning the FS management in the life cycle. They are related also to issues of human and organizational factors (Kosmowski 2006). The aim of FS management is to reduce the risk associated with operation of hazardous installations to an acceptable or tolerable level, introducing a set of safety functions that are implemented using the programmable control and protection systems (Kosmowski 2011).

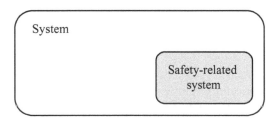

Figure 8.8 The concept of FS.

8.7.2   Safety integrity (SI)

An important term related to the FS concept is the SI, understood as the probability that given SrS will satisfactorily perform required safety functions under all stated conditions within a given period of time (IEC 2000). SI involves levels of protection against systematic failure in the specification of the functions allocated to the SrSs (Sojka 2018).

The SI is an attribute of a SrS with regards to safety functions. It is defined by a probability of a SrS satisfactorily performing specified safety functions. SI level (SIL) is defined as a relative level of risk reduction provided by a safety function, or to specify a target level of risk reduction. It is a measure of the safety risk of a given process. A SIL is based on a number of quantitative factors within qualitative factors, such as development process and safety life cycle management. This is a temporal map, which is important for the application of the standards' content because it establishes the technical framework for dealing in a methodical way with all the actions needed to realize the entailed SI for the safety functions.

The SILs are classes, ranging in SI from SIL 1 (for the lowest integrity level and least dependable) to SIL 4 (for the highest integrity level and most dependable). The higher the SIL level, the better the impact of a failure and the lower the satisfactory failure rate. Precisely, it is correct to say a device is suitable for use within a given SIL environment. For example, an X device is certified as suitable for use in a SIL 3 environment.

8.7.3   Safety requirement specification (SRS)

In general, a SRS is a core document created for two major purposes. First, it directs the design and creation of a safety system depending on the requirements of the workplace using the system. Second, it gives the employees in that workplace a clear idea of the safety potentials with which they are working. The SRS is used as the main reference to be followed by designers, installers, and operators of a FS.

The SRS defines the SrS requirements in terms of safety functions and SI requirements. SRS describes the safety functions and their required FS performances (which includes SI) in non-specific terms to the equipment. Actually, the equipment designers can use the SRS as a basis for selecting the equipment items and architectures. (Brissaud and Turcinovic 2015).

SRSs are associated with two major international standards. The first is the International Organization for Standardization (ISO) 13849, a standard which describes all parts of a FS analysis, including SRS, for the purposes of machine safety. The second is the IEC 61511 (International Electrotechnical Commission), a process FS standard which mandates the creation of SRSs for all safety systems including electrical, electronic, and programmable electronic safety-related systems. The SRS falls into two types: a preliminary conceptual SRS, often called the process safety SRS; and a detailed design SRS, which contains all the detailed design information.

8.7.4   Safety instrumented system (SIS)

A SIS is a system that provides an independent and predetermined emergency shutdown path in case a process runs out of control due to inherent risks and owing to the presence of dangerous material like gases and chemicals. SIS are specifically designed to protect personnel, equipment, and the environment by reducing the likelihood (frequency) or the impact severity of an identified emergency event. Typically, SISs consist of three components: a sensor, a logic solver, and a control system. It is essential that all three elements of the SIS system operate as designed in order to safely separate the process in the event of an emergency.

Safety is usually provided by layers of operation, safety, and protection (Figure 8.9). These layers start with safe and effective process control, extend to manual and automatic prevention layers, and continue with layers to mitigate the impacts of an event. The first layer is the basic process control system, which provides significant safety through proper design of process control. The next layer of protection is also provided by the control system and the system operators. Automated shutdown sequences in the process control system combined with operator intervention to shut down the process are the next layer of safety. The third layer is the SIS.

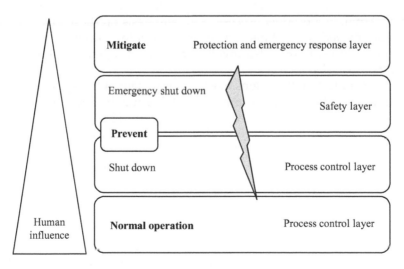

Figure 8.9 Layers of protection in a system safety scenario.

It has sensors, valves, and a logic system. The fourth layer is an active protection layer. This layer may have means to provide a relief point that prevents a break, large spill, or other uncontrolled release that may cause an explosion or fire. If a large safety event occurs, this layer responds in a way that minimizes ongoing damage, injury, or loss of life.

The regulating standards for SISs state that operators must determine and document that equipment is designed, maintained, inspected, tested, and operated in a safe manner. The IEC 61511 standard, for example, requires the user to create a SRS for a SIS that incorporates all the analysis done during the RA process.

8.8 Safety analysis

Rules are parts of systems and systems serve humans not humans serve systems. Unfortunately, safety engineers seem to think that humans serve systems.

Rob Long

Safety analysis techniques are well established and are used extensively during the design of safety-critical systems. In spite of this, most of the techniques are highly subjective and dependent on the skill of the practitioner.

8.8.1 Failure mode and effects analysis (FMEA)

FMEA is a step-by-step approach for identifying all possible failures in a design, a manufacturing or assembly process, or a product or service. FMEA defines the term "failure mode" to identify defects or errors, potential or actual, in a product process, with emphasis on those affecting the customer or end user. "Effects analysis" refers to studying the impacts of those failures. FMEA also involves documenting current knowledge about failure risks.

FMEA reflect malfunctions of each component of the system, including the modes of failure (McCormick 1981). Tracing the effects of each failure reveals their ultimate effects on the system. FMEA is both tedious and time-consuming, so much so that an FMEA analysis on the design of a system is often only completed after a first prototype has been constructed. There have been proposals to apply fuzzy techniques to FMEA (Pelaez and Bowles 1996).

8.8.2 Fault tree analysis (FTA)

FTA is one of the most common techniques used by safety engineers, yet different safety engineers will often produce fault trees for the same system that differ in substantive ways. FTA was introduced by Bell Laboratories in 1962 for the United States Air Force for use with the Minuteman system. It is one of the most widely used methods in system reliability, maintainability, and safety analysis. The main purpose of FTA is to help identify potential causes of system failures before the failures actually occur.

FTA is a technique based on information synthesized from several sources, including informal design models and requirements documents, by which many events that interact to produce other events can be related. FTA follows the concept of Boolean logic, which permits the creation of a series of statements based on True and False events. Events are related to electronic, software, or mechanical components used in the design of the product. The basic symbols used in an FTA logic diagram are called logic gates. The two most commonly used gates are "AND" and "OR" gates and are similar to the symbols used by logic circuit designers. The basic constructs in a FTA diagram are gates and events, where the events have an identical meaning as a block in a logic graph and the gates are the conditions. These relationships permit a methodical building of a structure that represents the system. The output of an AND gate exists only if all the inputs exist. The output of an OR gate exists provided that at least one of the inputs exists. Fault tree construction is even more tedious and time-consuming than FMEA, and computer programs ease the process. Figure 8.10 shows an example of a vehicle headlamp (Marshall 2012). To make a fault tree, the following steps may be followed:

- State the undesired event.
- Determine the event's immediate causes.
- Step back through events until the most basic causes are identified.
- Build a fault tree diagram.
- Evaluate the FTA.

8.9   Safety factor and design margin

> *For safety is not a gadget but a state of mind.*

Eleanor Everet

In engineering, developers add extra strength in order to safeguard against both safety risks and potential engineering changes by keeping a "margin" or "reserve" on key parameters. These safety margins serve to protect individuals and society from the consequences of failure. Safety margins are set to ensure that the product operates reliably under all use conditions, and they cover potential misuse by the customer. The practice of adding margins to a system is called safety factor, which is a ratio between the maximal load not leading to failure and the maximal load for which the construction is intended. SF can be seen as an insurance against design risks.

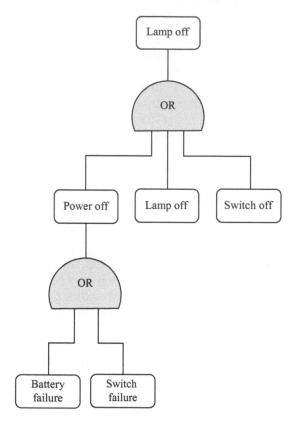

Figure 8.10 An example of a vehicle headlamp.

Safety and the avoidance of risk are key concerns in the design of products and services. Not only the health and well-being of human users and operators are major concerns, but also ensuring that the product or system can operate reliably for its intended life are decisive in the design (Eckerta and Isakssonb 2017). Attempts have been made to replace safety factor by probabilistic calculations. Probabilistic RA is now increasingly used as a tool for dimensioning safety measures. With these methods, safety margins are calibrated to achieve a certain, sufficiently low, calculated probability of failure. Both the SF approach and the probabilistic approach to engineering design employ numerical limits to draw the line between sufficiently safe and too unsafe designs (Vose 2000). These limits are different in nature, but in both cases they are, in practice, determined within the community of safety experts in a process that does not distinguish between RA and RM (Doorn and Hansson 2011).

Safety factors are not the only techniques in safety engineering that take uncertainties into account. The same applies to safety principles such as inherent safety and multiple safety barriers. These principles have in common that they introduce some degree of redundancy in the system, which is often a useful way to protect also against dangers for which probability estimates are not available.

The use of safety factors is a well-established method in the various branches of engineering. Safety factors play a huge role in the certification and licensing of products. They are added to requirements to handle known risks, whereas design margins are added to design parameters to deal with design uncertainties that arise from changes in the requirements. Design margins play a very significant role in responding to engineering change and generating engineering change. They can absorb change so that no action is required, or if they are exceeded, they can multiply the change so that many other components need to be changed in effect (Eckert et al. 2004). Today, companies simulate and test products to see whether they are meeting the requirements that are specified in the requirement documentation. Running simulations regularly to the point of distraction would generate helpful insights to margins at little additional cost (Eckerta and Isakssonb 2017).

Both safety factors and design margins cater against risk of some kind. They are generally kept confidential by companies. If disclosed, they could be misused in trials, hence leading to liability in case of an accident. Usually, these related factors are internally documented for product traceability and play a significant role in the certification and licensing of products.

8.10   Human factors and/or ergonomics

It takes leadership to improve safety.

Jackie Stewart

In general, human factors and ergonomics are two terms for almost the same meaning. The word "ergonomics" comes from the Greek "Ergon", meaning work, and "Nomos", which means law. Therefore, the term has been used historically in the European tradition. On the other hand, the term human factors was more commonly used in North America (Canas et al. 2018). So both terms can now be considered as synonyms and are used interchangeably.

The International Ergonomics Association defines these terms as "the scientific discipline concerned with the understanding of interactions among humans and other elements of a system, and the profession that applies theory, principles, data, and other methods to design in order to optimize human well-being and overall system performance". Briefly, human factors and ergonomics is the study of how humans interact with the objects, interfaces, and spaces around us, and how to design the world around us to increase usability in terms of ease and efficiency (Clawson 2018).

The terms represent a discipline concerned with the development and application of human system interface technology to systems analysis, design, and evaluation. They commonly refer to designing work environments for maximizing safety and efficiency (de Vasconcelos et al. 2009). Ergonomics is the practice of designing products, systems, or processes to take proper account of the interaction between them and the people who use or operate them. It is a scientific, user-centered discipline which plays a major role in design, but it is also a philosophy and a way of thinking. It is used to designate equally a body of knowledge, a process, and a profession.

Biometrics and anthropometrics play a key role in this use of the concept of ergonomics. The importance of ergonomics nowadays is because companies have learned that designing a safe work environment can also result in greater efficiency and productivity (de Vasconcelos et al. 2009).

Safe design also incorporates ergonomics principles. An ergonomic approach ensures that the design process takes into account a wide range of human factors, abilities, and limitations affecting end users. Ergonomics considers the physical and psychological characteristics of people, as well as their needs in doing their tasks – how they see, hear, understand, make decisions, and take action. User safety, efficiency, productivity, and comfort are indicators of how effective the design is in fulfilling its purpose (Australian Government 2006).

As a profession, ergonomics includes a range of scientists and engineers from several disciplines that are concerned with individuals and small groups at work. The field has seen contributions from numerous disciplines, such as psychology, engineering, biomechanics, industrial design, physiology, and anthropometry. In essence, it is the study of designing equipment and devices that fit the human body and its cognitive abilities (OGP 2011) (Figure 8.11).

Once the objective of analysis is defined, Figure 8.12 can be used as an overview of the possibilities of integration of the human factors, the life cycle step of the project (design, implantation, operation, or decommissioning), the target (quality, occupational health and safety, or environmental management), and the focus of analysis (safety, reliability, or risk). These later attributes will be evaluated, taking into account the applicable principles and criteria.

When analyzing the need for a designed product or space, an ergonomic approach will address five main elements, as shown in Table 8.4.

8.11   *Standards in professional practice*

Good design should be honest.

Ferdinand Porsche

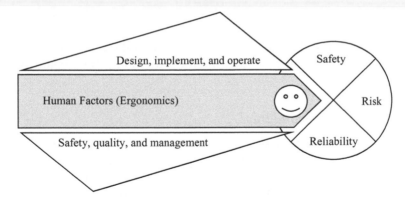

Figure 8.11 Framework for human factors integration.

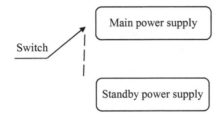

Figure 8.12 Power supply system.

Table 8.4 Ergonomics principles of safe design

Element	Summary
User	Characteristics, including physical, psychological, and behavioral capacities, knowledge, and skills.
Job and task features	Task demands, competence, work organization, and time constraints.
Work environment	Space, lighting, noise, and thermal comfort.
Equipment design and the interface with the user	Hardware required to perform the work, including equipment, protective clothing, furniture, and tools.
Work organization	Variations in workload, timing of work, and the need to communicate and interact with others.

Standards are developed through a set of processes to safeguard the general public. These benefits derive from interoperability between people and organizations that share a common vocabulary, compatible work processes, and the ability to benchmark individuals and organizations (Coallier 2007).

8.11.1   What are standards?

Using the ISO definition as a reference, standards are "guideline documentation that reflects agreements on products, practices, or operations by nationally or internationally recognized industrial, professional, trade associations or governmental bodies". Standards are referred to as guideline documents because they are not compulsory unless mandated by an individual, an organization, or the market. They are agreements because they often reflect a specific level of consensus (Coallier 2007).

Standards are an important part of society, forming the base for the introduction of new technologies and innovation, facilitating business collaboration, empowering industry to conform with appropriate laws and regulations, and serving as rules to measure or estimate size, quantity, content, amount, value, and quality. They are usually developed through an agreement practice. Others set criteria for use and practice in industry and for products and services used in everyday life. Such standards set a level of competence for the characteristics of products and services. It is these standards, above all others, which must be addressed before any engineering design project is implemented and operated.

8.11.2   Why standards?

The basic process of developing and obeying standards aims to ensure proper performance to assure safe operation of systems; to reduce cost by allowing manufacturers use of standard parts; to make sure that the product, system, or process is consistent and repeatable; to simplify maintenance and repair; and to provide for interfacing with other standard-compliant equipment.

Standardization is concerned with the use of common components, products, or processes to satisfy heterogeneous needs. It necessitates designing an overly robust product or the use of a robust process. Tarondeau (1998) argues that standardization results in higher productivity, larger lot sizes, a decrease in the number of reference points to be managed, decrease in the stock level, and the reduction of complexity of a manufacturing system. Relevant standards are consulted early in the design process since it is reasonable to assume many companies will want their products to be accepted in the global market. Standardizing design work also involves defining and implementing best practices for each design environment. Standardizing does not suppress speed or creativity.

The relationship between engineering practice and standards is therefore obvious. Because standards facilitate reuse and, usually, document proven and generally acceptable practices, they are an intimate part of every engineer's professional practice. Standards also constitute a significant part of an engineer's teaching and training curriculum. In software engineering, for example, the relationship with standards goes deeper. While the foundations of software engineering include fields such as computer science, systems engineering, and project management, standards play a significant role in the development and codification of this young engineering discipline (Coallier 2007).

8.11.3 Standardization guidelines

Standards are documents that describe the important features of a product, service, or system. Design standards encapsulate what has become accepted best practice for the design of particular types of product. Almost all the engineering products are prepared by following a series of guidelines including standards, codes, specifications, and technical regulations (Table 8.5). Almost all the engineering products implicitly use components prepared based on these guidelines and/or explicitly designed by

Table 8.5 Brief description of standardization guidelines

Standard	Document approved by a recognized body that provides for common and repeated use, rules, guidelines, or characteristics for products or related processes and production methods, with which compliance is not mandatory. It may also deal exclusively with terminology, symbols, packaging, marking, or labeling requirements as they apply to a product, process, or production method.
Code	Collections of laws, rules, and standards which provide correct procedures to maintain uniformity and safety. Codes are usually set forth and enforced by a local government agency for the protection of public safety, health, etc.
Specification	An explicit set of requirements to be satisfied by a material, design, product, or service. Standards may be referenced or included in specifications.
Technical regulation	Document which lays down product characteristics or their related processes and production methods, including the applicable administrative provisions, with which compliance is mandatory. It may also include terminology, symbols, packaging, marking, or labeling requirements as they apply to a product, process, or production techniques.

considering one or more of the established guidelines. For example, sport diver watch manufacturers design watches explicitly to satisfy ISO 6425 standards. Only after that can they call the watch a diver's watch.

8.11.4   Types of standards

There are three types of documentary standard: formal, informal, and private. Formal standards are published by (Hatto 2010):

- National Standards Bodies (NSB) include the Standards Council of Canada (SCC), the Canadian Standards Association (CSA), the Canadian Commission on Building and Fire Codes (CCBFC), the American National Standards Institute (ANSI), the Deutsches Institut für Normung (DIN), the Association Française de Normalisation (AFNOR), the British Standards Institute (BSI), the Japanese Industrial Standards Committee (JISC), etc. A list of the approximately 160 NSB that are members of ISO, together with links to each of them, is available at www.iso.org/iso/about/iso_members.htm.
- Regional standards bodies: CEN, European Committee for Electrotechnical Standardization (CENELEC), European Telecommunications Standards Institute (ETSI for Europe), Pacific Area Standards Congress (PASC), the Pan American Standards Commission (COPANT), the African Regional Organization for Standardization (ARSO), the Arabic Industrial Development and Mining Organization (AIDMO), and others.
- International standards bodies: ISO, IEEE, IEC, and the International Telecommunication Union (ITU), the International Council on Systems Engineering (INCOSE), the IT Service Management Forum (*it*SMF) International, and the Organization for the Advancement of Structured Information Standards (OASIS).

Informal standards are standards published by the Standards Development Organizations (SDOs), for example, the American Society for Testing and Materials (ASTM), IEEE, the Society of Automotive Engineers (SAE), the virtual desktop infrastructure, and others. Meanwhile, private standards are developed by a company or trade association.

8.12   Knowledge acquisition

Attempting to answer the following questions involves acquisition of knowledge from this book and other books, documents, and the Internet.

- Define the main responsibilities of the following specialties: (a) safety engineer, (b) human factors engineer, (c) fire protection engineer, (d)

risk manager, (e) physician in occupational medicine, (f) industrial hygienist, (g) health physicist.
- Define safety, hazard, control, and risk.
- How should engineering schools teach design?
- How can you achieve safety in engineering and computing?
- How is risk analysis defined?
- What is risk, RA, and RM?
- What are the value and benefits of RM for engineers and computing specialists?
- What unique risk aspects should computing specialists consider?
- Can today's RA techniques measure tomorrow's top risks?
- Why is RM necessary for engineers and computing specialists?
- What does FS mean?
- What is SIL 4?
- What standard(s) do you recommend for the specification, design, installation, operation, and maintenance of SISs?
- What is the main purpose of FTA?
- What are human factors and ergonomics?
- What is the difference between standards and codes?

8.13 Knowledge creation

Collaborate with peers on learning or work with others outside the class to narrow down the objectives of each activity. You may access class and online resources and analyze data and information to create new ideas and balanced solutions. High-level digital tools may be used to develop multimedia presentations, simulations or animations, videos and visual displays, digital portfolios, reflective practice (online publishing and blogging), or well-researched and up-to-date reports.

8.13.1 Handling risk

Which three of the following are approaches to handle risk: avoid the risk; challenge the risk; control the risk; hide the risk; or transfer the risk? After identifying the three right approaches, try to apply them in a real-life case.

8.13.2 Hierarchy of safety standards

The IEC is an international standards organization that prepares and publishes international standards for all electrical, electronic, and related technologies, collectively known as "electrotechnology". For this task, a group of students may investigate safety regulations, norms, and standards related to IEC. An e-Poster may be produced that summarizes at least 10 standards related to various topics in an artistic way. Areas of interest may include automation, medicine, nuclear energy, renewable energy, military, aviation, process industry, etc.

8.13.3 Power supply system with standby unit

Consider the configuration of an electrical supply system with a switch control between a principal and a standby power supply, as shown in Figure 8.12. The switch is originally connected to the main and will instantaneously connect to the standby when the main fails. The system fails if the main and the standby fail; in the second case, the switch fails first, and then the main fails. In the second case, the standby cannot be used because the switch has failed before the failure of the main. Draw the fault tree with "AND" and "OR" gates representing the sequence of the switch failure and then the main failure.

8.13.4 How to become a design entrepreneur

The current role of the engineer designer is changing; more than ever before, designers are becoming more valued for their naturally entrepreneurial mindset. Designers contribute new and alternative ideas to solve problems. For this task, collaborate with peers or work with others outside the class to narrow down the objectives. You may access online resources to create a three-minute video that reflects the above subject and answer the following three questions:

- How does the mindset apply if a designer is working in-house or in an organization?
- Can engineer designers be successful entrepreneurs?
- What stops designers from becoming entrepreneurs?

8.13.5 Write-up of a professional cover letter

Consider a firm that performs engineering design safety and/or RM. Look at the "career" section of the firm website. Find two job descriptions for engineering positions and identify the discipline, background, and skills of the individuals they intend to hire in these positions. Based on the job description, develop a cover letter for an application to the above two jobs.

References

Amyotte, P. R., and D. J. McCutcheon. 2006. Risk administration: Risk management: An area of knowledge for all engineers. Research Committee of the Canadian Council of Professional Engineers, Dalhousie University, Canada.

APEGGA. 2006. Guideline for management of risk in professional practice. The Association of Professional Engineers, Geologists and Geophysicists of Alberta. https://www.apega.ca/assets/PDFs/risk.pdf.

Australian Government. 2006. Safe design for engineering students and educational resource for undergraduate engineering students. Australian Safety and Compensation Council. https://www.safeworkaustralia.gov.au/system/files/documents/1702/safedesignforengineeringstudents_introduction_2006_pdf.pdf.

Brissaud, F., and D. Turcinovic. 2015. Functional safety for safety-related systems: 10 common mistakes. https://hal.archives-ouvertes.fr/hal-01199081/document.

Buchanan, R. 1992. *Wicked Problems in Design Thinking*. Boston, MA: The MIT Press.

Buchanan, R., and V. Margolin. 1995. *Discovering Design, Explorations in Design Studies*. Chicago, IL: The University of Chicago Press.

Cañas, J. J., B. B. Velichkovsky, and B. M. Velichkovsky. 2018. Human factors and ergonomics. https://pdfs.semanticscholar.org/dc92/2c866215ba5610adfa65fb3e48cf26001305.pdf.

CAE. 1999. *Evolution of Engineering Education in Canada*. Ottawa, ON: Canadian Academy of Engineering.

CEAB. 2005. Accreditation criteria and procedures. Canadian Engineering Accreditation Board, Canadian Council of Professional Engineers, Ottawa, ON.

Clawson, K. 2018. What is human factors and ergonomics? https://sites.tufts.edu/kateclawsonenp61/2018/02/02/what-is-human-factors-and-ergonomics/.

Coallier, F. 2007. Standards, agility, and engineering. *IEEE Computer* 40(9): 100–102.

de Vasconcelos, V., E. M. P. da Silva, A. C. L. da Costa, and S. C. dos Reis. 2009. Safety, reliability, risk management and human factors: An integrated engineering approach applied to nuclear facilities. International Nuclear Atlantic Conference – INAC 2009, Rio de Janeiro, RJ, Brazil, Sep 27–Oct 2. https://inis.iaea.org/collection/NCLCollectionStore/_Public/41/064/41064219.pdf.

Doorn, N., and S. O. Hansson. 2011. Should probabilistic design replace safety factors? *Philosophy and Technology* 24(2): 151–168.

Eckert, C., P. J. Clarkson, and W. Zanker. 2004. Change and customization in complex engineering domains. *Research in Engineering Design* 15(1): 1–21.

Eckerta, C., and O. Isakssonb. 2017. Safety margins and design margins: A differentiation between interconnected concepts. *Procedia CIRP* 60: 267–272.

Habash, R. 2017. *Green Engineering: Innovation, Entrepreneurship, and Design*. Boca Raton, FL: CRC Tylor and Francis.

Hatto, P. 2010. Standards and standardization handbook. European Commission. http://www.iec.ch/about/globalreach/academia/pdf/academia_governments/handbook-standardisation_en.pdf.

Horvath, I., and J. S. M. Vregeest. 2000. Engineering design research. International Design Conference-Design, Dubrovnik, Croatia, May 23–26.

HSE. 2009. Integrating risk concepts into undergraduate engineering courses. Health and Safety Laboratory and the University of Liverpool. http://www.hse.gov.uk/research/rrpdf/rr702.pdf.

IEC. 2000. IEC 61508: Functional Safety of Electrical/Electronic/Programmable Electronic Safety-Related Systems, Parts 1–7. International Electrotechnical Commission, Geneva, 2000.

IOSH. 2013. The business case for engineering in health and safety: A paper provided by the Inter Institutional Group on Health and Safety. Inter Institutional Group on Health and Safety Risk Management.

Kosmowski, K. T. 2006. Functional safety concept for hazardous systems and new challenges. *Journal of Loss Prevention in the Process Industries* 19(1): 298–305.

Kosmowski, K. T. 2011. Functional safety analysis including human factors. *International Journal of Performability Engineering* 7(1): 61–76.

Lacasse, S. 2016. Hazard, reliability and risk assessment: Research and practice for increased safety. Proceedings of the 17th Nordic Geotechnical Meeting Challenges in Nordic Geotechnic, Reykjavik, May 25–28.

Marshall, J. 2012. An introduction to fault tree analysis (FTA). The University of Warwick. http://s3.spanglefish.com/s/22631/documents/safety-documents/fta-an-intro.pdf.

Matthews, B. 2015. Safety in design. GCG Health Safety Hygiene. https://www.airah.org.au/Content_Files/DivisionMeetingPresentations/QLD/21–07-15-AIRAH-Qld-Brad-Matthews.pdf.

McCormick, N. M. 1981. *Reliability and Risk Analysis: Methods and Nuclear Power Applications*. San Diego, CA: Academic Press.

OEERE. 2000. From invention to innovation. Office of Energy Efficiency and Renewable Energy, US Department of Energy.

OGP. 2011. Human factors engineering in projects. International Association of Oil and Gas Producers, Report 454.

Pelaez, C. E., and J. B. Bowles. 1996. Using fuzzy cognitive maps as a system model for failure modes and effects analysis. *Information Sciences* 88(1–4): 177–199.

Renz, S. 2009. Influence of dynamic soil-structure interaction analyses on shear buildings. PhD Dissertation, Braunschweig University. http://rzbl04.biblio.etc.tu-bs.de:8080/docportal/servlets/MCRFileNodeServlet/DocPortal_derivate_00014948/Renzi_Dissertation.pdf.

Reymen, I. M. M. J. 2001. Improving design processes through structured reflection: A domain-independent approach. PhD Thesis, University of Technology, Eindhoven, the Netherlands.

Sojka, M. 2018. Introduction to safety engineering. Czech Technical University in Prague, Faculty of Electrical Engineering, Department of Control Engineering. https://support.dce.felk.cvut.cz/psr/prednasky/safety/safety-intro.pdf.

Tarondeau, J. C. 1998. *Stratégie Industrielle*. Second Edition. Collection Gestion, Vuibert.

Vose, D. 2000. *Risk Analysis*. Second Edition. New York, NY: Wiley.

module nine

Design for sustainability practice

9.1 Knowledge and understanding

Having successfully completed this module, you should be able to demonstrate knowledge and understanding of:

- Sustainability and quality movement overlaps
- Movement from a typical design approach into a sustainable engineering design approach
- The triple bottom line approach and its 3Ps and 3Es processes
- The green engineering practice and its 3Rs process
- The 12 principles of green engineering to incorporate elements of design for sustainability throughout all phases of project development
- Design for sustainability as an eco-design practice
- The Hannover Principles as a platform upon which designers can consider how to adapt their work toward sustainable ends
- Life cycle engineering as a discipline that focuses on a systematic approach to design an entire life cycle of a product
- Life cycle-based sustainability assessment and its four phases
- Eco-efficiency versus eco-effectiveness and life cycle sustainability assessment
- Cradle-to-cradle design framework
- Sustainability as an ethical principle in professional practices

9.2 Sustainable engineering design (SED)

> Quality is always sustainable.

Thomas Sandell

Quality, in the sense perceived in the quotation above, is not just meant as the technical quality of a product but also the less tangible desirability of the product, the pleasure of use of the product, as well as the attachment of a user to the product.

Sustainability, like quality, is a mega-trend for corporations for which adoption moved from defense to offensive tactics. The sustainability movement (Figure 9.1), like the quality movement, will follow four stages:

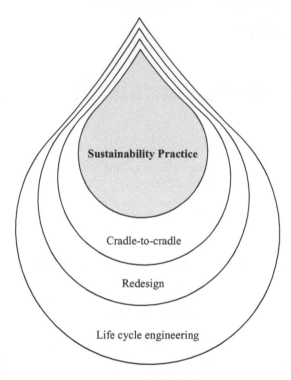

Figure 9.1 Main attributes of sustainability.

cost and risk reduction, redesigned products and processes, revenue growth strategies, and differentiated value propositions that provide sustained competitive advantage (Bair 2010).

The sustainability concept is both very ancient and relatively modern. It has been a design concept throughout history, although many consider it a contemporary movement. Design for sustainability (DfS) frameworks and tools provides important insights for thinking about the outcomes or analytical processes of designing sustainably (BSR 2008).

Sustainable means "capable of being sustained", which links to the capacity of durability, stability, permanence, or even eternalness. It means meeting needs without compromising the ability of future generations to meet their needs. It involves the interactions and relationships among environmental, social, and economic parameters.

Designers can stimulate desirability, increase pleasure, and deepen attachment by designing products that not only function better, are more aesthetically pleasing than comparable products, but are also tailored to better suit the individual needs of the user. Govers and Mugge (2004) argue that if an object is highly desirable, its longevity is extended and its negative impact on the environment is therefore reduced.

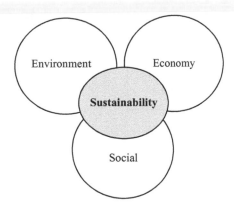

Figure 9.2 Three overlapping goals of sustainability.

Sustainability is a current design topic of both interest and concern. It is often thought of as composed of three overlapping, mutually dependent goals, as shown in Figure 9.2. It is clear from the current understanding that sustainability is a system property and not a property of individual elements of systems. Therefore, achieving sustainability requires a process-based, multi-scale, and overlapping systemic approach to planning for sustainability guided by a target/vision instead of traditional goal-based optimization approaches (Bagheri and Hjorth 2007).

Design is increasingly being viewed as a critical enabling component for sustainability because the design function is a concentration point for decisions about a large set of human and material resource flows (BSR 2008). Moving from a typical linear system of design to a closing loop system of sustainability is a growing idea in the world of sustainable design and manufacturing. Closing the loop means moving from traditional design, which looks at the linear model for design and production (make, use, and dispose), to how the disposal stage can be fed back into the creation of a new product (Smith 2012). To move towards a sustainable practice, the design process needs to be modified in order for engineers to effectively challenge the related issues. By reviewing the conventional design process and SED, Figure 9.3 identifies the differences between both approaches and shows how typical design can be shifted into sustainable design.

9.3   Triple bottom line (TBL)

> *The conventional design criteria is tripod: ecology, equity, and economy*
>
> **William McDonough**

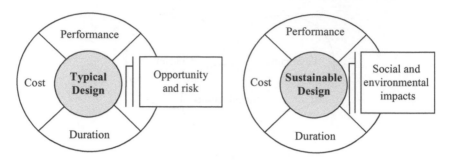

Figure 9.3 Shift from typical design into sustainable design.

TBL is a framework that incorporates three dimensions of performance: social, environmental, and financial. The key idea is that human society is only sustainable if it can be sustained in all the above dimensions. This view is incorporated into the TBL approach, where companies account not just for financial benefits but also for benefits and impacts in the social and environmental spheres (Elkington 2004).

In the late 1990s, John Elkington, the founder of a British consultancy called SustainAbility (Elkington 1997, 2004), coined the phrase TBL as a method for measuring sustainability. His argument was that companies should be preparing three different (and quite separate) bottom lines. One is the traditional measure of corporate profit, the "bottom line" of the profit and loss account. The second is the bottom line of a company's "people account", a measure in some shape or form of how socially responsible an organization has been throughout its operations. The third is the bottom line of the company's "planet" account, a measure of how environmentally responsible it has been (Onyali 2014), as shown in Figure 9.4. These elements are often called the "3Ps" of the TBL concept. "People" means employees within and outside corporations; the company pays fair wages and takes steps to ensure humane working conditions and work environment. "Planet" covers the impact on the environment to reduce its ecological footprint as much as possible. "Profit" means economic impact of products and services. Sustainable organizations recognize that profit is not entirely opposed to people or planet. The 3Ps do not have a common unit of measure.

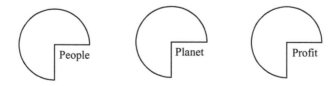

Figure 9.4 The 3Ps approach.

In Elkington's view, the ecological, economic, and social factors had to be brought into a direct and balanced relationship to each other to achieve sustainable development. The ecological measure of TBL refers to engaging in practices that do not compromise the environmental resources for future generations (Alhaddi 2015). The economic measure of the TBL framework refers to the impact of the organization's business practices on the economic system. It includes the organization's financial performance, the flow of capital, and their economic involvement in society. The social measure of TBL refers to conducting beneficial and fair business practices with the labor, human capital, and in the community (Elkington 1997). Measuring performance against these measures is a complicated task. Shareholder value, market share, and customer satisfaction are relatively easy to quantify, and measures developed by one organization are readily transferable to others, but social and environment performance are almost certainly unique to each organization, or at least each industry, and they are often very difficult to quantify (Hubbard 2009).

Inspired by Elkington's 3Ps approach, Braungart and McDonough (2002) introduced the strategy of the TBL, better known as Economy, Ecology, and Equity (3Es), as outlined in Figure 9.5. "Economy" means economic impact of products and services. "Ecology" involves the environment in which we live in. "Equity" is related to people, animals, and plants.

Both approaches bring ecological, economic, and social factors into a direct and balanced interrelationship. An important difference between the two approaches is in the concepts of people and equity. The 3Es strategy is not only about people, but about equality of people, animals, and plants.

9.4   Green engineering (GE) practice

> The best things in life aren't things.

> **Art Buchwald**

Although engineering is not directly one of the three components of sustainability, it is indirectly linked to each. Given the intimate ties between engineering and the key components of SD, it is evident that the attainment of sustainability in engineering is a critical aspect of achieving SD (Rosen 2012).

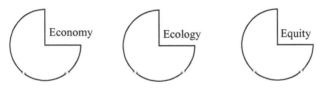

Figure 9.5 The 3Es approach.

9.4.1 The three Rs of GE practice

GE, an approach to product development that balances environmental compatibility with economic profitability, is fast becoming a necessary business practice. Several factors are pushing companies toward GE: environmental legislation, rising waste-disposal costs, and (to a lesser degree) corporate image and public perception (Hedberg 1996). From design to disposal, GE is finding ways to extend a product's life cycle through the "3R" processes: Reuse, Remanufacturing, and Recycling, as shown in Figure 9.6.

Reuse means using a functional component from a retired product. It means additional use of a component, part, or product after it has been removed from a clearly defined service cycle. It is applied to a product that has been used previously. The product will retain the problems it acquired during its previous life, as it will not have been repaired (Gray and Charter 2006). Reused products usually have no warranty of any kind.

Remanufacturing means bringing a product to "like-new" condition through replacing components and re-conditioning. It may be understood as the refurbishment or upgrading of the product or of recoverable components. The remanufacturing process involves returning a used product to its original specifications or even better through inspection, disassembly, cleaning, reprocessing, reassembly, and testing (Habash 2017).

Recycling is the process of collecting and processing materials that would otherwise be thrown away as trash. Recycling returns a product to raw material form, which can be used as raw material for a future manufacturing process. It is generally applied to consumable goods such as newspapers, glass bottles, and aluminum cans but can also be applied to durable goods such as engines (Gray and Charter 2006). Recycling involves the separation and collection of materials for processing and remanufacturing into new products, and the use of the products to complete the cycle (Barker and Andrew 2007).

9.4.2 The 12 principles of GE

The 12 principles of GE have been developed by Anastas and Zimmerman (2003) to provide a framework for engineers to implement when designing

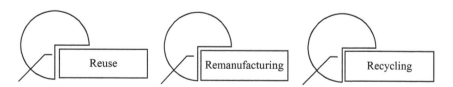

Figure 9.6 The 3Rs of GE.

new materials, products, processes, and systems. These principles have been developed with broad statements so they can be applied over a wide variety of engineering and science fields; the purpose of this paper is to illustrate how they can be applied to the water and wastewater industry. Table 9.1 shows the principles as a toolbox that can be used systematically to optimize a system or its components. This approach builds on the technical excellence, scientific rigor, and systems thinking that have addressed the issue of science and technology for sustainability in recent years (McDonough and Braungart 2003; Anastas and Zimmerman 2003; Gagnon et al. 2008).

A design based on the 12 principles of GE moves beyond baseline engineering quality and safety specifications to consider sustainability factors and allow designers to consider them as fundamental factors at the earliest stages as they are designing a material, product, process, building, or system. These principles provide an outline to guide engineers into considering suitability though all stages of design. They encourage the redefinition of the task to consider the full life cycle, inputs, and outputs.

9.5   Design for sustainability (DfS)

Be the change you wish to see in the world.

Mahatma Gandhi

DfS is an eco-design concept that has evolved to include both the social and economic elements of production. It has evolved from general cleaner production methods to focus on products and to reduce risks to humans and the environment (Clark et al. 2009).

9.5.1   The Hannover Principles

The Hannover Principles aim to provide a platform upon which designers can consider how to adapt their work toward sustainable ends. Designers include all those who change the environment with the inspiration of human creativity. Design implies the conception and realization of human needs and desires.

The Hannover Principles are a set of maxims that encourage the design professions to take sustainability into consideration. They are descriptive of a way of thinking, not prescriptions or requirements. The guidelines shown in Figure 9.7 demonstrate the German City of Hannover's intention to apply these principles as elements of the overall design competitions associated with EXPO 2000, where the City of Hannover has been designated as the site of the world exposition in the year 2000. In order to ensure that the design and construction related to the fair will represent SD for the city, region, and world, the City of Hannover has commissioned "the

Table 9.1 The 12 principles of GE

Principle 1	Designers need to strive to ensure that all material and energy inputs and outputs are as inherently nonhazardous as possible in terms of toxicity, minimal energy, and material inputs to complete the process.
Principle 2	It is better to prevent waste than to treat or clean up waste after it is formed. This principle steers the focus of design towards using materials and processes that generate minimal waste, thereby removing costs and risks associated with wastes that would otherwise have to be processed, treated, and disposed of.
Principle 3	Separation and purification operations should be designed to minimize energy consumption and materials use. Designing products and/or processes for self-separation can decrease waste, save costs, and reduce processing times.
Principle 4	Products, processes, and systems should be designed to maximize mass, energy, space, and time efficiency. Principle 4 guides the designer to consider the overall efficiency of the system over its lifetime, thus achieving sustainability whilst still providing a financial incentive.
Principle 5	Products, processes, and systems should be "output pulled" rather than "input pushed" through the use of energy and materials. Approaching design using this principle requires the designer to minimize the amount of resources consumed to transform inputs into the desired outputs.
Principle 6	Embedded entropy and complexity must be viewed as an investment when making design choices on recycling, reusing, or beneficial disposition. Recycling components that have high complexity in many cases come at a loss of value, where materials of minimal complexity are more favorable for recycling.
Principle 7	Targeted durability, not immortality, should be a design goal. Products that last beyond their useful life can often be the cause of environmental problems in disposal due to their persistence and bioaccumulation. By designing products/processes that withstand the typical operating conditions but still possess a targeted lifetime, such issues can be avoided.
Principle 8	Design for unnecessary capacity or capability solutions should be considered a design flaw. Over-designing processes or products to have significant flexibility and the ability to meet worst-case scenarios can often result in high costs in terms of capital and operation. Processing and plants should target the specific demands of the user, not only minimizing waste and cost.
Principle 9	Material diversity in multicomponent products should be minimized to promote disassembly and value retention. Less material diversity means more options for recyclability and reuse.

(Continued)

Table 9.1 (Continued) The 12 principles of GE

Principle 10	Design of products, processes, and systems must include integration and interconnectivity with available energy and materials flows. This means to use local materials and energy resources as close to the source as possible to minimize efficiencies and consumption associated with transport.
Principle 11	Products, processes, and systems should be designed for performance in a commercial "afterlife". This means designing such that their components can be reused or reconfigured to maintain their value and usability for new products.
Principle 12	Material and energy inputs should be renewable rather than depleting. The use of materials from a finite source has significant environmental effects due to its inability to be cycled back to the source for resources. Renewable materials by their nature can be recycled to replenish the source and provide a virtually infinite service with minimum waste.

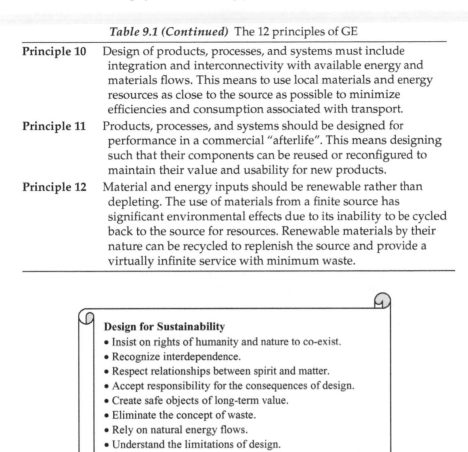

Design for Sustainability
- Insist on rights of humanity and nature to co-exist.
- Recognize interdependence.
- Respect relationships between spirit and matter.
- Accept responsibility for the consequences of design.
- Create safe objects of long-term value.
- Eliminate the concept of waste.
- Rely on natural energy flows.
- Understand the limitations of design.
- Seek constant improvement by the sharing of knowledge.

Earth   Air   Fire   Water   Spirit

Figure 9.7 The Hannover Principles, 1992, based on the enduring five elements.

Hannover Principles" to inform the international design competitions for EXPO 2000. They took the form of a framework, based on the enduring elements of Earth, Air, Fire, Water, and Spirit, in which design decisions may be reviewed and evaluated. The guidelines offer critical instruction on the responsibility of designers (McDonough and Partners 1992). The principles are to be considered by designers, planners, government officials, and all involved in setting priorities for the built environment.

Most of the environmental impacts of products throughout their life cycle are determined at the design phase. Thus concepts and methods, such as design for recycling (DfR), design for environment (DfE), or DfS in general, have come to the fore. Their aim is to reduce material and energy consumption and waste throughout the product life cycle (PLC) (Medini et al. 2015).

The challenges for DfS are to generate knowledge supporting the innovation and design engineering of products and service systems with superior sustainability and to make optimal use of networking and entrepreneurship as success factors for implementation (Clark et al. 2009). The key DfS approaches are: redesign, benchmarking (incremental design), new product design, product service system, and product innovation.

9.5.2   DfS redesign

Redesign is defined as the action of successive changes or improvements to a previously implemented design. An existing design is modified to meet the required changes in the original requirements. The goal of redesign is to sustainably redesign an existing product for which the specific market and manufacturing conditions are already known, taking into account its primary function and the associated services provided. A product's improvement potential can be determined relatively as the product already exists, so d manufacturing and market information is available.

It is important to realize that redesign for sustainability could again mean going back to the roots of a specific problem in design and then finding an improved solution, for example, practicing radical design strategy. In addition, redesign was recommended to be started by practicing radical design (Jarvenpaa and Stoddard 1998).

The redesign process uses a project team to harness expertise to incorporate sustainability aspects into products, but also company employees who can often provide valuable insight. When choosing an initial product for redesign, companies should focus on the interventions that have the potential for the greatest impact while being simple and timely to implement, and in line with overall company goals. The finished, redesigned product should be compared against the initial product to consider and estimate the sustainability advantages of the new product versus the original; after the product is launched, the company must do a follow-up to evaluate overall sustainability, which will spawn new implementation ideas for future products (Crul and Diehl 2006; Clark et al. 2009).

9.5.3   Benchmarking

A thoroughly connected approach, DfS benchmarking, promotes learning from competitors' efforts and experiences to improve a company's own products, and is especially suitable for companies that develop products by emulating existing products. The methodology for benchmarking is closely connected to redesign (Crul and Diehl 2006).

Benchmarking and other approaches based on replication are still the predominant way in which products are designed worldwide. DfS benchmarking is a structured approach to compare the environmental performance of a company's products against competitors' products and to generate improvement options. The goal of DfS benchmarking is to learn from the best practice of competitors by comparing one's product to those of competitors to determine how to make that product more sustainable. The methodology is a structured approach in which improvement options are generated by looking at the environmental, social, and economic aspects of a particular product. Benchmarking differs from DfS redesign in that it starts with comparing existing products in the market before moving into the design phase. Like redesign, DfS benchmarking also uses a project team to decide the goals for the process, including, but not limited to, entering new markets, improving competitiveness, and making environmental improvements (Crul and Diehl 2006; Clark et al. 2009).

Since individual competitors often use different solutions to resolve the same design problems, like a different product architecture, components, or technology, DfS benchmarking offers a reflective approach and advises learning from others' products.

9.5.4 New product design

The DfS new product development approach applies "out-of-the-box", or radical, innovation strategies, which can lead to more sustainable impacts while providing the breakthroughs necessary to ensure an company's continued competitiveness. New product development involves a higher level of technical, market, and organizational uncertainty than redesign but can be an inventive and iterative process where new ideas on how to meet needs are converted to products and services. Eco-friendly materials, SD practices, and innovative ICT are all concepts that can help inspire new product design (Clark et al. 2009).

The stages and processes involved with new product design can be viewed as three-fold: policy formulation, idea generation, and product development. Policy formulation addresses the company's goals and strategies; idea generation allows the company to brainstorm and develop ideas for new products, taking into account the ability to harness developing technologies, materials, and consumer needs; and finally, product development involves debating and testing concepts against the decisions in the idea finding phase. The key challenge with respect to new product design is market demand. Without consumer need, even the most sustainable product will fail (Crul and Diehl 2006; Clark et al. 2009).

New product development comprises a higher level of technical, market, and organizational uncertainty than redesign but can be an inventive and iterative process where new ideas on how to meet needs are converted to products and services (Crul and Diehl 2006). The process sets out the typical sequence of phases that new products typically go through, starting with ideation and concept initiation, and concluding with launching the product.

9.6 Life cycle engineering (LCE)

We never know the worth of water till the well is dry.

Thomas Fuller

LCE is an approach that analyzes the potential ecological, economic, technical, and social impacts of products, processes, and services throughout an entire life cycle (Fraunhofer IBP 2014). One of the major characteristics of the LCE approach is its close affiliation to the principles of sustainability as they were defined by the Brundlandt commission in 1987. LCE as an approach analyzes the potential ecological, economic, technical, and social impacts of products, processes, and services throughout an entire life cycle. It is an engineering activity that includes the application of technological and scientific principles to manufacture products with the goal of protecting the environment, conserving resources, encouraging economic progress, and keeping in mind social concerns while optimizing the PLC and minimizing pollution and waste (Jeswiet and Szekeres 2014). It focuses on a systematic approach to design an entire life cycle of a product in order to avoid unwarranted iterations in the following stages of the development path.

The LCE methodology presents the results clearly, guaranteeing maximum transparency along with a solid basis for decision-makers (Fraunhofer IBP 2014). Several methods, such as life cycle assesment (LCA), life cycle costing (LCC), and eco-design are applied in order to analyze the data and make decisions during the upstream and downstream of the product development. LCE is an iterative process for continuous improvement of the sustainable performance of the product, process, system, and the facility involved during the PLC. It is also a process to develop specifications to meet a set of performance, cost, and environmental requirements and goals that span the product, system, process, or facility life cycle. It presents the results clearly, guaranteeing maximum transparency along with a solid basis for decision-makers. The life cycle embodies material and energy use and waste throughout four conceptual stages, as shown in Figure 9.8.

Material production includes material acquisition and processing. Material acquisition includes activities related to the acquisition of natural resources. This includes mining non-renewable material and harvesting biomass. Manufacturing and construction involve the creation of

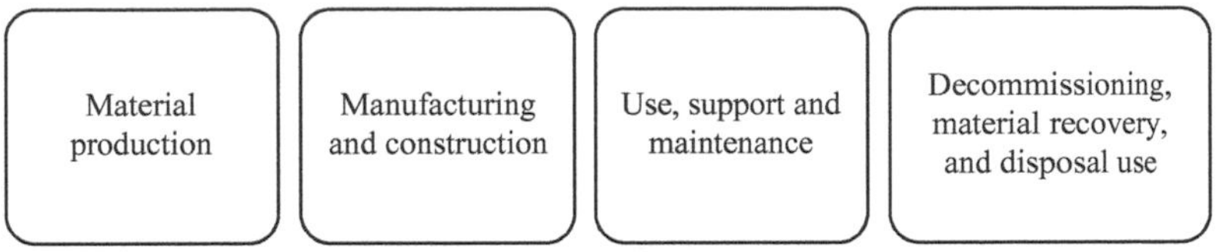

| Material production | Manufacturing and construction | Use, support and maintenance | Decommissioning, material recovery, and disposal use |

Figure 9.8 The four conceptual stages of LCE.

parts and their assembly into products. Products, systems, processes, and facilities are used, maintained, and repaired. Retirement and disposal of products, systems, processes, and facilities includes decommissioning; disassembly; the recovery of usable components, materials, and energy; and the treatment and disposal of residual materials (Cooper and Vigon 2001). To map the ecological, economic, technical, and social impact of a product, process, or service, LCE combines an array of methods that will be discussed in the following sections.

9.7 Life cycle-based sustainability assessment approaches

> *A society is defined not only by what it creates but also by what it refuses to destroy.*

John Sawhill

Numerous assessment methods and tools for environmental and sustainability performance have been developed along the past several years. They are grouped in Figure 9.9 according to an adapted pyramid of needs (Maslow 1943). While the original Maslow pyramid has the basic physiological needs at the bottom, followed by safety needs, love and belonging, through esteem to self-actualization at the very top, the adapted version starts with the basic approach of life cycle thinking (LCT), followed by single-issue methods like carbon or water footprinting, LCA, resource or eco-efficiency assessment, up to life cycle sustainability assessment (LCSA) at the top of the pyramid.

9.7.1 Life cycle thinking (LCT)

The main objective of LCT is to reduce a product's resource use and emissions into the environment as well as to improve its socio-economic performance throughout its life cycle. LCT is also a highly opportunity-driven thinking mode, because this approach can help identify important business opportunities by reducing resource consumption and improving the performance of products (Brazdauskas 2015).

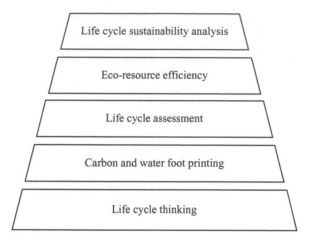

Figure 9.9 Adaptation of Maslow's pyramid of human needs.

LCT is a qualitative concept that represents the basic concept of considering the whole PLC from "the cradle to the grave". It aims to prevent individual parts of the life cycle from being addressed in a way that just results in the environmental burden being shifted to another part (EC 2015). Product LCT is essential in the path to sustainability by expanding the focus from the production site to the whole PLC. This facilitates the links between the economic and environmental dimensions within a company. LCT is about widening views and expands the traditional focus on manufacturing processes to incorporate various aspects associated with a product over its entire life cycle. The producer becomes responsible for the products from cradle to grave and has, for instance, to develop products which have improved performance in all phases of the PLC (Jensen and Remmen 2006). The approach aims at incorporating LCT in products, working with the market by the use of incentives, involving stakeholders, using a variety of policies in order to cover most sectors and stakeholders, as well as aiming at the continuous improvement on the environmental impact of products.

9.7.2   Carbon footprint (CF) and water footprint (WF)

The CF concept has become popular over the past few years and is currently widely accepted and used by the public and media despite its lack of scientifically accepted and universally adopted guidelines: it describes greenhouse gas (GHG) emission measurements from the narrowest to the widest sense. Several calculation methods and approaches for CF accounting have been proposed and are being used. Since about 2008, WF has also become a popular term.

With the next level in the pyramid, the approaches start to be quantitative. More recently, evaluation approaches for single environmental issues like CF (Berger and Finkbeiner 2010) and WF (Finkbeiner et al. 2006) have received considerable attention. The WF and CF concepts have similarities; however, their roots and intended purposes differ. CF was formulated to quantify the contribution of various activities to climate change. Concern about climate change started with the scientific recognition of the relationship between CO_2 emissions and global warming. Despite its popularity and use in commerce, there is no universally accepted definition of CF. Today it describes the narrowest to the widest interpretation of GHG emission measurement (East 2008; Finkbeiner 2009).

The WF concept is primarily rooted in the desire to illustrate the hidden links between human consumption and water use and between global trade and water resources management (Hoekstra 2008). Unlike CF, which emerged in practice, WF was born in science. WF started to gain broad interest from about 2008, the year in which the WF network was established, a network of academic institutions, governments, nongovernmental organizations, companies, investors, and UN institutions. One of the aims of the network is to ensure the establishment of one common language and a coherent and scientifically sound framework for WF assessment that serves different interests.

9.7.3   Life cycle assessment (LCA)

LCA is one of the most important techniques for the implementation of a process or product development in the framework of sustainability. It is an analytical tool designed to quantify the ecological impacts or sustainability performance of a system. It is a tool designed to account for all of the inputs and outputs of a system.

LCA is a decision-making tool that is built around the principle of comprehensiveness and therefore aims to address all environmental interventions, not just one. It is a well-established environmental management tool for which international standards are available in their second generation (Finkbeiner et al. 2010). LCA is a tool that includes extraction, processing, and quantifying materials and energy use, manufacturing, distribution, recycling, and final disposal. It is a complex environmental assessment tool that requires enormous amounts of data, which are often hard to find or expensive to purchase. There are a few variants of LCA, namely cradle-to-grave, cradle-to-gate, cradle-to-cradle (C2C), or gate-to-gate (Zimoch 2012).

The most widely used theory of the LCA analysis is an approach described in International Standards ISO 14040 that assumes four phases of the LCA: goal and scope definition, inventory analysis, impact assessment, and interpretation (Zimoch 2012). The first phase is goal and scope definition, where goals, system boundaries, and intended uses are established.

The second step is called a LCI analysis. This is a data-based quantification of energy and raw material requirements, air emissions, waterborne effluents, solid waste, and other environmental releases through the life of a product or process. In this phase, the goal is to examine all the inputs and outputs in a PLC, beginning with what the product is made of, the source of the materials, the operations involved in making those materials, where they go, and all of the inputs and outputs related to those component materials during their lifetime. The third phase is life cycle impact assessment (LCIA) to evaluate the effects of the environmental information collected in the inventory. A full impact assessment addresses ecological and human health, as well as the range of social, cultural, and economic effects. The fourth phase is interpretation, including identification of important issues arising from the LCI and LCIA phases, evaluation of completeness, sensitivity and consistency, and conclusions, limitations, and recommendations. Figure 9.10 shows the four phases of the LCA.

To carry out an LCA for a product, five stages of a PLC are analyzed (Skrainka 2012):

- Pre-manufacturing: performed by suppliers who extract in most cases virgin materials employed for manufacture
- Manufacturing: processes related to the transformation of the virgin materials into usable products
- Product delivery: the transport of the product to the customer
- Use: the intensity and frequency of the use of the product
- Disposal: a product that is no longer needed could be reused or remanufactured to use it once again, recycled or incinerated if materials permit, or landfilled

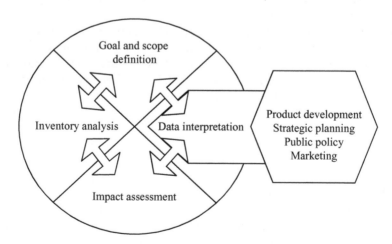

Figure 9.10 The four main phases of LCA.

Several software tools are available to analyze LCA. For example, SimaPro is a LCA software tool used to analyze the environmental impacts of products following ISO 14040 guidelines. SimaPro allows the quantification of the burden carried at each stage of a PLC. SimaPro is a convenient tool because it makes a complex analysis, such as an LCA, into a more straightforward analysis.

9.7.4   Eco-efficiency versus eco-effectiveness

Eco-efficiency is an important solution that leads to a more sustainable environment; it is only a partial solution. It starts with the assumption of a one-way, linear flow of materials through industrial systems: raw materials are extracted from the environment, transformed into products, and eventually disposed of. However, eco-efficient techniques seek total solutions by minimizing the volume, velocity, and toxicity of the material flow system. The relation of eco-efficiency and eco-effectiveness is an important goal in sustainable design, as the relation between short-term strategy and long-term strategy are important in every product development project. Both eco-efficiency and eco-effectiveness are identified as important indicators in SD (Habash 2017).

In contrast to the eco-efficiency approach of minimization and dematerialization, the concept of eco-effectiveness proposes the transformation of products and their related material flows such that they create a supportive relationship with ecological systems and future economic growth. The objective is not to minimize the cradle-to-grave flow of materials, but to generate cyclical, C2C breakdown that allow materials to maintain their status as resources and gather intelligence over time (upcycling).

9.7.5   LCSA

Andersson et al. (1998) examined the feasibility of incorporating the concept of sustainability principles into each phase of LCA. Four socio-ecological principles were identified:

- Substances from the lithosphere must not systematically accumulate in the ecosphere (i.e. the use of fossil fuels and mining must be radically decreased).
- Society-produced substances must not systematically accumulate in the ecosphere.
- The physical conditions for production and diversity within the ecosphere must not systematically deteriorate.
- The use of resources must be efficient and must meet human needs.

Kloepffer (2008) developed the LCSA framework into the following conceptual formula, which was improved into its current form:

$$LCSA = LCA + LCC + SLCA$$

LCA represents the state of the art in science and applications relating to the environmental dimension of sustainability. LCC is the total costs of a system or product, produced over a defined lifetime. The social LCA (SLCA) dimension of sustainability captures the impact of an organization, product, or process on society. The social benefits can be estimated by analyzing the effects of the organization on stakeholders at local, national, and global levels (GRI 2002). This is based on the well-known depiction of sustainability, where the three dimensions of environment, economy, and society intersect, as depicted in Figure 9.11.

The majority of social indicators measure the degree to which societal values and goals in the particular areas of life or politics can be achieved. However, many social issues on which a performance measurement takes place are not easy to quantify. Therefore, a number of social indicators contain qualitative standards of systems and activities of the organization, including operating principles, procedures, and management practices. These indicators address needs specific to social issues, such as forced labor, working hours, or the existence of trade unions (Finkbeiner et al. 2010).

9.8   Cradle-to-cradle (C2C) design framework

Cradle to Cradle is like good gardening; it is not about "saving" the planet but about learning to thrive on it.

Michael Braungart

"Cradle-to-cradle" is a phrase invented by Walter R. Stahel in the 1970s and popularized by William McDonough and Michael Braungart in their

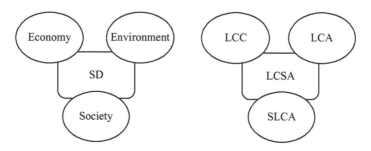

Figure 9.11 Domains of sustainability and LCSA.

2002 book of the same name. In the book *Cradle to Cradle: Remaking the Way We Make Things*, the authors present a "C2C'" approach in which biological and technical cycles are closed without damaging effects on the environment. In August 2010 an exclusive, worldwide license was granted to the C2C Product Innovation Institute as a third-party not-for-profit organization to manage the certification program.

C2C is a biomimetic approach to the design of products and systems. It is a valuable design approach integrating multiple attributes: safe materials, continuous reclamation and reuse of materials, clean water, renewable energy, and social fairness. This framework seeks to create production techniques that are not just efficient but are essentially waste-free. C2C is a science- and values-based vision of sustainability successfully applied over the past decade that articulates a positive, long-term goal for engineers. C2C is a helpful design approach integrating numerous attributes, including safe materials, continuous reclamation and reuse of materials, clean water, renewable energy, and social fairness. C2C designs industrial systems to be commercially productive, socially beneficial, and ecologically smart. It is also a revolutionary approach to the redesign of human industry based on the conviction that thoughtful design, mirroring the safe, regenerative productivity of nature, can create an industry that is sustaining, not just sustainable.

The C2C framework suggests a new way of designing human systems to eliminate conflicts between economic growth and environmental health resulting from poor design and market structure. In addition, the C2C design framework embraces the pursuit of maximum value (economic, ecological, and social) through the practice of intelligent design. It is the foundation of an emerging world in which all human industry is designed to celebrate interdependence with other living systems, transforming the making and consumption of things into a regenerative force.

C2C is model of industrial systems in which material flows cyclically in appropriate, continuous biological or technical nutrient cycles. All waste materials are productively re-incorporated into new production and use phases, for example, "waste equals food". In this approach, waste materials are turned into "nutrients" for a following cycle. To achieve this, the C2C approach uses the principles shown in Figure 9.12.

Waste virtually does not exist in nature because each organism's processes contribute to the health of the whole ecosystem. The closed-cycle biological system of C2C has for millions of years led to a flourishing planet with a varied abundance of food. Every being on the planet has formed part of it, and it provided good conditions for growth. Resources are extracted from the earth's crust and concentrated, changed, and synthesized, leading ultimately to unlimited amounts of waste. This process means that valuable resources are lost (Cohen 2007).

- **Principle 1:** Waste is food (everything is a nutrient for something else).
- **Principle 2:** Use the sun (use renewable energy only).
- **Principle 3:** Enjoy diversity (species, cultural and innovative diversity).

Figure 9.12 Principles of C2C.

9.9   *Ethical context of sustainability*

What seeds are you planting?

Lailah Gifty Akita

Unlike the concept of ethics, which has about a 2,000-year history of usage, sustainability as a powerful, yet abstract, concept entered the public dictionary relatively recently (Horn 2013). Sustainability, on the other hand, cannot be understood or achieved without careful attention to its ethical dimensions (Kibert et al. 2012). Ethical sustainability involves new knowledge needed to understand the complex interactions between society and nature. It is an ethic of diversity in which there is interplay among the ethos of diverse cultures. Addressing this challenge is the topic of this textbook, and it is a theme which this module elaborates with perspectives provided by philosophical traditions of ethical thinking.

9.9.1   *Sustainability as an ethical principle in practices*

Basically, sustainability is a guide to practice as well as ethical and moral principles; the question arises as to how this principle can be concretized and contextualized with respect to ethical reflection and decision-making. Another question arises as to which dimensions stand for the principle of sustainability and SD in professional engineering and/or computing practice.

    The practice of engineering and/or computing continues to evolve over time through a process of constant improvement. This includes not only the technological aspects but the human aspects as well. In practice, professionals use their expertise and experience to develop strategies and tactics to deliver solutions to their clients (WFEO 2013). This places a potential burden on them to consider not only narrow problems and the immediate solutions as may be requested but also whether there are implications for other stakeholders that must be considered within a wider context, including the environmental, economic, and social.

    The social dimension of sustainability should be understood as both the processes that generate social health and well-being now and in the future, and those social institutions that facilitate environmental and economic sustainability now and for the future (Dillard et al. 2008). Environmental ethics, a sub-discipline of ethics as a whole, focuses on human thought and behavior in relation to nature, nonhuman animals, plants, ecosystems, air and water quality, and so on. The social impact is an integral part of the environmental impact. Since its emergence in the 1970s, environmental ethics has been helpful in shifting the conversation about ethics toward a more inclusive understanding of human relationships to and values regarding others. However, in many ways the conversation about the human relationship to nature is as old as our species: how should we behave in relation to other creatures, the land, and our places, and what is our vision for the goodness of the whole? How do we best care for others and represent them in our decision-making, including the soils, waters, and creatures from whom we derive our physical sustenance, psychological wellbeing, and spiritual fulfillment?

Economic ethics is concerned with the moral grounds, characteristics, and consequences of economic activities and institutions. Economic ethics may look at specific business practices or industries, or at broader issues such as the moral values, implicit or explicit, that undergird economic policies and practices. When considering the ethical dimensions of economic systems, institutions, and decisions, a number of significant questions related to sustainability must be taken into account. One question concerns the definition of economic goals such as productivity, efficiency, and security.

In addition to the benefits that must be passed on to future generations, risky consequences must not be passed on. Many of the today's technologies are likely to pose warning threats to future generations, such as genetic engineering, nanotechnology, chemicals, antibiotics, pesticides, nuclear reactors and their fuel cycles, and others. Consequently, if sustainability suggests a responsibility to the well-being of future generations, how we deal with technology development and application must be an issue of great concern.

To conclude, ethical policies, which have been developed over time for certain situations, provide engineers and computing professionals with a structured approach for applying sustainability as an ethical principle reliably and to reach conclusions derived from ethical considerations which are applicable to those situations. To reinforce that, supporting procedures are necessary.

9.9.2   Sustainability in codes of ethics

The obligation of social responsibility is embraced in the codes of ethics of professional engineering societies. For example, the first canon of the ASCE states, "Engineers shall hold paramount the safety, health and welfare of the public and shall strive to comply with the principles of SD in the performance of their professional duties". The statement in this canon does not manifest the scope for social sustainability of engineering projects. The concept of sustainability in the codes of engineering ethics, for example Rule Four in the code of ethics of the Institution of Civil Engineers (ICE), UK, refers to the sustainability of the environment. However, the ASCE definition of sustainability embraces some factors of social sustainability, such as natural resources, energy, food, shelter, transportation, and waste management, essential for social sustainability (Moonasingha 2018).

The World Federation of Engineering Organizations (WFEO) presents a model code of practice and its interpretive guide that explains the link between ethics and professional practice by considering engineering in the wider context of SD and environmental stewardship. SD is development that meets the social, economic, and environmental needs of the present without compromising the ability of future generations to meet their needs. However, environmental stewardship is the prudent use of the finite resources in nature to produce the greatest benefit while maintaining a healthy environment for the foreseeable future (WFEO 2013).

9.10   Knowledge acquisition

Attempting to answer the following questions involves acquisition of knowledge from this book and other books, documents, and the Internet.

- When and where is sustainability practice important?
- What does it mean for an engineering design to be sustainable and of high quality?
- Should engineers be committed to, engaged in, and lead sustainability practices?
- What are the tools needed for the design of sustainable engineered systems?
- Who uses the TBL?
- What is SD? What are the key requirements for SD?
- What is design for sustainability, and why should we do it?
- What does it mean to design sustained technology that becomes part of a user's life and not a disruption from it?
- What are the objectives and focal areas of design for sustainability benchmarks?
- Why is life cycle costing important to a utility?
- Describe the difference between recycling and reuse.
- What are the principles of the cradle-to-cradle approach?
- What is eco-efficiency?
- What is life cycle assessment? What is its purpose?

- What are the principles of the cradle-to-cradle approach?
- Explain what is meant by life cycle considerations in the design of engineering applications.
- What is design in the context of remanufacture?
- How do we incorporate sustainable principles and concepts into engineering design?
- What are the social benefits of sustainable design? What defines a socially sustainable product?

9.11   Knowledge creation

Collaborate with peers on learning or work with others outside the class to narrow down the objectives of each activity. You may access class and online resources and analyze data and information to create new ideas and balanced solutions. High-level digital tools may be used to develop multimedia presentations, simulations or animations, videos and visual displays, digital portfolios, reflective practice (online publishing and blogging), or well-researched and up-to-date reports.

9.11.1   Dimensions of sustainability

Consider the overlapping of environmental, economic, and social sustainability aspects so that it is possible to measure sustainability as a wide phenomenon. In an e-Poster, make three boxes, as shown below in Figure 9.13, and itemize the variables of each aspect of sustainability into 12 related items. These 36 items should be based on SD strategies from different aspects.

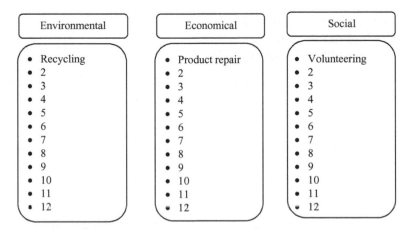

Figure 9.13 Proposed arrangement for sustainability dimensions.

9.11.2 Electronic waste

Consumer electronics have become an integral part of daily life and have revolutionized the way we communicate, retrieve information, and view entertainment. As a result, electronic waste (e-waste), which is defined as any piece of electronic equipment which has reached the end of its useful life, has become the fastest growing component of the solid waste stream worldwide. This life fact requires effective solutions.

Question: Is remanufacturing of consumer electronics consistent with the goals of sustainable design?

In this empirical research proposal, investigate the electronics industry, examining the implications of domestic e-waste and considering the economic, environmental, and societal aspects of consumer electronics production, use, reuse, and remanufacturing. The research on economic and societal aspects is largely literature-based. The research on environmental aspects is largely LCA-based, drawing from direct observation of consumer electronics production and remanufacturing activities as well as the literature. Apply sustainable design tools at an early design concept stage so that eco-design is integrated in the outcome. Design outcomes should be assessed for observance to the "Ten Golden Rules of Eco-Design" (Luttropp and Lagerstedt 2006).

9.11.3 Water system

Apply brainstorming to develop an idea and/or solution for an innovative product or system for the human need that is inspired by imitating nature (design to model nature: biomimicry.org) to help better manage the water issue. The idea can be applicable or specific to a region or climate. The design must either:

- Obtain water from the environment;
- Produce usable water; or
- Promote efficient water use.

Water accessibility projects are the focus of several organizations, such as the alliance for water stewardship (www.allianceforwaterstewardship. org), and competitions, such as the NAE's Grand Challenges (www.engin eeringchallenges.org/cms/8996/9142.aspx). The project idea reflects the notion of how nature inspires innovative solutions to water management issues.

9.11.4 The 12 Principles of GE

Read the 12 principles of GE given in Table 8.1. Create 12 logos and arrange them in a poster format that correspond to the 12 principles, and arrange them in a table format.

9.11.5   Green buildings and LEED system

In 1993 the U.S. Green Building Council (USGBC) was established to promote sustainability in the building and construction industry (USGBC 2014). Once the USGBC was formed, discussions with over 60 firms and non-profit organizations surrounding a sustainable construction industry began and ultimately led to the development of a new green building rating system. In 2000, the Leadership in Energy and Environmental Design (LEED) program was created by the USGBC to precipitate change in the construction industry by providing guidance on how to implement green building practices within the framework of a green rating system (Vanry 2015).

LEED has quickly become the industry standard for green buildings. Today, LEED buildings can be found in many countries and states. There are currently over tens of thousands of LEED-accredited professionals trained in this rating system and thousands of buildings on their way to certification. This represents a good percent of the new construction market, and this number is growing quickly.

The LEED system works by dividing the building into five categories: sustainable sites; water conservation; energy and atmosphere; materials and resources; and indoor environmental quality. LEED lists opportunities for a building to earn points in each. The final number of points determines the green level of the building, rated as Certified, Silver, Gold, or Platinum (Rabin 2005).

For this task, first investigate green buildings and the related five categories. Second outline the LEED accreditation procedure, including a foundational credential for professionals. This includes exam format, study material, credential maintenance, etc. You may present the outcomes of your investigation to the class in the form of an oral presentation, e-Poster, or a video.

References

Alhaddi, H. 2015. Triple bottom line and sustainability: A literature review. *Business and Management Studies* 1(2): 6–10.

Anastas, P. T., and J. B. Zimmerman. 2003. Design through the 12 principles of green engineering. *Environmental Science and Technology* 37(5): 94A–101A.

Andersson, K., M. H. Eide, M. Lundqvist, and B. Mattsson. 1998. The feasibility of including sustainability in LCA for product development. *Journal of Clean Production* 6(3–4): 289–298.

Bagheri, A., and P. Hjorth. 2007. Planning for sustainable development: A paradigm shift towards a process-based approach. *Sustainable Development* 15(2): 83–96.

Bair, P. 2010. Where the quality and sustainability movements converge. https://www.greenbiz.com/blog/2010/07/06/where-quality-and-sustainability-movements-converge.

Barker, S., and K. Andrew. 2007. Organising reuse: Managing the process of design for remanufacture (DFR). Department of Mechanical Engineering, University of Bristol, UK, Paper No. 007-0769. http://citeseerx.ist.psu.edu/v iewdoc/download?doi=10.1.1.454.1651&rep=rep1&type=pdf.

Berger, M., and M. Finkbeiner. 2010. Water footprinting: How to address water use in life cycle assessment. *Sustainability* 2: 919–944.

Braungart, M., and W. McDonough. 2002. *Cradle to Cradle: Remaking the Way We Make Things*. New York, NY: North Point Press.

Brazdauskas, M. 2015. Promoting student innovation-driven thinking and creative problem solving for sustainability and corporate social responsibility. *Journal of Creativity and Business* 1: 75–87.

BSR. 2008. Aligned for sustainable design: An A-B-C-D approach to making better products. https://www.bsr.org/reports/BSR_Sustainable_Design_Repo rt_0508.pdf.

Clark, G., J. Kosoris, L. N. Hong, and M. Crul. 2009. Design for sustainability: Current trends in sustainable product design and development. *Sustainability* 1: 409–424.

Cohen, D. 2007. Earth's natural wealth: An audit. *New Scientist* 2605: 35–41.

Cooper, J. S., and B. Vigon. 2001. Life cycle engineering guidelines. National Risk Management Research Laboratory Office of Research and Development, U.S. Environmental Protection Agency. http://infohouse.p2ric.org/ref/12/1 1932.pdf.

Crul, M., and J. Diehl. 2006. *Design for Sustainability: A Practical Approach for Developing Economics*. Paris, France: UNEP and TU Delft.

Dillard, J., V. Dujon, and M. King. 2008. *Understanding the Social Dimension of Sustainability*. New York, NY: Routledge Taylor and Francis Group.

EC. 2015. The circular economy: Connecting, creating and conserving value. European Commission. http://www.eesc.europa.eu/resources/docs/the-circular-economy.pdf.

East, A. J. 2008. What is a carbon footprint? An overview of definitions and methodologies. Vegetable industry carbon footprint scoping study: Discussion Paper 1. Sydney, NSW: Horticulture Australia Ltd.

Elkington, J. 1997. *Cannibals with Forks: The TBL of the 21st Century Business*. Oxford, UK: Capstone Publishers.

Elkington, J. 2004. Chapter 1: Enter the triple bottom line. *The Triple Bottom Line: Does It All Add Up*. pp. 1–16. http://www.johnelkington.com/archive/TBL elkington-chapter.pdf.

Finkbeiner, M. 2009. Carbon footprinting: Opportunities and threats. *The International Journal of Life Cycle Assessment* 14(2): 91–94.

Finkbeiner, M., A. Inaba, R. B. H. Tan, K. Christiansen, and H. J. Kluppel. 2006. The new international standards for life cycle assessment: ISO 14040 and ISO 14044. *The International Journal of Life Cycle Assessment* 11: 80–85.

Finkbeiner, M., E. M. Schau, A. Lehmann, and M. Traverso. 2010. Towards life cycle sustainability assessment. *Sustainability* 2: 3309–3322.

Fraunhofer IBP. 2014. Life cycle engineering. Fraunhofer Institute for Building Physics. Institute Stuttgart, Stuttgart, Germany. https://www.ibp.fraunhofe r.de/content/dam/ibp/en/documents/Areas-of-Expertise/Lifecycle-en gineering/IBP%20Abteilungsbrosch%C3%BCre_uk_neu.pdf.

Gagnon, B., R. Leduc, and L. Savard. 2008. From a conventional to a sustainable engineering design process: Different shades of sustainability. Working paper. Groupe de Recherche en Economie et Developpement International, University of Sherbrooke, Sherbrooke, QC.

Govers, P. C. M., and R. Mugge. 2004. I love my jeep, because it's tough like me: The effect of product-personality congruence on product attachment. International Conference on Design and Emotion, Ankara, Turkey.

Gray, C., and M. Charter. 2006. Remanufacturing and product design: Designing for the 7th generation. The Centre for Sustainable Design University College for the Creative Arts, Farnham, UK. http://cfsd.org.uk/Remanufacturing% 20and%20Product%20Design.pdf.

GRI. 2002. *Sustainability Reporting Guidelines*. Boston, MA: Global Reporting Initiative.

Habash, R. 2017. *Green Engineering: Innovation, Entrepreneurship, and Design*. Boca Raton, FL: CRC Taylor and Francis.

Hedberg, S. R. 1996. Green engineers: AI pioneers cutting a trail. *IEEE Intelligent systems* 11(3): 4–6.

Hoekstra, A. Y. 2008. Water neutral: Reducing and offsetting the impacts of water footprints. Value of Water Research Report Series No. 28. Delft, the Netherlands, UNESCO-IHE.

Horn, G. V. 2013. Ethics and sustainability: A primer with suggested readings. https://iseethics.files.wordpress.com/2013/09/ethics_and_sustainability_ primer.pdf.

Hubbard, G. 2009. Measuring organizational performance: Beyond the triple bottom line. *Business Strategy and the Environment* 18(3): 177–191.

Jarvenpaa, S. L., and D. B. Stoddard. 1998. Business process redesign: Radical and evolutionary change. *Journal of Business Research* 41(1): 15–27.

Jensen, A. A., and A. Remmen (eds.). 2006. *Background Report for a UNEP Guide to Life Cycle Management – A Bridge to Sustainable Products*. United Nations Environment Programme (UNEP). Paris, France: Life Cycle Initiative.

Jeswiet, J., and A. Szekeres. 2014. Definitions of critical nomenclature in environmental discussion. In Lien, T. K. (ed.). Proceedings of the 21st CIRP Conference on Life Cycle Engineering, Trondheim, pp. 14–18.

Kibert, C. J., L. Thiele, A. Peterson, and M. Monroe. 2012. The ethics of sustainability. http://rio20.net/wp-content/uploads/2012/01/Ethics-of-Sustainabil ity-Textbook.pdf.

Kloepffer, W. 2008. Life cycle sustainability assessment of products (with comments by Helias A. Udo de Haes, p. 95). *International Journal of Life Cycle Assessment* 13: 89–95.

Luttropp, C., and J. Lagerstedt. 2006. EcoDesign and the ten golden rules: Generic advice for merging environmental aspects into product development. *Journal of Cleaner Production* 14: 1396–1408.

Maslow, A. H. 1943. A theory of human motivation. *Psychology Review* 50: 370–396.

McDonough, W., and M. Braungart. 2003. Towards a sustaining architecture for the 21st century: The promise of cradle-to-cradle design. *Industry and Environment* 26(2): 13–16.

McDonough, W., and Partners. 1992. The Hannover principles. Design for sustainability. EXPO 2000. The World's Fair, Hannover, Germany.

Medini, K., J. Le Duigou, C. Da Cunha, and A. Bernard. 2015. Investigating mass customization and sustainability compatibilities. *International Journal of Engineering, Science and Technology* 7(1): 11–20.

Moonasingha, A. D. 2018. Ethics, engineering, and social sustainability. https://moonasingha.yolasite.com/anand_civil-engineering_ethics.php.

Onyali, C. I. 2014. Triple bottom line accounting and sustainable corporate performance. *Research Journal of Finance and Accounting* 5(8): 195–209.

Rabin, E. 2005. Ask the green architect: Top ten green building questions. https://www.greenbiz.com/blog/2005/09/15/ask-green-architect-top-ten-green-building-questions.

Rosen, M. A. 2012. Engineering sustainability: A technical approach to sustainability. *Sustainability* 4: 2270–2292.

Skrainka, M. S. 2012. Analysis of the environmental impact on remanufacturing wind turbines. MSc Thesis, Rochester Institute of Technology, Rochester, NY.

Smith, T. 2012. Closing the loop: Designing for a sustainable future. http://www.climatechangenews.com/2012/02/28/closing-the-loop-designing-for-asustainable-future/.

USGBC. 2014. United States green building council. http://www.usgbc.org/about/history.

Vanry, J. 2015. A case study assessment of the energy consumption of LEED certified academic buildings in Ontario: Is LEED certification necessarily better? MSc Thesis, Waterloo University, Ontario, Canada.

WFEO. 2013. Model code of practice for sustainable development and environmental stewardship. World Federation of Engineering Organizations. http://www.wfeo.org/wp-content/uploads/code-of-practice/WFEOModelCodePractice_SusDevEnvStewardship_Interpretive_Guide_Publication_Draft_en_oct_2013.pdf.

Zimoch, E. 2012. Life-cycle assessment (LCA) of existing bridges and other structures. http://citeseerx.ist.psu.edu/viewdoc/download?.

part four

---

*Contemporary issues in
management, AI, and
career development*

module ten

Project management practice

10.1 Knowledge and understanding

Having successfully completed this module, you should be able to demonstrate knowledge and understanding of:

- The project and its domains, scope, and constraints
- Management as practice and practice management
- Key project management phases
- Project manager, project team, and project portfolio management
- Quality management practice, principles, and processes
- Risk management practice and related processes
- Key drivers of change management practice, challenges, and related tools
- Major project management models to guide design life cycle including waterfall, concurrent engineering, and V-cycle
- Systems thinking as a foundation for understanding interpreting relationships within complex systems
- Project management practices like Lean and Agile to achieve business goals; management methodologies like Scrum, Kanban, and XP; and tools like sprints, boards, and tests
- Lean and green project management, Lean manufacturing, and Lean product development
- Agile project management and Scrum methodology

10.2 Project

There is nothing permanent except change.

Heraclitus

Management, with reference to Heraclitus in the quotation above; is not just about the process of completing activities but also about how to manage ongoing needs. Change is not the same as movement. However, it is evolutionary, with a new structure, strategy, teamwork, procedure, organization, motivation, improvement, and measurement (Figure 10.1).

The word "project" seems to be in popular use all around the world whether it is a work-related effort or a personal endeavor (Niemi 2015). A project is a sequence of unique, complex, and connected activities that

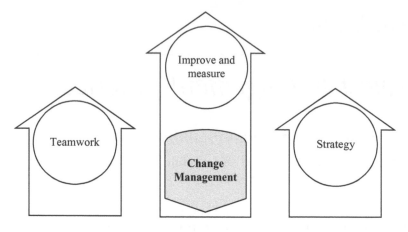

Figure 10.1 Project as a cycle of changes.

must be completed within a specific timeframe and budget to accomplish an ultimate objective. As shown in Figure 10.2, a typical project follows a set of processes.

According to Turner (2007), "a project is an endeavor in which human, financial and material resources are organized in a novel way to undertake a unique scope of work, of given specification, within constraints of cost and time, so as to achieve beneficial change defined by quantitative and qualitative objectives".

"Project" is perceived to be a means through which modern societies achieve social and economic ends to generate new values (Winch 2010). It is a set of unique tasks that need to be completed in order to reach a specific outcome. The temporary nature of projects implies that a project has a specific beginning and end. Projects can range from simple to large and can be managed by one person or by many. They may have social, economic, and environmental impacts that far endure the projects themselves.

A project is identified by a scope which classifies items and activities that are required to meet the project goals and objectives. A project's

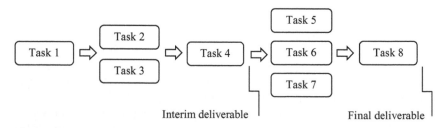

Figure 10.2 A typical project process.

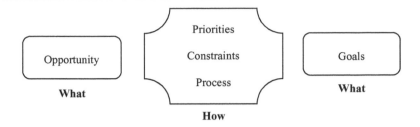

Figure 10.3 The project scope.

scope involves the specific goals, deliverables, and tasks that define the boundaries of the project. Examples of deliverables are plans, schedules, milestones, completion times, design details, specifications, drawings, and expenses (Oberlender 2000). Figure 10.3 outlines a typical project scope.

Projects are limited by their product quality, time, cost, and process quality requirements as shown in Figure 10.4. Project constraints are anything that restricts or dictates the actions of the project team. The three most significant project constraints – scope, goal, and cost – are sometimes known as the triple constraint or the project triangle. Project constraints are usually thought to be somewhat mutually exclusive.

Project activities can either take short or long amounts of time to complete. Completion of tasks depends on a number of factors, such as number of people working on the project, their experience, and their skills. It is also imperative to have an estimated cost when undertaking a project. Finally, quality is not a part of the triangle, but it is the eventual objective of every delivery. Scope consists of all deliverables. All the above constraints are tradeoffs. If the budget is constrained, the project may be low-quality. If time is constrained, the project will face risks of goal accomplishment.

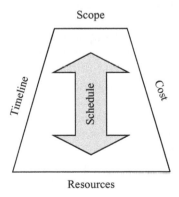

Figure 10.4 Project constraints.

10.3   Management

Practice Golden-Rule 1 of management in everything you do. Manage others the way you would like to be managed.

Brian Tracy

Management is a universal discipline and a widely-used term. It is a distinct act and/or a social process of getting people together to achieve desired goals and objectives by the use of human beings and other resources efficiently and effectively.

10.3.1   Functions of management

The essence of management is to achieve a goal as professionally and effectively as possible. Management is effective when targets are achieved, and it is efficient when these targets are not only being achieved but achieved with minimum resources at its disposal. Therefore, management entails the acquisition of managerial competence and efficiency in problem-solving, administration, human resources, and leadership.

Henri Fayol, a French engineer, was the first to attempt to classify managerial activities into specific functions. He established the first principles of the classical management theory at the start of the last century. Fayol is considered the founding father of concepts such as the line and staff organization (Anastasia 2017). Fayol also defined the five core functions of management, which are still used, and which form the basis of many of the later theories. These functions were organized later by Koontz and O'Donnell (1976) as planning, organizing, staffing, leading, and controlling.

Planning involves selecting missions and objectives and the actions to achieve them. This function is about creating a detailed plan towards achieving a specific organizational objective. The focus is about achieving objectives but requires knowledge of the organization's objectives and vision.

Organizing involves establishing an intentional structure of roles for people to fill in an organization. It is about employing the plan to bring together the physical, financial, and other available resources and to use them to achieve the organizational goal.

Staffing involves filling the positions in the organization structure. The focus is on people and their labor in relation to the organizational objectives. The function aims to ensure the organization always has the right people in the right positions.

Leading means influencing people so that they contribute to goals; it has to do with the interpersonal aspect of managing. It is about the actuation of methods to work efficiently to achieve set organizational objectives. This function involves ensuring that employees are able to perform tasks through a variety of means. Leading in essence is looking after productivity.

Controlling is the most important function, which means the risk-reduction ability. It involves measuring performance through feedback and adjustment processes to ensure that events conform to established plans and standards. Control is a critical determinant of organizational success since it focuses on results. It is one important aspect of management to ensure that things are done in an orderly fashion. This order entails the development of bureaucracy that derives its importance from the need for strategic planning, coordination, and controlling of large and complex decision-making processes.

10.3.2 Management practice

Management, like all other practices including medicine, engineering, nursing, accountancy, and others, is an art; it is know-how. Rigby (2001) considers management practices to be a set of concepts, processes, and exercises. It is doing things in light of the realities of a situation.

The development of management has gone through six phases, for example classical, humanistic, systems, contingency, post-modernistic, and scientific values phases (Mullins 2013). In line with the aims of this module, the focus is on the use of management practices, which are recognized as an important driver of competitiveness and performance. Therefore, scientific value would matter, when managers can work better by using the organized knowledge about management. It is this knowledge that constitutes science. However, the science underlying management can certainly improve managerial practice. Managers who attempt to manage without management science must put their trust to luck, intuition, or past experience (Fleet and Peterson 1994). Management science is increasingly focusing on the impact of ICT on performance. ICT usage infuses virtually every sector of modern economies, and for decades the world IT industry has been undergoing considerable growth with especially enhanced levels of ICT diffusion.

In managing, as in any other field, unless practitioners learn by trial and error, there are no places they can turn for guidance other than the accumulated knowledge underlying their practices. Today, there is a huge spread of management practices across firms worldwide. However, for practical purposes all managers must develop three general sets of skills, namely: conceptual, technical, and human. Conceptual skills allow the manager to develop relationships between factors that other people may not see (Olum 2004). For a manager to be technical, it implies ICT knowledge and professionalism. Also, managers should be able to see members of the organization as human beings who have needs and emotions to be positively harnessed for the advancement of the organization.

10.3.3   Practice management

Practice management encompasses multiple topics including governance, finance, medical, architecture, engineering and computing, transcription, marketing, etc. Its main objectives are to maintain high standards of technical competence and professionalism; ensure a consistency of performance; acquire skills and knowledge as required; and conduct its practice in accordance with the code of ethics.

Practice management for engineering and computing businesses comprises using data, tools, and systems to develop business decisions, allocate resources, rationalize revenue and costs, and to enhance growth and efficiency across the business. Effective practice management enables firms to achieve business objectives and meet the needs of customers while maintaining control and visibility of business trajectory. As with individual projects, the main goals of the practice are to deliver projects on time, to budget, and to meet or exceed client expectations.

The crucial goals of the practice should be determined by the head and could focus on sustainable projects, innovative designs, and growing and taking on increasingly large projects. These goals establish the practice forward strategy. Figure 10.5 shows the key elements of practice management to help operate related business more effectively and profitably. Job costing is about understanding that behind every project is a series of transactions representing the business model that encapsulates the business. Forecasting ultimately helps firms see what income could come in alongside the resources. Resource planning ultimately helps firms reduce empty time and maximize utilization and efficiency. Investing in technology is an effective way to attract and keep efficient people (Synergy 2018). Good communication with clients makes a strong professional

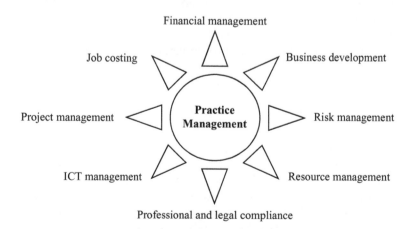

Figure 10.5 Key elements of practice management.

relationship. Also, practices need a clear focus on the work they are capable of and want to do. More importantly, they must understand the work that they are equipped to do. They need to decline any work outside their experience, knowledge, and capability.

Practice management is the powerhouse that forms the foundation of the organization. It is about taking responsibility for operation processes including document policy, authentication, client information and relationship, and IPs. Also, practice management requires complying with regulatory codes and standards as applicable.

10.4   Project management (PM)

*Trying to manage a project without project management
is like trying to play a football game without a game plan.*

K. Tate

The PMI defines PM as "the application of knowledge, skills, tools, and techniques to meet project requirements". PM may also be defined as the discipline of planning, organizing, motivating, and controlling resources to achieve specific goals.

10.4.1   Phases of PM

The main challenge of PM is to achieve all project goals and objectives while honoring scope, time, quality, and cost (Newton 2015). A key factor of successful PM is to see the project as a series of interrelated tasks. From the perspective of PM, any series of activities that go through the project cycle are projects. The project cycle consists of project phases. An organization should already have a well-defined strategy from which it can begin to assess relevant needs and opportunities in its field (Nebiu 1990). The PM process can be divided into several phases (Figure 10.6):

- **Initiation phase:** To define a new project idea or a new phase of an existing project to pinpoint what issue the project is actually supposed to resolve and to obtain an authorization or approval (if needed) to begin the project.
- **Planning phase:** To establish the project scope and goal; to improve the objectives and define the course of action required to achieve the

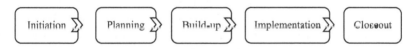

Figure 10.6 Phases of PM.

project objectives; and to define fundamentals – identify problems that require solving and what can be achieved.

- **Build-up phase:** To complete the work defined in the PM plan to fulfill the project requirements. This phase includes assembling the team, planning assignments, creating schedules, and developing the budget.
- **Implementation phase including monitoring and controlling:** To track, review, and control the progress of the project tactics and logistics; to recognize any areas in which changes to the project plan are required and initiate those changes; and to manage problems.
- **Closeout phase:** To wrap outcomes, review, and evaluate all activities across the entire process.

Each of the above phases contains critical decision points including functions like "proceed, cancel, revise, scope, goal, cost, schedule, quality".

10.4.2   Project manager

A project manager is the person accountable for performing the five basic functions of management: planning, organizing, staffing, directing, and controlling. Therefore, understanding the mission and vision of the organization is a priority. The project manager needs to acquire a solid understanding of business cases and risk management processes, strong leadership skills, communication and negotiation skills, and the ability to monitor and control a budget. The task of the project manager typically involves ensuring progress of the project according to defined metrics, identifying and monitoring risks, ensuring progress toward deliverables within time and resource constraints, running coordination meetings, and other related activities.

Since the project manager's job is mostly about dealing with people, it is important to exercise leadership as well as management skills. The significant skills a project manager needs are people skills, therefore exercising leadership is essential, since the project manager has no absolute authority to ensure a quality project within time, budget, and scope constraints, as outlined in Figure 10.7. Based on management skills, the project manager must achieve the end results despite all the risks and problems that are encountered. Success depends on carrying out the required tasks in a logical sequence, utilizing the available resources to the best advantage (Oberlender 2000).

The project manager acquires and manages required human and other resources. Personal traits and behaviors can also help the project manager select team members with specific roles in mind. As a project advances through its life cycle, the number of people involved typically increases. A critical task of the team is to manage risks and opportunities.

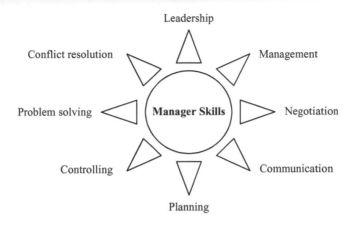

Figure 10.7 Skills needed by a project manager.

By comparing costs and benefits of various courses of action, the team can select which sequence of actions to take and obtain agreement from necessary parties.

The key to handling projects is not to resist changes but to manage them. Managing change makes good practical sense. It helps the project manager as well as the team to maintain control by providing feedback on what is and should be happening at each development step. Finally, it allows them the opportunity to adjust or modify plans so the goals remain realistic (Kleim and Ludin 1998). The project manager's job at the end is to ensure that everyone in the project team has what he needs to successfully perform the task.

10.4.3 Integrated project team

The work of most engineering projects is carried out in teams. Effective teams are vital to the success of engineering organizations, beginning with the project's conception, continuing through development, and extending into delivery. Engineers may form or work with a variety of teams, including overall project teams and subsets of those teams.

An integrated project team brings together the project team and the team of workers, consultants, developers, and suppliers, as shown in Figure 10.8. Team-working is characterized by mutual trust and openness, where problems and risks are shared and resolved collectively by the integrated project team. The team-working ethic must be demonstrated by senior management, by acting as exemplars of professional practice and behavior and showing commitment to collaboration and partnering throughout the project. Partnering involves the integrated project team working together to improve performance through agreeing on mutual

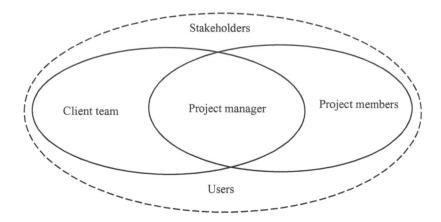

Figure 10.8 Components of a project team.

objectives, devising a way to resolve any disputes, committing themselves to continuous improvement, measuring progress, and sharing the gains (OGC 2003). Project partnering facilitates building an integrated team with a common goal, which in turn enhances quality, reduces costs, and increases efficiency. It is applicable to all projects, even those that are very simple and limited in scope.

10.4.4 *Project portfolio management (PPM)*

The line between PM and PPM is often blurred because people attempt to accomplish all of the tasks discussed under the heading of PM. The purpose of PPM is to prioritize projects, plan and staff with qualified and available employees (resource management), monitor them, and keep all involved parties informed about their status. For organizations that work on a large number of projects, it makes sense to clearly delineate between PPM and PM.

PPM focuses on the high-level, strategic decisions for the entire project portfolio (doing the right projects), while PM focuses on the execution of individual projects (doing the projects right). PPM places great value on resource planning and resource conflict resolution, which in turn increases value creation in a business. In general, PPM tasks may include (Holicky 2017):

- Selecting and prioritizing projects that align with strategic objectives
- Initiating, planning, staffing, implementing, and completing the projects
- Training and coaching project managers and teams

- Maintenance of PM methods, tools, and technologies
- Monitoring and evaluating project progress
- Communication and support for project teams

10.5   Project quality management (PQM)

Quality is not act. It is a habit.

Aristotle

The ISO defines quality as the totality of characteristics of an entity that bear on its ability to satisfy stated or implied needs. Other experts define quality as "the characteristic of a product or service that bear on its ability to satisfy stated or implied needs" (Hoang 2017). Quality in general implies fitness for the intended purpose including performance, safety, reliability, handling, etc.

QM is a continuous process for ensuring that all project activities required to design, plan, and implement are effective and efficient with respect to the objective and performance. The primary focus of QM is to meet or exceed customer requirements (ISO 2015). Leaders at all levels establish directions and create conditions in which people are engaged in achieving the organization's QM objectives.

PQM includes all the processes and activities needed to achieve project quality. It involves the skill of forming and managing a team of people to accomplish a qualitative goal within an effective cost and time frame, which will result in the production of a quality product or service. Its main purpose is to satisfy the needs for which it is being done and to enable realization or exceeding the needs and expectations of stakeholders.

10.5.1   PQM principles

PQM principles are a set of fundamental beliefs, norms, rules, and values that are accepted as true and can be used as a basis for quality management. These principles can be used as a foundation to guide an organization's performance improvement. They were developed and updated by international experts of ISO/TC 176, which is responsible for developing and maintaining ISO's quality management standards.

ISO 9001 is underpinned by the eight principles of quality management (Figure 10.9). They have been the guiding principles for the most popular quality standard: ISO 9001. But they are also useful resources for any management professionals who want to implement or improve their existing quality management program. QPM principles top management systems as guidance in running an organization with the aim of continual improvement (BAB 2017).

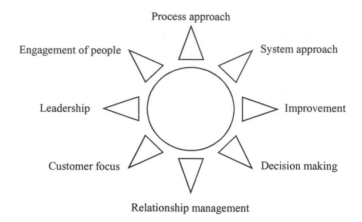

Figure 10.9 8 PQM principles based on ISO 9001: 2015.

Customer focus is Principle 1, which covers both customer needs and customer service. This principle underlines that a business should understand its customers, what they need, and when by attempting to understand and meet their current and future requirements and anticipations.

Principle 2 is concerned with strong leadership. The organization should have clear goals and objectives to ensure its employees are actively involved in achieving the organization's unified objectives.

Principle 3 is all about people engagement to reduce costs, improve consistency, eliminate waste, promote continuous improvement and empowerment, encouraging engagement, and recognizing achievements.

Principle 4 is about consistency and understanding that good processes also speed up activities as well as the inputs and outputs that tie these processes together.

Principle 5 is about understanding and managing interrelated processes as a system which should lead to greater efficiency. Organizations maintain success when processes are managed as one coherent QM system.

Principle 6 is about increased ability to embrace new opportunities, organizational flexibility and improved performance, and creation and exploitation of new opportunities when they establish and sustain an ongoing focus on improvement.

Principle 7 is about establishing an evidence-based decision-making process that entails gathering input from multiple sources, identifying facts, objectively analyzing data, examining cause/effect, and considering potential consequences.

And Principle 8 deals with supply chains, which promotes a productive relationship between the organization and its suppliers.

10.5.2   PQM process

PQM consists of three main processes, as shown in Figure 10.10. These processes are required to ensure that the project will satisfy the needs for which it was undertaken. It is all about the synergy of continuous improvement of the project and its delivery. The three processes associated with PQM are quality planning, quality assurance, and quality control.

Quality planning includes the identification of quality standards relevant for the project and deciding how to meet them. These standards are defined depending on the project nature and the corresponding activities. The crucial step in this process is to develop a quality plan based on quality standards that will be used during the project implementation phase.

Quality assurance is all the planned and systematic activities implemented within the quality system to ensure that appropriate quality standards are used. It occurs during the implementation phase of the project and includes the evaluation of the overall performance of the project on a regular basis to provide confidence that the project will satisfy the quality standards defined by the project. Performing quality assurance centers on the processes that are in place to supply the project deliverables at the relevant level of quality. The most popular tool used to determine quality assurance is the Shewhart cycle (PM4DEV 2016). This cycle consists of four steps: Plan–Do–Check–Act. These steps are commonly abbreviated as PDCA.

Quality control comprises supervising particular results with a view of progressing the total quality. It involves monitoring specific project results to determine if they meet relevant quality standards; to evaluate performance and recommend required modifications; and to recognize approaches to abolish causes of undesirable results. The goal of quality control is to improve quality and meet quality standards or designations based on the project stakeholder's expectations.

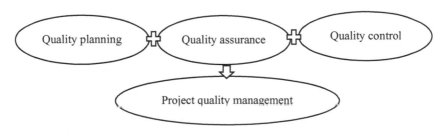

Figure 10.10 Three main processes of PQM.

10.6   Project risk management (PRM)

Being able to be repeated controllably is one key element
in risk management.

Toba Beta
[from Master of Stupidity (2011)]

Risk is an uncertainty that matters. It can affect project objectives negatively or positively. Where negative risk implies something unwanted that has the potential to irreparably damage a project, positive risks are opportunities that can affect the project in beneficial ways (Landau 2016).

RM is an integral part of a good management practice. It is the process of identifying, classifying, assessing, and controlling threats to an organization's capital and earnings. These threats or risks could stem from several sources, including financial uncertainty, legal liabilities, managerial errors, accidents, and natural disasters. Therefore, it is important to understand how RM practices occur in different types of projects.

10.6.1   Reactive, predictive, and proactive PRM

RM techniques have contributed greatly to improving reliability and safety in projects. Therefore, a clear understanding of the risks must be established. The sources of project risk are almost limitless, emphasizing the need for a well-thought-out, detailed, responsive plan.

Reactive PRM consists of responding to risk events as they occur to mitigate negative impacts to the organization. Managing risk is not only reactive; it should be part of the planning process to figure out risks that might happen in the project and how to control those risks if they in fact occur (Landau 2016). The objective of PRM is to identify project risks and develop strategies to prevent them from occurring or minimize their impact to the project if they occur.

Predictive PRM actions attempt to forecast future and potential hazard/risk occurrence. This happens solely by reviewing existing systems and processes. Predictive PRM is largely possible due to the use of indicators or past historical performance, which is used to predict possible future performances (Britton 2016).

PRM should be proactive rather than reactive or predictive and should be managed at the earliest prospect within the project life cycle. Proactive RM is often upheld as the highest form of PRM. It can be described as an adaptive, closed loop feedback control approach based on measurement and observation of the desired present safety level. Proactive PRM combines a mixed method of past, present, and future prediction before finding solutions to avoid risks. It focuses on mitigating the risks of threat events before these might possibly occur and negatively impact the organization. It begins early in the life cycle.

Technology plays an intrinsic role in building on effective and proactive PRM approaches. Many organizations leverage software solutions to minimize risk inconsistencies and to establish a single risk taxonomy and culture across the organization (MetricStream 2016).

In general, PRM should begin early in the process and continue through the life cycle. A key to success in dealing with risk is to start early and lay the foundation for PRM; be proactive, not reactive; manage risks formally with a process; and be flexible.

10.6.2   PRM Process

PRM, basically, is the process of conducting RM planning, identification, analysis, response planning, monitoring, and control. The expanded six-step process to establishing a project risk plan includes making a list of potential risks; determining the probability of risk occurrence; determining its negative impact; preventing or mitigating the risk; considering contingencies; improving the efficacy of the entire plan; and finally communicating risk with all stakeholders.

This six-step PRM process is outlined in Figure 10.11.

Step 1: Brainstorm
Make a list of potential risks to the project.

Step 2: Probability of risk occurrence
Prioritize all identified threats to the project information.

Step 3: Mitigate the risk
Eradicate the risk before it has a chance to grow.

Step 4: Consider contingencies
Preventive measures are those steps taken before the risk becomes reality.

Step 5: Risk mitigation plan
Project managers should improve the efficacy of the entire plan.

Step 6: Risk communication
Project managers should improve the efficacy of the entire plan.

Figure 10.11 PRM process.

It is a common and practical approach to establishing PRM. This process should not be created in a vacuum but typically involves a great deal of research and collaboration with the project team. Making a list of potential risks to the project should not be an analysis but a formal brainstorming session, where all ideas are captured (Heagney 2012). Steps 2 and 3 of the process allow for a vetting of these ideas. Preventive measures are the steps taken before the risk becomes reality. Therefore, a risk mitigation plan is designed to eliminate or minimize the impact of the risk occurrences on the project. Usually, the project team mitigates risks by following the sequence of risk avoidance, risk sharing, risk reduction, and risk transfer. Each of these mitigation techniques can be an effective tool in reducing individual risks and the risk profile of the project.

Contingencies represent certain actions that will be taken if the risk arises. The PRM balances the investment of the mitigation against the benefit for the project. Contingency funds are set aside by the project team to address unforeseen events that cause the project costs to increase. Most project managers, especially on large projects, manage contingency funds at the project level.

Today, RC is an interactive two-way process to exchange information and opinions throughout the PRM process concerning risk, risk-related factors, and risk perceptions among risk assessors, risk managers, and other related stakeholders. Successful RC is a prerequisite for effective PRM and RA. Finally, RC contributes to the transparency of the PRM, and it promotes a better understanding and acceptance of the risk management decisions.

10.7   Change management (CM) practice

Slowness to change usually means fear of the new.

Philip Crosby

CM is a practice that helps ease organizational transitions. It involves a range of tools, techniques, and processes aimed at successfully implementing change. More specifically, it aids the people side of change. These tools and techniques can be employed in a variety of contexts. Typical tools and techniques that a CM practitioner might use during a change initiative include: questioning skills, PM, problem-solving, and negotiation skills (Downey 2008). The two major areas of CM for consideration are: organizational CM and change control.

10.7.1   Organizational CM

Change is not only part of life, it is required for life. Change of any sort succeeds or fails on the basis of whether the people affected do things differently (Bridges and Bridges 2009). Change can occur in an organization in many ways, strategic, leadership, or technological. As things mature and grow, changes occur naturally and are often healthy. Organizational change in general minimizes resistance, increases engagement, improves performance, reduces costs, and enhances innovation. Figure 10.12 shows the environment of organization change and its attributes.

There are various CM models that force change into an organization. ADKAR (Awareness–Desire–Knowledge–Ability–Reinforcement), first introduced as a practical tool by Prosci in 1998, is one of the models which may help in the development of an organization change program. Change happens on two aspects: the organization and the employees. All five building blocks of the model are sequential where each block provides knowledge and skills for creating an understanding and desire for change, and how to create the right environment for those impacted by change and/or resisting change. In general, the ADKAR model is used as a learning platform in teaching and coaching CM.

Change may take different approaches including production, managing, and operating practices, use of resources, physical resources, development life cycles, procedures and standards, applications and networks, etc. It may take different forms, such as downsizing, growing the organization, or introducing a new technology. Whatever the reason for change, a well-structured approach is always essential. It will help employees to

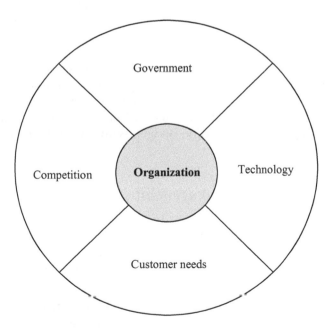

Figure 10.12 Environment of organization change.

understand, accept, embrace, and commit to the changes without resistance (Smith 2014). To help minimize the impacts and effects of change, from having unintended negative outcomes, it is necessary to have CM methodologies in place with skilled resources delivering and executing on those methodologies, principles, and processes. Without such CM, organizations could experience problems and unnecessary difficulties, mostly those resulting from resistance to change.

Resistance to change, which can include valid questioning of the need for the change, is a natural part of almost all organizations, especially since those that move through change without a plan always have a hard time making employees accept the new ideas to implement. Without managing the change to the agency and its people's work patterns, the potential benefits of a project are unlikely to be fully realized. Therefore, CM is significant because it helps an organization to be efficient.

10.7.2   Change control

Change usually involves three overlapping aspects: people, processes, and culture. The change control process can vary but usually includes a number of important and mandatory steps. For people, EQ has been identified as one predictor of a person's career adaptability (in addition to life satisfaction and positive interactions with each other) (Coetzee and Nisha 2014). Figure 10.13 outlines the five steps of the project change control process.

Change should not be a source of fear but needs to be embraced and managed. This does not have to be a difficult task while investing in a project team and a formidable plan. Changes often represent necessary adjustments to the original project plan. The idea of change control is how to manage those changes, which makes all of the difference and helps deliver the project on time and on budget, with an excellent deliverable (Heagney 2012).

10.8   Configuration management

> *Security is always going to be a cat and mouse game because there'll be people out there that are hunting for the zero day award, you have people that don't have configuration management, don't have vulnerability management, don't have patch management.*

> **Kevin Mitnick**
> *[from "An Hour with Kevin Mitnick, Part 2 – Page 2" (interview with InternetNews, 2009)]*

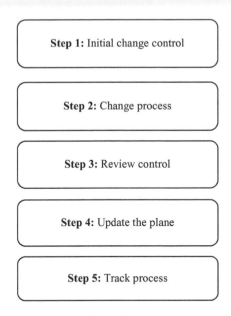

Figure 10.13 Project change control process.

Configuration management incorporates the administrative activities concerned with the creation, maintenance, and quality control of the work scope. A configuration is a set of functional and physical characteristics of a final deliverable defined in the specification and achieved in the execution of plans. A configuration management system is used to keep track of an organization's hardware, software, and related information. It may be regarded as asset control and is essential whether or not multiple versions of a deliverable will be created.

In software development , configuration management signifies to the items that need to be configured and managed in order for the project to be successful. Software configuration management is a set of processes, policies, and tools that organizes the development process. It simultaneously maintains the current state of the software while enabling developers to work on new versions for features or fixes. This involves software versions and updates installed on the organization's computing systems.

Configuration management is the big picture encompassing PM and customer management, depending on what configuration management tools can manage. Configuration management and CM stand side-by-side. Though not independent, one cannot be considered a subset of the other. Managing change is an ongoing decision-making process that is closely tied to RM. Configuration management is an ongoing tracking process that provides the traceability and persistent access to information based on a specified context (Farah 2005).

A configuration management tool can improve the organization's change-impact analysis, reducing the outages caused by production changes. It deals with changes in product specifications and with the identification, maintenance, reporting on, and verification of items and their interrelationships. The configuration management process takes into consideration the following broad-set activities (Kaiser 2018):

- **Configuration identification:** Configuration that needs to be maintained must first be identified. It can either be a manual process, such as maintaining the source code on a common repository, or using discovery tools to automatically identify the configuration.
- **Configuration control:** Once the configuration items are identified, there is no guarantee that it will remain unchanged. In all probability, the configuration is likely to change. Thus, there needs to be an effective mechanism to control the changes that go into the configuration management system. In this regard, the CM process acts as a guardian for controlling the changes to the configuration management system.
- **Configuration audit:** Despite there being control mechanisms protecting against changes in configuration, means of bypassing exist. Therefore, configuration audits are necessary to keep an eye on configuration compliance.

10.9   *Project management (PM) models*

> *Most people spend more time and energy going around problems than in trying to solve them.*
>
> **Henry Ford**

PM plays a crucial role in achieving goals and following through with plans and expectations. Various projects benefit from various methodologies. Not every model of PM will work for every assignment.

10.9.1   *The waterfall model*

The waterfall model (Figure 10.14) is an approach which was initially developed for software development. It is called such because the model develops systematically from one phase to another in a downward fashion, like a waterfall. Often called linear, this approach includes a number of internal phases which are sequential and executed in a chronological order. The waterfall model is best suited to the user whose needs are fixed, or when the result is predictable. Currently it is applied most commonly to the construction or manufacturing industry, where little or no changes are required at every stage.

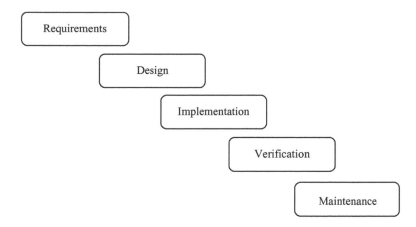

Figure 10.14 Waterfall model.

Throughout the development effort of the waterfall, it is possible for various members of the team to be involved or to continue with other work, depending on the active phase of the project. A business analyst may learn about and document what needs to be done while developers are working on other projects. Testers can prepare test scripts from requirements documentation while coding is under way (Habash 2017). Because design is completed early in the development life cycle, this methodology lends itself to projects where multiple components must be designed (often in parallel) for integration with external systems.

10.9.2   Concurrent engineering (CE) model

CE is a technique of designing and developing products where the different stages run simultaneously instead of sequentially. It decreases product development time and also the time to market, leading to improved productivity and reduced costs. The CE environment supports PM, the control of project information, and promotes collaboration in the building process. The approach of CE considers all the elements, starting from the design and including manufacturing and support, quality, cost, competitive advantage, schedule, and customer needs.

The concept of CE is not new. According to Ziemke and Spann (1993), CE was commonly used in the development of the US weapon and transportation arsenal in the WWII era. After this period, many US and Western producers forgot this good way of engineering as corporations grew, products became more complex, and greater specialization of the workforce took place. Its redevelopment began in the 1980s with the coining of the term "computer-supported cooperative work" by Grief and Cashman in 1984 (Shen et al. 2008). Shortly thereafter, the concept of CE was developed and defined as "a systematic approach to the integrated, concurrent design of products and their related processes, including manufacture and support" (Turino 1992; Shen et al. 2008). In particular, CE grew out of the American automobile industry's efforts to emulate the Japanese approach to product development. According to Hartley (1992), many Japanese companies have been using the basic elements of CE successfully for over 30 years. They did not call it CE, but the success of Japanese manufacturing, particularly in the automotive industry, created strong competitive pressure on American and European automobile manufacturers (Habash 2017).

CE is also an engineering management approach and a business strategy which enables the integrated development of products and processes with the goal of completing the entire cycle in a shorter time (Smith and Reinertsen 1995). CE is a non-linear product or project design approach during which all phases of manufacturing operate at the same time, simultaneously. Both product and process design run in parallel and occur in the same time frame. It removes the need to have multiple design reworks by creating an environment for designing a product right the first time around.

The CE approach is based on five key elements: a process; a multi-disciplinary team; an integrated design model; a facility; and a software infrastructure (Bandecchi et al. 1999). The design process is conducted in a number of sessions in which all specialists must participate. It is an iterative process that addresses all aspects of the system design in a quick and complete fashion.

An important aspect to the realization of the CE process is assembling a capable team to carry out the task. All disciplines that are concerned with hardware and software designs should be engaged. Typical engineering disciplines that may be represented on a CE team are: system hardware or software design, operations, manufacturing and assembly, machining, and safety. As shown on Figure 10.15, consideration of each of these disciplines, coupled with the user requirements, is important to a successful integrated design.

10.9.3   The V-cycle model

In terms of management processes, there are various methods within system engineering to guide the design life cycle, including the waterfall, spiral, and Agile models. However, the emergence of all the above design life cycle management processes is the design V (validation and verification)-model, which represents the different phases in design and the coordination activities that should occur across them at each step (Haskins et al. 2010). Validation is the process of demonstrating that the product satisfies the user needs, regardless of what the system specification requires. Verification is the process of proving that each product

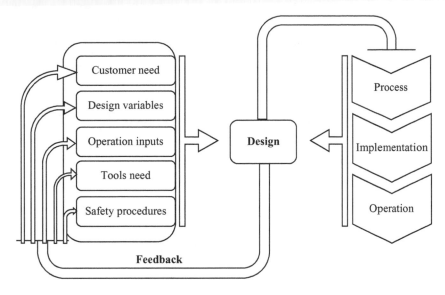

Figure 10.15 CE-integrated design.

meets its specification. Figure 10.16 shows an overview of project development within the V-model.

The V-model is a modified version of the common waterfall method. Its core involves a sequential evolution of plans, specifications, and products that are baselined and put under configuration management. The V-model is a sequential path of execution of processes. Each phase must be completed before the next phase begins. Testing of the product is planned in parallel with a corresponding phase of development in the V-model (Habash 2017). Unlike the waterfall method, there is no prohibition against doing detailed work early in the cycle. In fact, hardware and software feasibility models may be required at the very first stage.

The left side of the V-model represents the decomposition of requirements and creation of system specifications. The right side represents integration of parts and their validation. This developmental process is balanced and relies on verification from the previous steps before proceeding forward. At each level there is a direct correspondence between activities on the left and right sides of the chart. Note that at the bottom level on the V-model, the tasks break into three parallel efforts: operations (including manual operations), hardware, and software (Habash 2017).

Finally, the V-model should be used for small- to medium-sized projects where requirements are clearly defined and fixed. It should be chosen when sufficient technical resources are available with needed technical expertise. In the V-model, developer and tester work in parallel. Moreover, the model provides guidance for the planning and realization of projects.

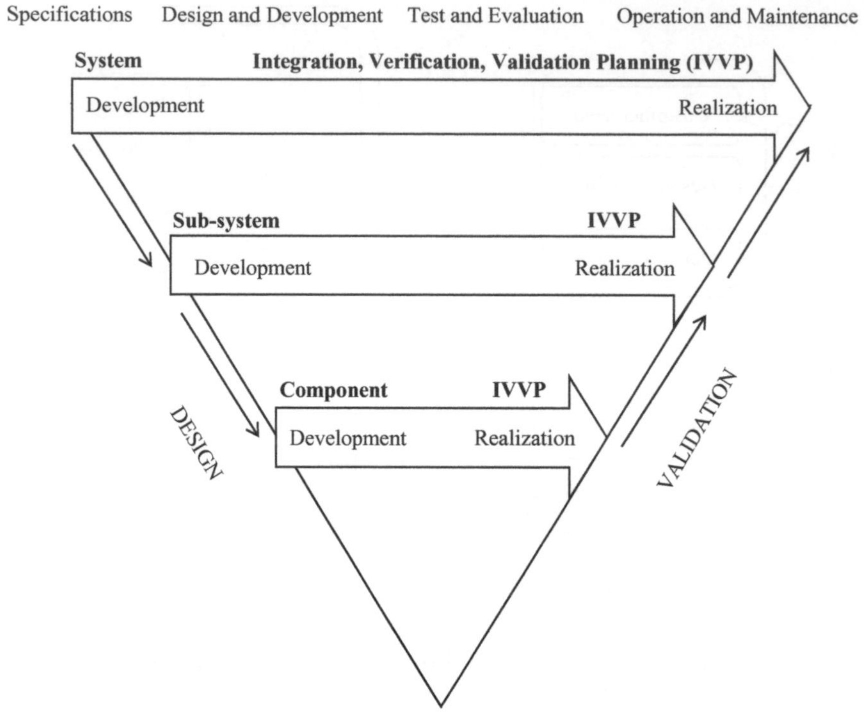

Specifications   Design and Development   Test and Evaluation   Operation and Maintenance

System   **Integration, Verification, Validation Planning (IVVP)**

Development   Realization

Sub-system   **IVVP**

Development   Realization

Component   **IVVP**

Development   Realization

DESIGN

VALIDATION

Figure 10.16 Design V-model for project development.

10.10   Lean practice

> *The most dangerous kind of waste is the waste we do not recognize.*

Shigeo Shingo

Over the past few decades, several management practices like Lean and Agile; management methodologies like Scrum, Kanban, and extreme programming (XP); and tools like sprints, boards, and tests have been steadily gaining acceptance in various fields. This scenario is reflected in Figure 10.17.

10.10.1   New paradigm of systems thinking (ST)

With roots in math, science, and philosophy, ST has emerged as a highly relevant concept in social and organizational contexts. ST is a mindset for understanding how things work. This means looking at the component parts of a complex system and their characteristics and relationships to better understand the whole, including the way they are interconnected

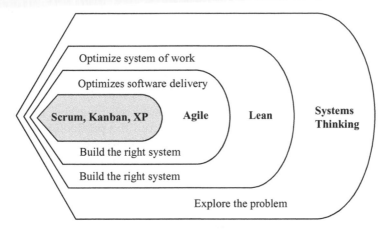

Figure 10.17 Scenario of management practices, methodologies, and tools in the paradigm of ST.

and interacting. When considering a whole system, the term complex is frequently used to describe it.

ST is the opposite of linear thinking in that it focuses on the relationships among system components as opposed to the components themselves. It may be used to solve complex problems that are not solvable using conventional reductionist thinking because it focuses on the relationships among system components as well as on the components themselves (Monat and Gannon 2015). Complex systems usually interact with their environments and are, therefore, open systems. A project is usually an open, complex social system made up of many subsystems including administrative and management functions, teams, and individuals, and operates within the larger system that comprises the performing organization.

ST provides an approach for managing complexity. It is an approach to help decision makers recognize and understand the cause-and-effect relationships among all types of subsystems by applying various tools. ST is an innovative means of the leader's activity; it has an impact on quality of leadership performance, which in turn enhances results of an organization. ST recognizes that the parts of any whole system may only exist or be understood in relation to the whole (Page 2011). This way of thinking about a system helps to move away from focusing on a simple and linear cause-and-effect relation to one that is multidimensional and emphasizes the parts of the system to the whole system.

10.10.2 Lean and green

Lean is a practice that eliminates waste, focuses on value creation, and improves cycle time. As a practice-oriented movement, Lean is by and large a way of abstract thinking and generalization. The practice of ST is the process of understanding how things regarded as systems influence one another within a whole. Without an understanding of both systems and design thinking, it is hard to get Lean right, and without the practice of Lean techniques, it is difficult to make ST a day-to-day reality to concretely improve system performance (Balle 2018).

Eliminating waste means eradicating ineffective meetings, tasks, and documentation. Lean as a concept started from the production environment, but now the concept has spread to all business areas. It puts a very strong emphasis on the system, the way that the team operates *as a whole*. Implementing Lean methodology is not a task with a start and an end; it is a continuous development process.

The principles of Lean thinking are an approach to manufacturing derived from the work of W. Edwards Deming in the 1950s. Enhancing value for the customer is the essence of Lean by providing what the customer needs when it is required and at the most affordable cost. One of the main aspects of Lean is continuous improvement. Minimizing waste and errors are recurring topics in Lean visions. Key factors are quality, cost, and time, as well as ability to adapt to changes. The application of Lean thinking has a significant impact in academia as well as in industry over the last decade.

Many leading companies have implemented Lean manufacturing programs, which yield increased efficiency, reduced costs, improved customer response time, and more. Others have adopted green programs resulting in reduced energy consumption, waste generation, and hazardous materials usage. Models for both Lean and green systems all include management systems, waste identification, and implementation of waste-reducing techniques to achieve desired business results (Bergmiller and McCright 2009). Figure 10.18 shows the main elements of a Lean/green system model. The separate models of Lean and green have many similarities, mainly their reliance on management systems

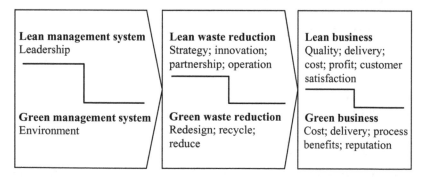

Figure 10.18 Lean and green system model.

to drive waste identification within the organization to achieve desired business results.

Both Lean models and green models may be recognized as similar structures. They emphasize the importance of the management system, the application of various waste reduction techniques, and the achievement of desired business results (Bergmiller and McCright 2009). Both systems are parallel by nature and have similar components and elements.

10.10.3   Lean manufacturing

Lean manufacturing is mostly understood from the examples of Henry Ford and the Western automotive industry which are applied to the manufacturing sector. It was a counteraction for the unproductive and slow manufacturing that was happening in craft production where each product was individually crafted. Leadership is one of the key practices in Lean manufacturing organizations.

Ford applied just-in-time (JIT) manufacturing (means to produce and deliver the right item, at the right time, in the right amount, at the right place) for car production that focused on reducing the carrying costs of inventory by eliminating as much inventory as possible. JIT uses several branches of tools, including the "pull" approach and "Kanban production" control, inventory reduction, quick setups and   orders, quality at the source (jidoka), supplier networks, teamwork and participation, and continuous improvement (Kaizen) that can be used to achieve the above efforts (Bruuna and Meffordb 2003). Kaizen is one well-known tool in Lean manufacturing that has been used for continuous improvement. Kaizen is a Japanese word that means "continuous improvement".

The modern principles of Lean manufacturing are derived from the success of the Japanese automobile industry, especially Toyota, which created a new revolution for Lean methods (Womack et al. 1990). Eiji Toyoda and Taiichi Ohno, Japanese industrial engineers and developers of TPS, were pioneers in the development of modern production methodology. TPS is a business philosophy that emphasizes continuous improvement, employee learning and empowerment, and standardized work methods (Heizer and Render 2014). TPS philosophy focuses on eliminating three types of inefficiency: non-value-adding work, overburdening of workers, and unevenness in productivity. In other industries, Lean methodology may be applied to identify sources of waste and eliminate them by establishing clear best practices (Womack et al. 2008).

One of the popular Lean principles developed by Womack and Jones (2003) suggested five steps for Lean manufacturing: value, value stream, flow, pull, and perfection, as shown in Table 10.1. The elimination of waste is a key underlying principle of Lean. It requires moving away from the

Table 10.1 The five principles of Lean manufacturing

Principle	Summary
Value	Specify and understand value from a customer perspective and by product family. This value is created by the producer, and this is what producers struggle with: how to create the ultimate value for their customer.
Value stream	Identify all the steps in the entire flow of a product's life cycle and eliminate any wastes that do not create value. Value stream means all the relevant activities needed to create and deliver a product.
Flow	Streamlining the value-creating steps to occur in a tight sequence that flows towards the customer or the next upstream process. The goal is that everything flows smoothly through the value stream in one common direction. Flow describes a situation where each individual's work keeps moving with no queues, waiting, or rework.
Pull	Let customers pull from the next upstream process. This requires flexibility and short cycle times of design and delivery of products. The main idea is to get one process to make only what the next process needs, only when it needs it.
Perfection	Repeat for ongoing system improvements and to continuously remove the root causes of poor quality from the production process. Continuously adapt to customer needs in order to deliver a product of the highest possible quality.

traditional approaches to process improvement and instead focusing on the product or service provided to the end consumer.

10.10.4   Lean product development (LPD)

Product development is one of the most innovative processes in manufacturing. It is mostly about finding a way to produce new products, unlike production where the same product is to be produced over and over again with a physical product as the output (Reinertsen 2005). The process is not foreseeable, and the success of the work is evaluated only later, from market reaction. Product development deals largely with knowledge, information, and creativity and not with actual products. The processes are complex, highly consistent, parallel, iterative, and less anticipated than production processes (Trapp 2018).

Waste in product development is not the same as waste in manufacturing. Waste in manufacturing has to do with physical things, such as over-the-top stocks. In product development, most of the waste is knowledge waste, invisible. There are three types of knowledge waste: scatter, hand-off, and wishful thinking. Scatter waste means when knowledge in

Table 10.2 Principles of LPD

Principle	Summary
Principle 1	Define precisely the customer's problem and identify the specific function to be performed to resolve the problem.
Principle 2	Identify more quickly the process by which the identified functions can be integrated into a low-cost and high-quality product.
Principle 3	Remove any waste item and redundant or unnecessary cost to reveal a great product solution.
Principle 4	Listen often and interactively to the voice of the customer throughout the development process.
Principle 5	Introduce methods and cost-reduction tools both in their business practices and in their culture to allow continuing cost-reduction.

the product development is spread all over the place, scattered for some reason. Hand-off waste is the result of the separation of responsibility, action, feedback, and knowledge. Wishful thinking is then the third main type of product development waste. This simply means that decisions are made without appropriate data and knowledge, and in this manner wishful thinking is what happens in development (Yliopisto 2015).

The adoption of Lean manufacturing principles into product development offers enormous potential for reorganizing flow in the process. LPD should be considered separately from Lean manufacturing, but both need to work together in order for the whole value stream of a product to work. Womack and Jones (1996) broaden the scope of understanding of Lean principles, emphasizing that the same that would apply to any company should be extended to the product development process. Table 10.2 outlines five principles for LPD.

Figure 10.19 shows a representation of the LPD innovation process. The process begins with the typical front end, where a number of ideas

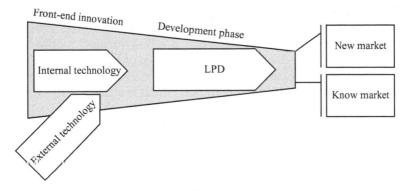

Figure 10.19 LPD within the innovation process.

are to be generated. These are then typically evaluated, selected, further developed, or tested in an iterative process. For highly innovative ideas, special projects are performed (platform or breakthrough projects, advanced development). The best ideas are then advanced to the subsequent development stage until they finally reach product maturity (Trapp 2018). The development phase is more structured and formalized than the front end, which is also reflected in greater process stages with a focus on LPD.

10.10.5 Lean six sigma (LSS)

Sigma (σ) is a Greek letter that is a statistical unit of measurement used to define the standard deviation of a population. As process variation decreases, so does the standard deviation. A σ level is defined as the number of standard deviations that fit between the process mean and the customer specification limit. As the process "σ level" increases, more process outputs, products, and services meet customer requirements, reducing production defects.

Six σ (6σ) is a problem-focused set of techniques and tools for process improvement. It has its foundations in controlling defects. If the 6σ process can be summarized in one term, it would be the acronym DMAIC: define; measure, analyze; improve, control. These process improvement methodologies are equivalent to Lean thinking principles outlined in Table 10.1. This statistical methodology pursues to improve the quality of a product or service by concentrating not on the output but on the process that creates the output. It is a process improvement methodology, originally used by Motorola in manufacturing in 1980s. Implementation of 6σ requires commitment of the organization and leaders. 6σ demands that concentrating on reduction of variation will solve process and problems. By using statistical tools to recognize the fluctuation of a process, management may begin to foresee the anticipated outcome of that process.

Fundamentally, 6σ and Lean systems have the same goal. While initially designed for manufacturing, Lean is a flow-focused methodology that works across all industries and in all types of operations. LSS combines the principles of Lean with 6σ to improve process effectiveness and alignment with the voice of the customer, which is related to the way the customer describe quality and tolerance for defects.

Lean focuses on reducing lead time by removing waste and non-value added steps and 6σ focuses on reducing variability and defects by identifying and controlling its causes. The main emphasis of Lean is on removing unnecessary and wasteful steps in the creation of a product so that only steps that directly add value to the product are taken. They both pursue eliminating waste and creating the most efficient system possible, but they follow different approaches toward how achieving this goal. The main difference between Lean and 6σ is that they recognize the root cause of waste differently. Lean practitioners think that waste comes from needless steps in the production process that do not add value to the final product, including overproduction, handling time, defects, and inspection practices; while 6σ proponents assert that waste results from variation within the process. Therefore in Lean, any process that does not add value to the end user of the product or service needs to be removed. Employed together (Figure 10.20), this hybrid methodology combines the best of both Lean and 6s to increase speed, process capability, and customer satisfaction.

Despite their different origins, it is obvious that Lean and 6σ comprise many common features, such as an emphasis on customer satisfaction, an environment of continuous improvement, the search for root causes, and full employee engagement. The two methodologies facilitate organizations with a management philosophy to become more efficient across all operations while also producing better quality products and services.

LSS is a scalable approach to support a broad spectrum of improvement initiatives and to repeatedly seek out and remove waste and wasteful practices. It is a synergistic, structured, disciplined, thorough approach to process improvement. Today, LSS is a worldwide endeavor at unceasing development to help organizations transform their processes in order to satisfy the customer and organizational requirements. Those with knowledge in Lean, 6σ, and LSS are in position to take a lead role in employing needed changes.

Management obligation to a LSS process in the portfolio of management improvement programs must be serious and go beyond motivational talks. The management team should be made accountable for both managing the organization and improving its effectiveness. Each LSS project should include three stages: project initiation, project implementation, and project communication. An improvement project should be initiated based on an organized project selection procedure and project team. The project team should include an experienced facilitator, representatives from each department through which the service flows, frontline employees, administrators from various contexts, and customers to introduce new ideas. The final project results should be provided to key leaders and affected administrators. It is advocated that recommendations made during project meetings that impact quality of work be discussed seriously and allowed to evolve naturally. As project begins, displaying the results internally using posters or digital media, is advisable.

LSS has embraced the roles from the Motorola 6s methodology, which derive the naming convention of the progression of mastery used within martial arts. Several organizations have developed their own ranks and designations of mastery.

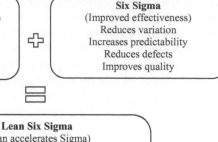

Figure 10.20 The formation of LSS.

10.11   Agile practice

> *Agile project management focuses on selecting the right skills for project team members and molding them into productive teams.*
>
> **Jim Highsmith**

Agile came from a need to deliver software projects better (Schneider 2017). Understanding the importance of ST and Agile is critical in order to gain a deeper understanding of Agile. Officially, Agile was born in 2001 from the Agile Manifesto to improve productivity in software development, and it was gradually expanded and widely used in many projects in other areas.

10.11.1   Agile Methodology

There are several methodologies that can be used to manage an Agile project; three of the best-known being Scrum, Kanban, and XP for technical practices (with new practices becoming popular, largely from Lean start-up, such as continuous deployment and testing in production). In general, an Agile project produces and delivers work in short bursts (or sprints) of anything up to a few weeks. These are repeated to refine the working deliverable until it meets the client's requirements (APM 2018; Fichtner 2018).

Agile methodologies take an iterative approach to product development. Unlike a straightforward linear waterfall model, Agile projects consist of a number of smaller cycles/sprints. Each one of them is a small-scale project: it has a backlog and consists of design, implementation, testing, and deployment stages within the predefined scope of work.

The objective of each Agile method is to adjust to change and deliver working software as quickly as possible. However, each methodology has slim variations in the way it defines the phases of software development. Moreover, even though the goal is the same, each team's process movement may vary depending on the specific project or situation. As an example, the full Agile software development life cycle (Figure 10.21) includes the concept, inception, construction, release, production, and retirement phases.

According to Highsmith (2012), "agility is the ability to both create and respond to change in order to profit in a turbulent business environment". There are different types of Agile methods that have emerged, and the most popular include crystal methods, scrum, dynamic systems development methodology (DSDM), feature-driven development (FDD), and XP (Shahidul Islam and Tura 2013).

Agile PM (APM) is a team-based approach centered on delivering requirements iteratively and incrementally throughout the project life cycle. This approach emphasizes the rapid delivery of an application in complete functional components. Rather than creating tasks and schedules, all time is "time-boxed" into phases called "sprints". Each sprint has a defined duration with a running list of deliverables, which are planned at the start of the sprint. APM is guided by a manifesto developed in 2001 by a group called the Agile Alliance (www.agilealiance.org). The group came up with the so-called Agile manifesto, which is based on four broad values (Folwer and Highsmith 2018):

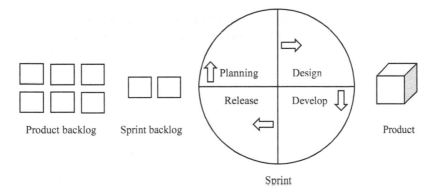

Figure 10.21 Agile development cycle.

- Individuals and interactions over processes and tools
- Working software over comprehensive documentation
- Customer collaboration over contract negotiation
- Responding to change over following a plan

10.11.2   Agile principles

The book *Agile Principles Unleashed: Proven Approaches for Achieving Real Productivity Gains in any Organization* (Cooke 2010) discusses the 12 core principles on which the success of Agile approaches depends. The author writes how these principles combined can create a business environment that produces high business-value output, motivates employees, encourages innovation, and delivers tangible results. The 12 Agile principles are outlined in Table 10.3.

10.11.3   Scrum and Kanban

Scrum and Kanban are Agile methodologies with few differences. Understanding these differences is key to selecting the path that will work best for the designated environment. Both Scrum and Kanban work for large and complex tasks to be divided and accomplished effectively.

Scrum, a time-boxed iteration, is one type of adaptive software development (ASD) methodology that was used and developed in the early 1990s by Ken Schwaber and Jeff Sutherland with later collaboration with Mike Beedle. It gets its name from the scrum in rugby and initially introduced by Takeuchi and Nonaka. It has been a core sub-methodology of Agile since 2001. Scrum values management tools and practices and deals with team-level processes to enable the team to work together effectively for good product delivery (Schwaber and Beedle 2002). Like other ASD methodologies, scrum is an iterative and incremental development method that gives more emphasis to PM values and practices rather than those in requirement, implementation, and so on (Larman 2004). The work is planned and divided into a set of smaller tasks. Scrum processes place heavy emphasis on schedule, and the stakeholders play one of the three roles: product owner, scrum master, and scrum team.

There are some challenges with scrum that may make Kanban a better choice for teams. The Kanban model, coined in Toyota (the name means billboard in Japanese), addresses these challenges with an event-driven approach to scheduling. It is great for improving workflow and minimizing the time cycle, but it also increases the process flexibility (Landau 2017). Kanban is simple and less structured than Scrum; its planning is optional – tasks can be added at any time – and it has no time restrictions.

Rather than working in time-boxed sprints, Kanban has no sprints and puts limits on how many features a team can work on at a given time.

Table 10.3 The 12 Agile principles

Principle	Summary
Responsive planning	This has to do with breaking down the whole system into shorter iterative delivery cycles, and depending on the outcome of the delivery cycle, one can adapt and continue.
Business-value-driven work	Involves prioritizing the organization's work according to primary and secondary business-value outcomes.
Hands-on business outputs	Making sure the business requirements are met and business values are delivered for the organization by checking outputs often.
Direct stakeholder engagement	Active participation of both the internal and external customers throughout the process in order to fulfill their expectations.
Immovable deadlines	Team members are more committed and have the urgency to work towards fixed deadlines rather than flexible deadlines; it helps the organization get ongoing business value.
Management by self-motivation	Trusting self-motivated and organized employees to do the job in their own way rather than telling them how to do it.
Just-in-time communication	Changing the traditional corporate meetings to regular and active face-to-face communication for better knowledge transfer and effective learning. Effective communication means much more than simply talking to someone. It means active participation by all those involved in sharing and understanding information.
Immediate status tracking	An ongoing activity expected from delivery team members to keep everyone in the organization, including business owners, aware of the progress of the work they are doing.
Waste management	Eliminating anything in the organization that cannot lead to high business-value outputs; anything which wastes the time, money, and resources of the organization.
Constantly measurable quality	Involves creating active checkpoints where organizations can assess outputs against both qualitative and quantitative measurements.
Rear-view mirror checking	Provides different tools, such as retrospectives, for the staff, for regularly monitoring and self-correcting their work.
Continuous improvement	To make sure organizations are keeping pace with the current technology, maintaining a competitive advantage, and fulfilling the customers' demand, the work being done is in continuous improvement in each iteration with the involvement of the stakeholders.

As soon as a feature is completed, two things happen: the feature is available for immediate release into production (should the team wish to do so); the team can start working on *whatever* the next highest priority item is (Fichtner 2018), even if that item was just learned today.

10.12   Knowledge acquisition

Attempting to answer the following questions involves acquisition of knowledge from this book and other books, documents, and the Internet.

- Describe the differences between project objectives and project scope definition.
- What are the responsibilities of the project manager?
- Why is project planning important?
- Think about the projects you are working on right now. What has caused you to modify your plan or make adjustments?
- What is the difference between PM and PPM?
- What is quality assurance?
- Why is RM important?
- What is the difference between reactive PMR and proactive PMR?
- What is CE? Why is it important?
- What is CM and its significance?
- Why do companies adopt CE practice?
- What are V-model- advantages and disadvantages, and when should it be used?
- What does ST involve?
- What is the relationship between ST, Lean, and Agile?
- How can Lean product development be used to improve the value stream for an ICT firm?
- How can managers benefit from combining Agile and Lean practices?
- What are the differences between Lean and Agile practices based on a stakeholder perspective?
- What are the differences between Scrum and Kanban?
- What are the good things and bad things about the waterfall approach?

10.13   Knowledge creation

Collaborate with peers on learning or work with others outside the class to narrow down the objectives of each activity. You may access online resources and analyze data and information to create new ideas and balanced solutions. High-level digital tools may be used to develop multimedia presentations, simulations or animations, videos and visual displays, digital portfolios, reflective practice (online publishing and blogging), or well-researched and up-to-date reports.

10.13.1   Project planning

Choose a course project that you are going to do or perhaps have just started. Look at PM phases shown in Figure 10.6 to prepare a three-page e-Portfolio. Consider the second phase of project planning, which may involve the following steps:

- Define the problem to be solved by the project.
- Develop a mission statement answering the two basic questions.
- What are we going to do, and for whom are we going to do it?
- Write statements of major objectives.
- Develop a project strategy that will meet all project objectives.
- Write a scope statement to define project boundaries.
- Develop a work breakdown structure and estimate activity durations, resource requirements, and costs.

10.13.2   PRM

Risk is part of the project planning process. When starting the planning process for a project, one of the first things to think about is: what can go wrong? For this task, continue the activity in 10.13.1 to develop a digital poster by considering a current or recent projects, and practice the six-step process of risk management (identify, analyze, prioritize, assign an owner, respond, and monitor).

10.13.3   CM

Continue the activity 10.13.2 to identify a recent change to your project that required a response. On the basis of what you have learned in this module, answer the following questions:

- Is it appropriate to accept the change?
- Should a change control document be triggered?
- How did this change impact the project triangle?
- To whom should the response be communicated?
- What change thresholds are appropriate to establish for this project?

10.13.4   Project objectives and activities

Once you have determined how you are going to implement your project, you can begin developing your objectives. Objectives are specific, measurable accomplishments designed to address the stated problems and attain your project goal. An objective is an endpoint, not a process, to be achieved within the proposed project period. Completion of objectives must result in specific, measurable outcomes that benefit the community and directly contribute to the achievement of the stated project goal.

10.13.5   Project summary

The project summary is the last component written but will be the first read by an application reviewer. The project summary should not exceed one single-spaced page and should reflect the essence of the entire project. The summary section should include the following:

- A clear statement of the priority area the application is submitted under
- Two or three pertinent facts about the community and the population to be served
- A brief discussion of the problem that exists in the community, relating it to the facts you presented in the first paragraph about your community (one paragraph maximum). This can include your problem statement
- The project goal
- The project objectives
- The impact indicators
- The number of people to be served or impacted by the project

References

Anastasia. 2017. Functions of management: Planning, organizing, staffing and more. https://www.cleverism.com/functions-of-management-planning-organizing-staffing/.

APM. 2018. Agile project management: The what and the why. https://www.apm.org.uk/blog/agile-project-management-the-what-and-the-why/.

BAB. 2017. The 8 principles of QMS. https://www.british-assessment.co.uk/guides/the-8-principles-of-quality-management/.

Balle, M. 2018. What is the relationship between systems thinking and lean? https://thesystemsthinker.com/%EF%BB%BFwhat-is-the-relationship-between-systems-thinking-and-lean/.

Bandecchi, M., B. Melton, and F. Ongaro. 1999. Concurrent engineering applied to space mission assessment and design. EESA Bulletin.

Bergmiller, G. G., and P. R. McCright. 2009. Parallel models for lean and green operations. Proceedings of the Industrial Engineering Research Conference. http://zworc.com/site/publications_assets/parallelmodels.pdf.

Bridges, W., and S. Bridges. 2009. *Managing Transitions*. Third Edition. Philadelphia, PA: Da Campo Press.

Britton, T. 2016. Difference between reactive, predictive and proactive risk management in aviation SMS. http://aviationsafetyblog.asms-pro.com/blog/understand-reactive-predictive-and-proactive-risk-management-in-aviation-sms.

Bruun, P., and R. N. Mefford. 2003. Lean production and the Internet. *International Journal of Production Economics* 89: 247–260.

Coetzee, M., and H. Nisha. 2014. Emotional intelligence as a predictor of employees' career adaptability. *Journal of Vocational Behavior* 84(1): 90–97.

Cooke, J. L. 2010. *Agile Principles Unleased*. Cambridgeshire, UK: IT Governance Publishing.

Downey, J. 2008. Change management. https://www.cimaglobal.com/Documents/ ImportedDocuments/48_Change_Management.pdf.

Farah, J. 2005. Configuration management versus change management – Who's in control. https://www.cmcrossroads.com/article/configuration-mana gement-vs-change-management-whos-control.

Fichtner, A. 2018. Agile versus Lean: Yeah yeah, what's the difference? https://ha ckerchick.com/agile-vs-lean-yeah-yeah-whats-the-difference/.

Fleet, D. D., and T. O. Peterson. 1994. *Contemporary Management*. Third Edition. Boston, MA: Houghton Mifflin Company.

Folwer, K. B. M., and J. A. Highsmith. 2018. Manifesto for Agile software development. http://agilemanifesto.org/.

Habash, R. 2017. *Green Engineering: Innovation, Entrepreneurship, and Design*. Boca Raton, FL: CRC Taylor and Francis.

Hartley, J. R. 1992. *Concurrent Engineering*. Cambridge, MA: Productivity Press.

Haskins, C., K. Forsberg, M. Krueger, D. Walden, and R. Hamelin. 2010. INCOSE Systems Engineering Handbook: A Guide for System Life Cycle Processes and Activities, Vol. 3.2. INCOSE-TP-2003-002-03.2. San Diego, CA: International Council on Systems Engineering.

Heagney, J. 2012. *Fundamentals of Project Management*. Fourth Edition. New York, NY: AMACOM.

Heizer, J., and B. Render. 2014. *Operations Management: Sustainability and Supply Chain Management*. Eleventh Edition. USA: Pearson education.

Highsmith, J. 2012. What is Agility? http://jimhighsmith.com/what-is-agility/.

Hoang, V. Q. 2017. Quality management: The importance of the collaboration between focal firm and first-tier supplier(s). Bachelor's Thesis, April 2017 School of Technology, JAMK University of Applied Sciences. http://doc uments.rec.org/publications/ProposalWriting.pdf.

Holicky, K. 2017. What is the difference between project management and project portfolio management? https://meisterplan.com/blog/difference-project-management-project-portfolio-management/.

ISO. 2015. Quality management principles. International Organization for Standardization. https://www.iso.org/files/live/sites/isoorg/files/archive/ pdf/en/pub100080.pdf; https://www.theseus.fi/bitstream/handle/10024/ 99697/Niemi_Elisa.pdf?sequence=1.

Kaiser, A. 2018. Role of configuration management in DevOps. https://www.plu ralsight.com/guides/role-of-configuration-management-in-devops.

Kleim, R. L., and I. S. Ludin. 1998. *Project Management Practitioner's Handbook*. Nashville, TN: AMACOM Books.

Koontz, H., and C. O'Donnell. 1976. *Management: A Systems and Contingency Analysis of Managerial Functions*. New York, NY: Mc-Graw-Hill.

Landau, P. 2016. What is risk management on projects? https://www.projectm anager.com/blog/what-is-risk-management-on-projects.

Landau, P. 2017. Kanban versus Scrum: Which is better? https://www.projectm anager.com/blog/kanban-vs-scrum-better.

Larman, C. 2003. *Agile and Iterative Development: A Manager's Guide.* Boston, MA: Pearson Education.

MetricStream. 2016. Proactive risk management: The key to business excellence. https://mtcbh.net/mt-content/uploads/2017/01/proactive-risk-mgmt.pdf.

Monat, J. P., and T. F. Gannon. 2015. What is systems thinking? A review of selected literature plus recommendations. *American Journal of Systems Science* 4(1): 11–26.

Mullins, L. 2013. *Management and Organizational Behaviour.* London, UK: FT Publishing International.

Nebiu, B. 1990. Project proposal writing. The Regional Environmental Center for Central and Eastern Europe, Szentendre, Hungary. http://documents.rec.org/publications/ProposalWriting.pdf.

Newton, P. 2015. Principles of project management. http://www.free-management-ebooks.com/dldebk-pdf/fme-project-principles.pdf.

Niemi, E. 2015. Lean project management. Bachelor's Thesis, Supply Chain Management, Hame University of Applied Sciences.

Oberlender, G. D. 2000. *Project Management for Engineering and Construction.* Boston, MA: McGraw-Hill Higher Education.

OGC. 2003. Procurement guide: The integrated project team teamworking and partnering. Office of Government Commerce. https://www.toronto.ca/ext/digital_comm/inquiry/inquiry_site/cd/gg/add_pdf/77/Procurement/Electronic_Documents/UK/UK_OGC_best_practices.pdf.

Olum, Y. 2004. Modern management theories and practices. Faculty of Social Sciences, Makerere University.

Page, S. E. 2011. *Diversity and Complexity.* Princeton, NY: Princeton University Press.

PM4DEV. 2016. Project quality management. Project Management for Development Organizations. https://www.youtube.com/watch?v=H-EioT5i6Jw.

Reinertsen, D. 2005. Let it flow. *Industrial Engineer* 37(6): 40–45.

Rigby, D. 2001. Management tools and techniques: A survey. *California Management Review* 43(2): 139–160.

Schneider, J. 2017. Understanding design thinking, Lean, and Agile. https://www.ami.org.au/imis15/librarymanager/understanding-design-thinking-lean-and-agile.pdf.

Schwaber, K., and M. Beedle. 2002. *Agile Software Development with Scrum.* Upper Saddle River, NJ: Prentice-Hall.

Shahidul Islam, M., and S. Tura. 2013. Exploring the difference between Agile and Lean: A stakeholder perspective. Department of Informatics and Media, Uppsala University. https://www.diva-portal.org/smash/get/diva2:632981/FULLTEXT01.pdf.

Shen, W., Q. Hao, and W. Li. 2008. Computer supported collaborative design: Retrospective and perspective. *Computers in Industry* 59(9): 855–862.

Smith, C. 2014. Understanding the importance of change management. https://change.walkme.com/understanding-the-importance-of-change-management/.

Smith, P. S., and D. G. Reinertsen. 1995. *Developing Products in Half the Time.* New York, NY: Van Nostrand Reinhold.

Synergy. 2018. Practice management. https://www.totalsynergy.com/docs/default-source/downloads/practice-management-guide.pdf?sfvrsn=2.

Trapp, S. 2018. Lean product development and radical innovations – Why Lean is not enough. http://www.stefan-trapp-consulting.de/downloads/leanpro ductdevelopment_engl.pdf.

Turino, J. 1992. *Managing Concurrent Engineering.* New York, NY: Van Nostrand Reinhold.

Turner, R. 2007. *Gower Handbook of Project Management.* Fourth Edition. Hampshire, UK: Gower Publishing Limited.

Winch, G. M. 2010. *Managing Construction Projects: An Information Processing Approach.* Hoboken, NJ: Wiley-Blackwell.

Womack, J. P., and D. T. Jones. 1996. *Lean Thinking: Banish Waste and Create Wealth in Your Corporation.* New York, NY: Simon and Schuster.

Womack, J. P., and D. T. Jones. 2003. *Lean Thinking: Banish Waste and Create Wealth in Your Corporation.* New York, NY: Free Press.

Womack, J. P., D. T. Jones, D. Roos. 1990. *The Machine that Changed the World.* New York, NY: Rawson Associates.

Womack, J. P., D. T. Jones, and D. Roos. 2008. *The Machine that Changed the World.* London, UK: Simon and Schuster.

Yliopisto, O. 2015. Using Lean principles to improve software development practices in a large-scale software intensive company. Master's Thesis, Department of Information Processing Science, University of Oulu.

Ziemke, M. C., and M. S. Spann. 1993. Concurrent engineering's roots in the World War II era. *Concurrent Engineering: Contemporary Issues and Modern Design Tools.* London, UK: Chapman and Hall.

module eleven

Professional practice in artificial intelligence

11.1 Knowledge and understanding

Having successfully completed this module, you should be able to demonstrate knowledge and understanding of:

- The substantial increase in the future applications of AI technologies
- Historical evolution of the many founding concepts of AI
- Current main enablers of AI focus technologies
- Major AI technologies and tools
- Examples from various applications of AI
- The main pillars of AI, namely accountability, responsibility, transparency, safety, and privacy
- The impact of widespread implementation of AI technologies on employment levels
- Ethical engineering of robotics and AI
- Ethical responsibility and international ethical initiatives
- Legal implications of AI technologies
- Ownership of intellectual properties generated by AI technologies

11.2 What is AI?

As a technologist, I see how AI and the fourth Industrial Revolution will impact every aspect of people's lives.

Fei-Fei Li
[from Wired interview (2017)]

AI is not just about technology (acting), but about cognitive science (feeling) and computing (thinking) as well as about all social, ethical, and legal impacts on humanity (Figure 11.1). AI as a science means cognitive science with a focus on intelligence theories (El-Attar 1997). Thinking rationally, including prediction and judgment, is information processing, which is basically computation. AI as a technology means designing systems that act intelligently. As this scenario evolves, what tasks will humans perform that underline their strengths in thinking while staying aware of their limitations in acting?

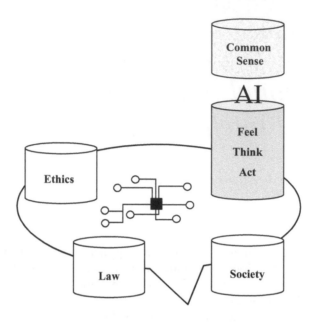

Figure 11.1 AI impact environment.

Rapid advances in the field of AI have deep economic implications as well as at-large societal implications. As important as these effects are likely to be, AI also has the potential to change the innovation process itself, with consequences that may be equally profound and that may, over time, come to dominate the direct effect (Cockburn et al. 2017). However, AI technologies are not about human elimination but the substitution of manual and repetitive tasks with automation.

According to John McCarthy, father of AI, "AI is the science and engineering of making intelligent machines, especially intelligent computer programs". AI has grown into a transdisciplinary field with applications in nearly every aspect of human life. In general, the goal of AI is to develop functioning systems capable of handling complex problems in ways similar to human logic and reasoning. Figure 11.2 outlines the AI functioning approach.

"Artificial" is a concept that refers to something that is made or produced rather than occurring naturally, often replicating something natural. Intelligence is a very complex term. It can be defined in many different ways like logic, understanding, self-awareness, learning, emotional knowledge, planning, creativity, and of course, problem-solving (Schultebraucks 2017). Intelligence is a cornerstone of the human condition, while human intelligence is a work of talents like learning, reasoning, understanding, perceiving, feeling, and the ability to interact with other humans.

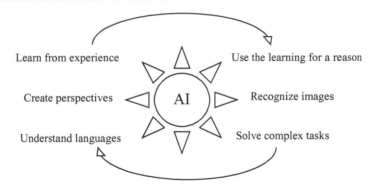

Figure 11.2 AI functioning approach.

Nils J. Nilsson (2010) has provided a useful definition: "AI is that activity devoted to making machines intelligent, and intelligence is that quality that enables an entity to function appropriately and with foresight in its environment". Today, AI is a term used to refer to both the field of research and software capabilities. While the field of AI encompasses a wide range of techniques dating back to the 1950s, the current state of the art uses machine learning, deep learning, and reinforcement learning to identify patterns, produce insights, enhance knowledge-based work, and automate routine tasks (Brookfield 2018). The term AI brings to mind the notion of replacing human intelligence with complex machines that possess the same characteristics as human intelligence. AI mimics certain operations of the human mind and is the term used when machines are able to complete tasks that require human intelligence. Such a philosophical view is relevant especially when looking at the risks of a society where artificial and human intelligence co-exist.

Technically, AI is software that exhibits analytical, decision-making, and learning abilities similar to those of humans. It is also a growing field in computer science that studies intelligent entities, not only from a technical perspective, but also from a philosophical and psychological perspective (Russell and Norvig 2016). AI refers to the ability of a computer program to think and learn like a human, and its snowballing impact on society is undeniable.

AI is not constrained to the digital world. Combined with advances in mechanical and electrical engineering, it has also enlarged the capacity for robots to perform cognitive tasks in the physical world. AI will enable robots to adapt to new working environments with no reprogramming. AI-enabled robots will become increasingly central to logistics and manufacturing, complementing and sometimes displacing human labor in many productive processes (OECD 2015).

The literature today classifies AI into three tiers, which can also be seen as three consecutive generations of AI (Brookfield 2018):

- Narrow AI: Machine intelligence that equals or exceeds human intelligence for specific tasks. Existing examples of such systems would be IBM's Deep Blue (Chess), IBM Watson, and Google's AlphaGo (Go).
- General AI: Machine intelligence meeting the full range of human performance across any task.
- Artificial superintelligence (ASI): A hypothetical type of AI that surpasses human intellect and abilities in nearly all areas.

11.3   History of AI

The question of whether a computer can think is no more interesting than the question of whether a submarine can swim.

Edsger W. Dijkstra
[from "The threats to computing science" (1984)]

Contrary to common perception, AI is not an entirely new discipline. Many of its founding concepts draw on over 2,000 years of insights accumulated in philosophy, logic, mathematics, theories of reasoning, cognitive psychology, and linguistics (Russell and Norvig 2010).

11.3.1   Early history

Historians trace the beginnings of the concept of AI all the way back to ancient times, where thinking machines and artificial creatures were used in myth and storytelling. Pamela McCorduck, in her book *Machines Who Think* (McCorduck 2004), references the Greek myth of Talos, a man created out of bronze by the god Hephaestus to patrol and protect the beaches of Crete. Throughout the next several centuries, inventors and mechanics from many cultures continued to build mechanical toys and tools of increasing complexity but were never able to capture real intelligence. In folklore and myth, artificially intelligent beings continued to be depicted, such as the clay golems from Jewish myth (Evans 2013).

In the eighteenth century, Thomas Bayes provided a background for reasoning about the probability of events. In the nineteenth century, George Boole proved that logical reasoning, dating back to Aristotle, could be implemented analytically in the same manner as solving a system of equations. Towards the end of the nineteenth century, significant milestones in computational machines and logic were reached, with notable mentions being George Boole, who invented Boolean algebra, along with Charles Babbage and Ada Lovelace, who created what is credited as the first mechanical computer.

The beginning of the twentieth century was an exciting time for mathematics and computer science and can be marked as a turning point for AI progress. In 1913, Bertrand Russell and Alfred Whitehead published the *Principia Mathematica*, which helped to create a foundation for mathematics, a landmark work in formal logic. The *Principia Mathematica* in part attempted to describe a set of symbolic logic rules that could be used to derive all mathematical truths. In 1936, a landmark achievement was reached, and the idea of the modern computer was born, with Alan Turing publishing his paper on computable numbers (Turing 1937).

While the early computer scientists and mathematicians of the twentieth century were building the foundations of what would later become modern computational theory, the authors and novelists of the time were imagining what the world might look like in the future.

In 1945, the electrical engineer Vannevar Bush published his essay "As We May Think" (Bush 1945), which was regarded as a visionary look at what the future of computers, AI, and information science might be (Evans 2013).

The prominent ideas behind computer science came from English mathematician Alan Turing in 1950, who proposed a formal model of computing. Turing's paper, entitled "Computing Machinery and Intelligence", imagines the possibility of computers created for simulating intelligence and explores many of the elements now associated with AI, including how intelligence might be tested and how machines might routinely learn. The paper itself began by posing the simple question: can machines think? This was years before the community adopted the term "AI", as coined by John McCarthy.

In 1951, Marvin Minsky and Dean Edmunds built the stochastic neural analog reinforcement calculator (SNARC), the first artificial neural network, using 3,000 vacuum tubes to simulate a network of 40 neurons. In 1952, Arthur Samuel developed the first checkers-playing computer program and the first computer program to learn on its own.

As early as the 1940s and 1950s, scientists in the fields of math, engineering, and computer science had investigated the potentials of artificial brains and were attempting to define the intelligence of the machine. Also, the concept of engineering a machine to implement sequences of inspiration, which had captured the imagination of pioneers such as Charles Babbage, had matured by the 1950s, and resulted in the construction of the first electronic computers.

11.3.2   Modern AI

The modern history of AI is traced back to the year 1956, when John McCarthy, a young computer scientist, proposed the term as a topic for a conference held at Dartmouth College. The goal was to investigate ways in which machines could be made to simulate aspects of intelligence, the essential idea that has continued to drive the field forward. McCarthy is credited with the first use of the term "AI" in the proposal he co-authored for the workshop (McCarthy et al. 1955). The Dartmouth Conference would mark the beginning of a decade of large investment in AI research with many promises for results and returns (Evans 2013). In 1959, Arthur Samuel coined the term "machine learning", and Oliver Selfridge described a model for a process by which computers could recognize patterns.

The years following the Dartmouth Conference were an era of discovery. In the 1960s and 1970s, the focus was primarily on the development of knowledge-based systems. By the late 1960s, the initial promises of AI researchers and theorists began to seem hollow. While progress in AI research had been made in a number of subfields after two decades, the progress was slower than some anticipated. High initial enthusiasm lent itself to a large letdown. In particular, true machine intelligence seemed out of immediate grasp (Evans 2013). Expert systems represented an approach in AI research that became popular throughout the 1970s. An ES uses the knowledge of experts to create a program and can answer questions and solve problems within a clearly defined arena of knowledge, and it uses "rules" of logic.

In the 1980s, knowledge-based and expert systems received big success, in which there were knowledge bases that involved high-level domain knowledge extracted from experts and expressed in specific structured formats. In the mid-1980s, neural networks become widely used with the backpropagation algorithm (first described by Werbos in 1974). During the above period, AI was utilized in several major subjects, including computer vision, natural language processing (NLP), cognition and reasoning, robotics, game theory, and machine learning.

In 1985, the autonomous drawing program, Aaron, created by Harold Cohen, was demonstrated at the Association for the Advancement of AI (AAAI) National Conference. The 1980s also saw military-funded research into autonomous vehicles, as well as continued efforts in robotics and machine vision. Neural networks also arose in academia, which helped pave the way for today's machine learning. Text search and speech recognition became real.

In the early 1990s, there were major advances in all areas of AI, with significant demonstrations in machine learning, intelligent tutoring, case-based reasoning, multi-agent planning, scheduling, uncertain reasoning, data mining, natural language understanding and translation, vision, virtual reality, games, and other topics. AI research shifted its focus to something called an intelligent agent. These intelligent agents can be used for news retrieval services, online shopping, and browsing the Web. Intelligent agents are also sometimes called agents or bots. With the use of big data programs, they have gradually evolved into personal digital assistants, or virtual assistants (Foote 2016).

In the 2000s, Web 2.0, Web services, and Web intelligence emerged in AI systems. The prevalence of the Internet resulted in large volumes of data available online. Also, individuals or organizations produce a great deal of structured and unstructured data which is in need of processing. The storing and processing of such large volumes of data reflects an urgent need and a great challenge in mining and processing this data as knowledge (Berman 2008). In addition, interactive robot pets become commercially available, realizing the vision of the eighteenth-century novelty toymakers.

The current wave of interest in AI started around 2010, promoted by three factors associated with each other (NSTC 2016): the sources of big data, including e-commerce, social media, research community, organization, and government; machine learning approaches and algorithms which have been dramatically improved based on raw material provided by big data; and the powerful computers which support the computing of big data.

11.3.3 Current enablers of AI

AI technologies will be the most disruptive technology over the next several years due to radical computational power, vast amounts of data, and other technologies. In the last two decades, AI grew heavily in every aspect of society. The AI market (hardware and software) has expanded heavily. This is all possible because of cloud infrastructures; the growth in the Internet of Things and big data, faster computers and advancements in machine learning techniques, and specifically the open-source availability of very large data sets. Furthermore, AI research has advanced enormously from a vast level, diversity, and sources of funding and talent, including from major players such as Apple, Amazon, Google, Facebook, IBM, and Microsoft (Desai 2018).

AI enablers are based on several principles, including open-source algorithms, support of local languages and industries, AI expertise and awareness, positive social attitudes and trust in AI, data literacy and policies, and reliable infrastructure. Currently, several competitors are flooding the market with AI offerings, as shown in Table 11.1. Some companies control the entire value chain, while other companies are selling a piece of software which includes AI with vertical and horizontal solutions. Vertical solutions supply the needs of a particular industry, whereas horizontal ones have no industry focus.

Table 11.1 Current main enablers of AI technologies

Enabler/ Platform	Summary
Google	DeepMind (machine learning tool), Cloud Machine Learning (cloud machine learning services).
Amazon	Amazon Machine Learning Services (creates models and finds patterns in data to make predictions on new data).
IBM	Watson (cognitive solutions platform: broad number of offerings spanning cognitive computing, machine learning, deep learning, predictive APIs, and NLP).
Microsoft	Cortana Intelligence Suite (vision, speech, language, knowledge, and search APIs), Microsoft Xiaoice (Chatbot).
Facebook	Facebook Artificial Intelligent Lab – research arm that publishes reports on advancements in collaborative effort, offers open-source software, engages in conferences, and workshops Torch – open-sourced AI modules.
Intel	Xeon Phi (parallel computing product specifically addressing deep learning with all instruction sets based on Intel homegrown solutions), acquired field-programmable gate array (FPGA) through Altera, acquired custom *application-specific integrated circuit* (ASIC) solutions through Nervana acquisition.
Qualcomm	Zeroth: Taking deep learning/AI to consumer devices by enabling localized computing and real-time analytics with a hardware that anticipates user needs and shares the perception of the world naturally.
Nvidia	Nvidia currently dominates the high-end graphics processing unit (GPU) market, today driven by PC/gaming.
Relx	Relx is transitioning from providing electronic reference tools to providing electronic decision tools; it is developing proprietary machine learning algorithms to electronically process articles, analyze data, and link relevant entities so that customers integrate these high-quality data sets to their critical work flows.
Babylon Health	Building the next generation clinic using AI; it is an example of a full-stack AI company.

11.4   *AI technology landscape*

> *Turn[ing] technical brute force into real artificial intelligence requires a deeper understanding of human thinking based on knowledge engineering and reasoning mechanisms.*
>
> **Stephane Nappo**

AI today includes a variety of focus technologies and tools, some already-tested, others relatively new, and more in development. Figure 11.3 outlines a few major AI domain technologies.

NLP is an area of computer science and AI concerned with the interactions between computers and human (*natural*) languages to produce text from computer data. It is currently used in customer service, report generation, and market summaries. Software like Amazon's Alexa, Apple's Siri, Microsoft's Cortana, and Google Assistant all employ NLP to recognize and respond to users' oral questions.

Speech recognition is the ability of a program to recognize and analyze spoken language words and phrases and convert them into data. Speech recognition can be employed by an enterprise for a variety of services, including call routing, voice dialing, voice search, and speech-to-text processing.

Machine learning is a core component within AI that provides computers with the ability to learn without being explicitly programmed. It involves programming computers that can teach themselves and learn from example data or past experience. It consists of the design of learning algorithms, as well as scaling existing algorithms to work with extremely large data sets. One of the most widespread uses of machine learning is image recognition.

AI-integrated hardware includes appliances combined with AI, chips, and GPUs. Google has embedded AI into its hardware to establish an end-to-end control and give it a drive into the future. The impact of integrating AI with hardware goes far beyond consumer applications, such as generating entertainment and bringing about the next level of gaming.

Deep learning is a class of learning procedures to facilitate object recognition in images, video labeling, and activity recognition. It is making significant inroads into other areas of perception, such as audio, speech, and NLP, often coupled with automatic speech recognition. It is quickly becoming a commodity for widely spoken languages with large data sets.

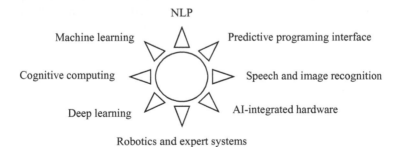

Figure 11.3 Major domains of AI.

Research is now shifting to develop refined and capable systems that are able to interact with people through dialogue, not just react to stylized requests.

Robotics is currently about how to train a machine to interact with the world around it in anticipated ways, how to facilitate manipulation of objects in interactive environments, and how to interact with people. Developments in robotics will rely on commensurate advances to improve the reliability and simplification of computer vision and other forms of machine perception. Deep-learning robots take a more perceptive approach to solving problems, which results in unpredictable behavior that is more human-like and less robotic. Convergence of AI, big data, and the cloud will enable a cloud-based brain that robots can use for high-powered intelligent and intuitive collaboration with humans.

ESs are computer programs aiming to model human expertise in one or more specific knowledge areas. They usually consist of three basic components: a knowledge database with facts and rules representing human knowledge and experience; an inference engine processing consultation and determining how inferences are being made; and an input/output interface for interactions with the user. ESs, as a subset of AI, initially emerged when LISP (programming language, originally specified in 1958), the later dominant programming language in AI and ESs, was invented by John McCarthy at MIT (McCarthy 1960).

11.5   Applications of AI

> To save the humanity compassionate AI is not an option
> but the destination.
>
> **Amit Ray**
> *[from Compassionate Artificial Superintelligence*
> *AI 5.0 – AI with Blockchain, BMI, Drone,*
> *IoT, and Biometric Technologies (2018)]*

In the past, AI was mainly used for robotics and solving complex problems. Today, AI is expected to improve many aspects of life and change several paradigms in industries including manufacturing, robotics, military, healthcare, transport, e-commerce business, governance, finance, and warehouse operations. Technological advances in AI promise to be pervasive, with impacts, implications, and promises of an even better role in the near future.

11.5.1   Intelligent automation

A definition of automation is offered by Balfe et al. (2015) as "the performance of tasks by machines (often computers) rather than human operators often to increase efficiency and reduce variability". Division in opinion is evident in regard to the impact of AI on automation. Some see that the combination of AI and automation is currently helping industries exceed conventional performance tradeoffs to achieve unprecedented levels of efficiency and quality. On the other hand, others believe in an irresistible march of AI and automation that will lead to mass automation of jobs, rising inequality, and economic strife, unless impending action is taken (Allianz 2018). AI is poised to replace people in certain kinds of jobs. However, in many realms, AI will likely replace tasks rather than jobs in the near-term and will also create new kinds of jobs. AI, robotics, and autonomous systems can bring prosperity, contribute to well-being, and help to achieve moral ideals and socio-economic goals if designed and deployed wisely.

11.5.2   Autonomous driving

One of the most advanced AI applications is autonomous driving. This technology offers the possibility of profoundly changing transportation. The recognition that autonomous driving is a prediction problem-solvable with machine learning meant that autonomous vehicles could start to become a reality in the marketplace years earlier than had been anticipated (Agrawal et al. 2017). This will change the way individual travel is used and organized and may blur the difference between private and public transport. Equipping cars and light vehicles with this technology will likely reduce collisions, energy consumption, and pollution; eliminate human errors; substantially affect safety and congestion; and increase mobility for those who are presently unable or unwilling to drive. Autonomous transportation will soon be commonplace and, as most people's first experience with physically embodied AI systems, will strongly influence the public's perception of AI.

As AI existing on a substrate of computing power, these machines will be open to attack and intromission. This gives rise to a range of important and hard moral and ethical questions. First, questions about safety, security, prevention of harm, and the mitigation of risks. Second, questions about human moral responsibility and ethical considerations located in dynamic and complex socio-technical systems with advanced AI and robotic components, and fundamental rights of privacy and data protection. Third, they give rise to questions about governance, regulation, design, development, inspection, monitoring, testing, and certification (EC 2018). With autonomous driving, the moral responsibility is shifting from a human driver to some programmed algorithm.

The question here is: are humans willing to give up the right and responsibility to make moral decisions in life-and-death situations to the engineers who design these machines? To answer this question, consumers, regulators, manufacturers, and the engineers who design these autonomous systems need to think hard about the social and ethical impacts of these new emerging technologies (Witten 2018).

11.5.3 Healthcare

AI technologies are rapidly advancing enablers in healthcare. These technologies seem promising in healthcare because they have the potential to improve quality of life and health consequences for a substantial number of patients in future years (Nadimpalli 2017). Healthcare is the sector where AI is probably expected to deliver the most societal benefit, but humans will still have an important role to play. Although AI can improve diagnosis, which is likely to lead to more effective treatments and better patient care, treatment and care will still rely on human judgment (Agrawal et al. 2017).

In healthcare, there has been an immense forward leap in collecting useful data from personal monitoring devices and mobile applications, from electronic health records in clinical settings and, to a lesser extent, from surgical robots designed to assist with medical procedures and service robots supporting hospital operations. This could improve health outcomes and the quality of life for millions of people in the coming years (AI100 2016). AI is also helping to speed up telemedicine. It is able to improve online consultations by recognizing patient history and symptoms more quickly and suggesting the finest course of action.

While AI improves healthcare, the adoption of these technologies is not without considerable potential risks. The clinical setting, healthcare provisions, and patient data necessitate the highest level of accuracy, reliability, security, and privacy. The data collected by these devices needs to be secured with the highest security standards (Hamid 2017). On the other hand, AI is replacing jobs that formerly needed humans with computers. It is being applied to repetitive types of jobs or actions in healthcare.

11.5.4 Education

Education is a domain mainly ruled by human-to-human interaction, and integration of AI has been slower to develop the necessary human-like attributes of responsiveness, adaptability, and understanding (Faggella 2017). Therefore, it is not uncommon for educators to fear how their role would be diminished by the use of technology. However, at the same time, it would be absolutely unwise to overlook the enhancements and potentials that AI can offer in education. In fact, AI is assumed to bring about a remarkable upgrade in the overall educational experience.

Though quality education will always require active engagement by human teachers, AI promises to enhance education at all levels, especially by providing personalized learning, which offers many benefits for students with different learning styles. Just like human tutors, intelligent tutoring systems are able to understand the style of learning preferred by students. NLP, machine learning, and crowdsourcing have boosted online learning and enabled teachers in higher education to increase the size of their classrooms while tailoring to the learning needs and styles of individual students.

Smart content creation, from digitized guides of textbooks to customizable learning digital interfaces, is being introduced at all levels, from elementary to post-secondary to corporate environments. Companies are creating smart digital content platforms, complete with content delivery, practice exercises, and real-time feedback and assessment (Faggella 2017).

Woolf et al. (2013) has proposed five key areas for ongoing research in using AI for the delivery of educational services. These areas include mentors for every learner; learning twenty-first century skills; interaction data for learning; universal access to global classrooms; and lifelong and life-wide learning. The above seems a useful framework for framing objectives and generating aligned ideas, as researchers and companies continue to move forward in developing AI applications in education.

11.5.5   Intelligent product design and smart manufacturing

Smart manufacturing is a general concept currently under continuous development. It is an emerging form of intelligent product design which can be viewed as the intersection of AI and manufacturing. An intelligent product has two major modules: the intelligent functions and the intelligent software components. The intelligent software makes all decision-making tasks. It retrieves the real world completely through the intelligent functions and services to generate intelligent products.

Smart manufacturing reflects the impact of smart technologies such as IoT, cloud computing, cyber-physical systems, and data science. It integrates manufacturing platforms with sensors, computing resources, communication technologies, control, simulation, data intensive modeling, and predictive engineering.

The digitalization and interconnection of products, value chains, and business models presents considerable market opportunities for companies (PWC 2018). Figure 11.4 outlines a chain of smart manufacturing

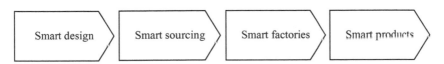

Figure 11.4 Smart manufacturing chain of activities.

activities. Smart design involves rapid prototyping and 3D modeling. Smart sourcing provides automated ordering services, just-in-sequence deliveries, route optimization, and condition monitoring. Smart factories involves flexible production, preventive maintenance and quality, remote and guided maintenance, and Lean manufacturing. Smart products provides new revenue models, forward-looking services, automatic parts ordering, and preventive maintenance.

11.5.6   Retail

AI influences the international business environment greatly, providing important benefits to both the sellers and buyers in retail. The technology taps into the retail domain's information pool associated with advertising, think-product development, and online search, among others. Since retailers embraced market research for many years, AI allows them to reengineer complicated data into streamlined and easier experiences for customers and retailers alike. Its machine learning and predictive instruments often offer relief to the buyer efforts (Nadimpalli 2017).

When discussing opportunities in AI, e-commerce is widely considered to be a space with a lot of potential, with AI trends explaining that many techniques are well-positioned to make a big impact on the industry. AI enables retailers to drive sales and predict demand, to gain a good understanding of consumer behavior, and to present highly precise personalized promotions. AI computerizes decisions through algorithms informed by machine learning, a technology that enables computers to observe and learn from large sets of data and make decisions without the need for human involvement. Figure 11.5 explores eight different ways AI can be used in e-commerce, with real-life examples where possible.

AI is used in retail to explore customer data, adapt the approach through which the business interacts with shoppers, and predict consumer demand to enable better inventory management. Amazon Echo is one of the best-known applications of AI by a retailer.

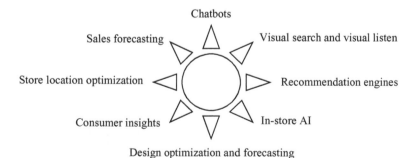

Figure 11.5 Retail applications of AI.

11.6   Concerns with AI

AI will probably most likely lead to the end of the world,
but in the meantime, there'll be great companies.

Sam Altman

In simple terms, AI aims to extend and augment the capacity and efficiency of mankind in tasks of remaking nature and governing society through intelligent machines, with the final goal of realizing a society where people and machines co-exist harmoniously together (Bench-Capon and Dunne 2007). With AI technologies set to transform the way that we live and work, it raises the inevitable question of how much these technologies will impact businesses, consumers, and the economy more generally.

11.6.1   Elements of concern

AI may be thought of as a comprehensive concept that may answer the following question: is it possible to build a machine that has intelligence, specifically a human level of intelligence? AI may be capable of substituting for humans because of several characteristics which are progressively more sophisticated. These include the processing of large amounts of data; learning from example data; recognizing objects; inferring the future state of an object or situation; and identifying decisions based on past, present, and future states. Does all that carry any risk or concern?

Risks and benefits can appear in the short- or long-term depending on how long it takes for strong AI applications to be deployed in the real world. The rate of adoption depends on the level of investment in R&D in each application field. AI comes with both massive potential benefits and enormous risks. With the increasing know-how of AI, consumers are concerned of the AI capabilities and potential associated with taking over all aspects of life.

It is noteworthy that most of the well-informed consumers view AI in a positive light (Kristin 2017). Advocates of AI anticipate that it will promote time-saving, offer relevant and improved information access, and allow engagement in dangerous tasks (Kaplan 2017).

Several areas of concern are crucial for identifying emerging AI risks, namely software accessibility, safety, accountability, liability, and ethics, as outlined in Figure 11.6. By addressing each of these areas, responsible development and introduction of AI becomes less risky for society.

11.6.2   Technology

Currently, AI technology is the most significant topic of concern that is dominating society, alongside other important issues such as climate

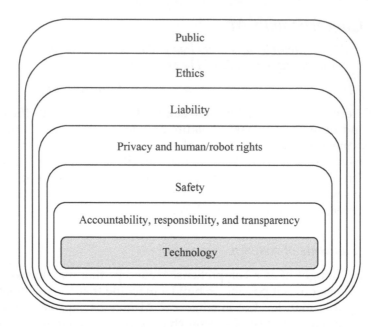

Figure 11.6 Elements of concern about future AI.

change and even terrorism. The unprecedented technological advances in AI may occur very quickly and without adequate management and controls.

Today, there is much speculation regarding the future situation where AI systems will become more intelligent, perhaps even able to understand their own design and create more intelligent successor systems. Eventually, machines may become super intelligent, that is, more intelligent than humans (Bostrom and Yudkowsky 2011). For instance, AI could publish outstanding academic papers, patents, or make money on the stock market. Furthermore, super intelligent machines would be able to self-modify their goal systems, meaning they would acquire a level of autonomy. While current AI technologies are not intelligent enough to overshadow humans, some scientists warn of the danger of losing control over machines (for example, highly intelligent drones/lethal autonomous weapon machines) in the future (Russell et al. 2015).

According to the IEEE Global Initiative, AI technologies can be narrowly conceived from an ethical standpoint; be legal, profitable, and safe in their usage; and yet not positively contribute to human well-being. This means technologies created with the best intentions but without considering well-being metrics can still have dramatic negative consequences on people's mental health, emotions, sense of themselves, their autonomy, their ability to achieve their goals, and other dimensions of well-being.

11.6.3   Accountability, responsibility, and transparency

Responsible AI rests on three main pillars: accountability, responsibility, and transparency (Dignum 2017). "Accountability" refers to the need to explain and justify decisions and actions to partners and users of AI systems. To ensure accountability, decisions must be derivable from, and explained by, the decision-making algorithms used. This includes the need for representation of the moral values and societal norms held in the context of operation, which the agent uses for deliberation. Accountability for an algorithm and how it is applied begins with those who design and deploy the system that relies on it (Dignum 2018). Responsible innovation requires designers to anticipate, reflect, and engage with users of AI. Therefore, through education and awareness, citizens, lawyers, and governments have a role to play in developing accountability structures.

"Responsibility" refers to the role of people themselves and to the capability of AI systems to make decisions and identify errors or unexpected results. As the chain of responsibility grows, means are needed to link an AI system's decisions to the fair use of data and to the actions of stakeholders involved in the system's decision.

"Transparency" refers to the need to describe, inspect, and reproduce the mechanisms through which AI systems make decisions and learn to adapt to their environment, and to the governance of the data used or created. Current AI algorithms are basically black boxes. However, regulators and users should demand explanation and clarity about the data used. Methods are needed to inspect algorithms and their results and to manage data, their provenance, and their dynamics (Dignum 2018). When people are able to understand how something works, they are more likely to use the system appropriately and to trust those who develop and deploy it (Zicari 2018).

11.6.4   Safety

AI is enormously transformative, but that is not to say everyone sees it in a positive and safe light. In the context of AI, safety means the ability of AI systems to operate without causing harm to humans. As AI is gradually embedded in all features of life, both noticeably and unnoticeably, ensuring safety becomes a challenge. AI may help create and enforce parameters of safety by codifying a set of behaviors that are known to boost safe practices.

Public security and safety are instrumental to guarantee development. Owing to this, many cities and countries around the world are integrating AI technologies to aid in fighting crime. These technologies are in the form of surveillance cameras, which easily identify anomalies that may result in crime, predictive policing applications, and drones (Nissan 2012).

On the other hand, safety may become jeopardized due to technical bugs or errors within the system, biased data, neglect of maintenance, lack of privacy, use in unintended contexts, or if the AI learns unsafe behavior once it is operating. In order to foster safety and controllability, AI systems that are intended to have their capabilities improved to the point where the above issues begin to apply should be designed to avoid those issues preemptively.

11.6.5   Privacy and human/robot rights

AI may challenge different dimensions of human rights, for example in terms of freedoms (privacy and data protection, ownership, autonomy, personality), equality (more specifically, non-discrimination), and justice (fair trial, access to justice) (van Est et al. 2017).

Privacy is an individual's right to have control over their own data. It refers to the condition of being unobserved and the confidentiality of an individual or group's personal and behavioral data. The collection, analysis, sharing, and use of personal data is becoming an increasingly important feature for AI systems (Campolo et al. 2017). Generally, AI systems collect a lot of information from human users. This presents a potential risk of breaking data protection rules and, ultimately, human privacy and trust (Luxton 2014), partly because AI systems can gather data and move around in the real world because they can be perceived by humans as social actors.

Personal data is often collected, used, and shared on an opt-out basis, or without the option to consent. The increasing ease with which intelligent systems collect and analyze personal data, as well as the ability for companies to share this information, has been critiqued for challenging current understandings of privacy and straining the laws and regulations in place to protect personal information (Campolo et al. 2017).

According to the IEEE Global Initiative (IEEE 2018): to best honor human rights, society must assure the safety and security of AI so that they are designed and operated in a way that benefits humans. Accordingly, standards and regulatory bodies should be established to oversee processes and assure that the use of AI does not infringe upon human rights, freedoms, dignity, and privacy, and of traceability to contribute to building public trust in AI. For the foreseeable future, AI should not be granted rights and privileges equal to human rights: AI should always be subordinate to human judgment and control.

11.7   Impact of AI on employment

We're going to become caretakers for the robots. That's what the next generation of work is going to be.

Gray Scott

Major advanced economies have experienced various sectoral shifts in employment, first in agriculture and then in manufacturing. In the US, the agricultural share of total employment declined from 60 percent in 1850 to less than 5% by 1970, while manufacturing fell from 26% of total US employment in 1960 to below 10% in the 2010s. Other countries have experienced even faster declines. Fifty years ago, three-quarters of workers in China were employed in agriculture, but with the advent of technologies, agriculture now only accounts for around one-quarter of employment, which became dominated by manufacturing and services in turn. Throughout these large shifts of workers across occupations and sectors, overall employment has continued to grow. New industries and occupations have emerged to absorb workers displaced by technology (Felipe et al. 2016; Lund and Manyika 2017).

Another phase or shift is in the making: one of the most significant potential social impacts of the widespread implementation of AI technologies is on employment. Today, there are legitimate concerns that AI applications on a large scale may exacerbate inequality, especially via their impact on unskilled workers by acquiring robots and automated systems. Opinion is divided on the above topic, ranging from those who predict large-scale job losses through the automation of non-routine work, through to those who suggest that large-scale job losses are unlikely.

Fears of large-scale technological unemployment are nothing new, and in fact typically accompany every wave of radical technological development, dating back to the machine-breaking Luddites in eighteenth-century England. The Luddites attempted to sabotage the implementation of automated production technologies because of fears that they would eliminate the need for factory workers (Hislop et al. 2017). In the 1930s, John Maynard Keynes postulated his "technological unemployment theory" as technological change causes loss of jobs (Keynes 1937).

There is even fear that advances in AI will be so rapid as to replace all human jobs – including those that are largely cognitive or involve judgment – within a single generation. This scenario is highly unlikely, but AI will gradually invade almost all employment sectors, requiring a shift away from human labor that computers are able to take over.

Technological development, and in particular AI, has major implications for labor markets. It can affect employment in two major ways, first by directly displacing workers from tasks they were previously performing, and second by increasing the demand for labor in industries that arise or develop due to technological progress (Petropoulos 2018). There are clear examples of industries in which digital technologies have had profound impacts, good and bad, and other sectors in which automation will likely make major changes in the near future. Many of these changes have been driven strongly by routine digital technologies. It is clear that technology can substitute humans in routine tasks, whether manual or intellectual, but as yet cannot replace humans in non-routine tasks.

Understanding these changes should provide insights into how AI will affect future labor demand, including the shift in skill demands. To be successful, AI innovations will need to overcome understandable human fears of being marginalized. AI will likely replace tasks rather than jobs in the near term and will also create new kinds of jobs. But the new jobs that will emerge are harder to imagine in advance than the existing jobs that will likely be lost (Ashkenas and Parlapiano 2016). In general, changes in employment usually happen gradually, often without a sharp transition, a trend likely to continue as AI slowly moves into the workplace.

Equally important is that none of this industrial history, from car frames to AI, was the result of a planned evolution. The only kind of plan needed today is one to assist the few displaced workers whose livelihoods may get forever sidelined by the technological developments that help everyone else progress (Atikian 2018).

11.8 Ethical engineering of robotics and AI

> *Some people worry that artificial intelligence will make us feel inferior, but then, anybody in his right mind should have an inferiority complex every time he looks at a flower.*
>
> **Alan Kay**

A determination to adopt AI can raise important ethical and moral issues for society. Ethics is about how we relate to human beings; how we relate to community and to the world; how we even understand what it is to live a human life (Davey 2017). Today, there is a lot of power in robotics and AI, creating endless possibilities for the best and probably for the worst. The greatest ethical challenge humans face in this regard has yet to be realized.

11.8.1 Ethical issues and challenges

Ethics, in the context of AI, refers to whether, when, and how autonomous devices should make decisions, and what values should guide those decisions. The values embedded into AI systems will determine whether, and how, these systems will act in moral situations (Brookfield 2018). AI systems give rise to a range of important and hard ethical issues: first, issues about safety, security, the prevention of harm, and the mitigation of risks (EU 2018); second, issues about ways to implement AI including trust, fairness, and honesty in AI models. These issues require ethical analysis always, which depends on getting the facts first; only then can evaluation start. Figure 11.7 outlines these moral and ethical issues.

Machines may be super-capable, but do they possess the wisdom to choose what you or other humans believe is the right thing to do? How much scope do you want to give self-driving cars, or other autonomous systems, to act and make decisions on your behalf (Witten 2018)? In order to ensure that AI systems will uphold human values, design and manufacturing techniques should integrate ethical values and address social concerns. Greater autonomy must come with greater responsibility, even when these notions are necessarily different when applied to machines than to people (Dignum 2018). An ethical framework needs to underpin the building blocks of the AI and robotics ecosystem.

AI community should work to ensure that the tradition of openness and a safety mindset be maintained when it comes to safety research. AI researchers should be encouraged to freely discuss AI safety and security problems and share best practices with their peers across institutional, industrial, and national boundaries.

AI will never generate trust in the way humans do. Nevertheless, it is critical that users trust AI systems by building trustworthy algorithms; designing algorithms which are aware of their uncertainty; and making well-founded decisions. This can be achieved by improving fairness and removing unwanted bias in AI systems by improving data efficiency and methodologies for collecting and labeling data. However, inherent human biases threaten the integrity of the data that train AI systems and therefore undermine AI neutrality and ultimately erode the trust in AI platforms. This occurs when designers unwittingly introduce bias into the data on which the algorithm is trained, ultimately surfacing in AI systems (Cle 2018). Steve Adire, AI start-up advisor, suggests that "effective

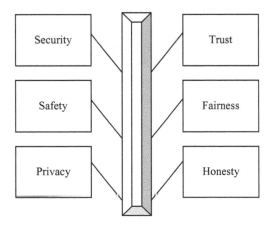

Figure 11.7 Ethical issues for AI.

mechanisms in algorithms must be developed to filter out biases and build ethics into AI with ability to read between the lines to get closer to common sense reasoning" (Cle 2018).

Today, there is a need for machine learning models to be embedded with the capability to read between the lines to understand what can be implied in addition to what is explicitly stated in the algorithms. Thus, to achieve effective AI outcomes, algorithms should be built and trained to be ethically-sound and neutral, requiring diversity among the researchers who design them. Algorithms are not born agnostic and therefore rely on human choices that must be accounted for during the product design process in order to prevent biased automated decision-making. In order to understand the basis on which decisions are made, algorithms must be honest about how they are making decisions, requiring them to be transparent and interpretable. This requires saliency techniques which explain causality from input to output and interoperability of black box models (Kendall 2018). Black box AI refers to the complex network of perceptions that are hidden between the input and output layers, making it very difficult to track the process on which the model bases its decisions.

Engineering education often incorporates components and even whole courses on professional ethics, which is the ethics that human practitioners should follow when acting within their profession. Advances in AI have made it crucial to expand the scope of how we think about ethics; the key questions of ethics, which have, in the past, been asked only about humans and human behaviors. These questions should be asked about human-designed or built machines, because these machines are capable of making their own decisions based on their own perceptions of the complex environment.

11.8.2 *Ethical responsibility*

The question of AI ethics is making everyone anxious. The main worry is about the lack of empathy, the way to know how to do the right thing, and how to judge and punish machine beings. While it is necessary to look at responsibility, this is not about punishment. The ability or inability to punish a machine is a matter of how to respond to unethical behavior, not how to assess it (Hammond 2016). The question of whether a machine has done something wrong is very different than the issue of what to do about it.

Ethical perspectives of AI and robotics should be addressed in at least two ways. First, the engineers developing systems need to be aware of possible ethical challenges that should be considered, including avoiding misuse and allowing for human inspection of the functionality of the algorithms and systems (Bostrom and Yudkowsky 2014). Second, when moving toward advanced autonomous systems, the systems should themselves be able to do ethical decision-making to reduce the risk of unwanted behavior (Wallach and Allen 2009).

The broader role and ethical responsibility of an engineer is to design solutions that take into account human values and the impact on society. A background in engineering and philosophy may help to talk about human values and understand how to translate human values into solutions. When good technology functions well, it is efficient and easy to use and incorporates a layer of ethics; it takes into account human values, and it respects the user's autonomy and preferences (Witten 2018).

Codes of ethics serve a role in any field that impacts human lives, including engineering. Technological organizations like the IEEE and the ACM also adhere to codes of ethics to keep technology beneficial, but no concrete ethical framework exists to guide all researchers involved in AI's development. By codifying AI research ethics, researchers can more clearly frame AI's development within society's broader quest of improving human well-being (Davey 2017).

As AI is one of the most ambitious scientific and engineering adventures of all time, there is an ethical requirement for engineers to broaden their professional duties to account for the social consequences of their technologies (Burton et al. 2017). Because engineers already function intentionally, or unintentionally, as *de facto* policymakers by introducing new technologies that often have strong social effects (whether they anticipate or think about these effects or not), they should be trained and develop the knowledge to fulfill the duties of a more robust public role. Companies and engineers should engage and seek input from the public on ethical and social issues to inform and influence their design solutions.

The role of an AI ethicist is not to block or roll back advances in technology, but to enhance the technology by giving users and society at large meaningful choices and control over its use and effects. Engineers can help make technology more user-friendly in an ethical way that respects the user's autonomy and preferences and takes into account social impact (Witten 2018).

11.8.3   Ethical initiatives

Organizations that develop and use AI systems require ethical principles to lead them through the experiment that is already upon us and that which lies ahead. These principles should be a practical and actionable guide (MacCarthy 2018).

Some of the most prominent initiatives towards the formulation of ethical principles regarding AI and autonomous systems have stemmed from industry, practitioners, and professional associations, such as the

IEEE's second version of "Ethically Aligned Design"; ITU's Global Summit "AI for Good" (ITU 2018), and the ACM major AAAI/ACM conference on "AI, Ethics, and Society" (ACM 2018). Within the private sector, companies such as IBM, Microsoft, and Google's DeepMind have established their own ethic codes on AI and joined forces in creating broad initiatives such as the "Partnership on AI: www.partnershiponai.org" or "OpenAI: www.openai.com", which bring together industry and non-profit and academic organizations.

One of the leading initiatives calling for a responsible development of AI has been launched by the Future of Life Institute and has culminated in the creation of the "Asilomar AI Principles": futureoflife.org/ai-principles. This list of 23 fundamental principles to guide AI research and application has been signed by hundreds of stakeholders, signatories representing predominantly scientists, AI researchers, and industry. A similar participatory process has been launched upon the initiative of the "Forum on the Socially Responsible Development of AI", held by the University of Montreal in 2017, in reaction to which a first draft of a potential "Declaration for a Responsible Development of AI" has been developed (EC 2018).

The European Group on Ethics (EGE) in science and new technologies (EGE 2018) calls for a wide-ranging and systematic public engagement and deliberation on the ethics of AI, robotics, and autonomous technology and on the set of values that societies choose to embed in the development and governance of these technologies. This process, in which the EGE stands ready to play its part, should provide a platform for joining together the diverse global initiatives outlined above. It should integrate a wide, inclusive, and far-reaching societal debate, drawing upon the input of diverse perspectives, where those with different expertise and values can be heard. The EGE urges the European Union to place itself at the vanguard of such a process and calls upon the European Commission to launch and support its implementation. Table 11.2 outlines EGE ethical principles and democratic prerequisites of AI.

11.9   Legal implications of AI

> *I know that lawyers are quite worried about [AI] and I*
> *think appropriately.*
>
> **Malcolm Gladwell**

Ethics and law are inseparably connected in modern society, and many legal decisions arise from the analysis of various ethical issues. Today, there has been much discussion about how to legally regulate robots and AI-related technologies.

Table 11.2 EGE ethical principles and democratic prerequisites of AI

Principle	Summary
Human dignity	Recognition of the inherent human state of being worthy of respect; must not be violated by autonomous technologies.
Autonomy	Freedom of the human being. This translates into human responsibility and thus control over and knowledge about autonomous systems, as they must not impair freedom of human beings to set their own standards and norms and be able to live according to them.
Responsibility	Autonomous systems should only be developed and used in ways that serve the global, social, and environmental good, as determined by outcomes of deliberative democratic processes.
Justice, equity, and solidarity	AI should contribute to global justice and equal access to the benefits and advantages that AI, robotics and 'autonomous' systems can bring. Discriminatory biases in data sets used to train and run AI systems should be prevented or detected, reported, and neutralized at the earliest stage possible.
Democracy	Key decisions on the regulation of AI development and application should be the result of democratic debate and public engagement.
Rule of law and accountability	Rule of law, access to justice, and the right to redress and a fair trial provide the necessary framework for ensuring the observance of human rights standards and potential AI-specific regulations.
Security, safety, bodily and mental integrity	Safety and security of autonomous systems materialize in three forms: (1) external safety for their environment and users, (2) reliability and internal robustness, e.g. against hacking, and (3) emotional safety with respect to human-machine interaction.
Data protection and privacy	In an age of ubiquitous and massive collection of data through digital communication technologies, the right to protection of personal information and the right to respect for privacy are crucially challenged.
Sustainability	AI technology must be in line with the human responsibility to ensure the basic preconditions for life on our planet, continued prospering for mankind, and preservation of a good environment for future generations.

11.9.1   Clarifying the legal status

As some types of robots begin to display characteristics that resemble those of human actors, some governmental entities and private commentators have concluded that it is time to examine how legal regimes should categorize and treat various types of AI. Should the law treat such systems as legal persons with all the rights and responsibilities that personhood entails, or should they be treated as products and tools of human developers? Such a status seems initially remarkable until consideration is given to the long-standing legal personhood status granted to corporations, governmental entities, and the like, none of which are human even though they are run by humans (IEEE 2008).

Society has historically placed a strong emphasis on the legal concept of a person; it determines the approach of rules on ownership and liability. Throughout history, personhood was attached to the human: individuals own items, commit crimes, or enter into contractual relations. The impact of personhood discussions for AI is easily seen in a couple of areas, including IP rights and liability (Monthly 2017).

As AI is still in its infancy, the ramifications of its advancement are not yet fully understood. Nonetheless, certain jurisdictions have been proactive at developing frameworks for AI regulation. As the One Hundred Year Study on AI report from Stanford University notes (Stanford 2016): "as a transformative technology, AI has the potential to challenge any number of legal assumptions in the short, medium, and long term. Precisely how law and policy will adapt to advances in AI, and how AI will adapt to values reflected in law and policy, depends on a variety of social, cultural, economic, and other factors, and is likely to vary by jurisdiction".

Systems that use AI technologies are becoming increasingly autonomous in terms of complexity, impact on the world, and the fading capability of humans to realize, predict, and control operation of their functioning. One area that deserves particular attention is autonomous driving for exploring a number of legal issues in the AI context. Its use has consequences in tort, contract, IP, and insurance law. In the context of personal injury, should the AI be programmed to protect the driver over a third party in an impending collision? If an injury does result from a collision with an autonomous vehicle, is the designer of the AI liable in tort (Ramsey 2017)? The legal problems run even deeper. A system that learns from information it receives from the outside world can act in ways that its creators could not have predicted, and predictability is crucial to modern legal approaches. What is more, such systems can operate independently from their designers or operators, thus complicating the task of determining responsibility (Karliuk 2018). These characteristics pose problems related to predictability and the ability to act independently while at the same time not being held responsible.

11.9.2 Will AI replace lawyers?

As AI technology improves, predictions by machines will increasingly take the place of predictions by humans. As this scenario unfolds, what roles will humans play that emphasize their strengths in judgment while recognizing their limitations in prediction (Agrawal et al. 2017)?

Technology has already transformed the way that law is practiced. As a transformative technology, AI has the potential to challenge any number of legal assumptions in the short, medium, and long-term. Precisely how law and policy will adapt to advances in AI and how AI will adapt to values reflected in law and policy depends on a variety of social, cultural, economic, and other factors, and is likely to vary by jurisdiction (Desai 2018).

The use of AI in law will be an evolution, not a revolution. AI is already changing almost every business and activity that attorneys deal with, some more quickly and radically than others, and the legal profession will not be spared from this disruptive change. Incorporation of AI into a law firm's systems and operations is a gradual learning process, so early adopters will have a major advantage over firms that lag in adopting the technology (Marchant 2018). AI is more than legal technology. It is the next great hope that will revolutionize the legal profession (Sobowale 2016).

While AI has many attributes for its many different applications, two are currently most important for legal applications. First, machine learning is the capability of computers to teach themselves and learn from experience. This means that AI can do more than blindly adhere to what it has been programmed to do, but can learn from experience and data to constantly improve its capabilities. This is how Google's DeepMind system was able to defeat the world's best human Go players. Second, NLP is the capability of computers to understand the meaning of spoken or written human speech and to apply and integrate that understanding to perform human-like analysis (Marchant 2018).

11.9.3 The role of AI in IP

Under the fourth Industrial Revolution, AI is pushing innovation in new ways and accelerating with technological advancements in computing power, data, and algorithms. As technology advances, so too does the ability to use AI tools in previously unachievable ways. This has led to a recent uptrend in AI innovation ranging from start-ups to long-established companies. IP protects and encourages innovation and creativity. As such, companies, investors, and entrepreneurs should be aware of key IP considerations as applied to AI innovation. IP relates to intangible assets, including inventions, brands, new technologies, source code, and artistic works. In particular, IP pertains to patents, trademarks, copyright, and industrial design (Medeiros and Sanft 2018).

When patent law and copyright law came into being, it was very clear that inventors and authors were natural persons, because there wasn't anything else that was up to the task. The world is different now, in that AI can do some things that might be considered inventive enough to patent and can create works that might be considered creative enough to be copyrightable (Albert and Block 2018).

In the IP domain, questions arise as to the ownership of IP generated by AI. Securing IP may be a major hurdle for new technologies at the best of times. However, AI and its technologies like machine learning, an evolving area of law, bring their own distinctive challenges, where machine learning by its nature constantly writes its own code to improve itself. In autonomous vehicles, for example, consider a situation where the vehicle's AI learns a new method of predicting potential accidents from the data it collects while transporting its passengers. Assuming the new invention is patentable on its own, to whom does that IP belong? It is likely that for now, these issues will be explicitly spelled out in the contracts governing the relationship between driver and manufacturer, but legislative changes may ultimately be required to eliminate the uncertainty.

Copyright is an important IP asset for AI, as it protects the technology product (code and data) from unauthorized use and reproduction. Contributors to the technology should be identified and tracked. Ownership and confidentiality of the copyright should clearly be set out in a written agreement. Companies should have policies for developers incorporating third-party copyright, even if unintentionally, as it may impact ownership of the technology and freedom to operate. (Medeiros and Sanft 2018).

AI involves software, which is increasingly difficult to patent. Patent offices, along with the courts, have struggled with establishing clear delineations of what is patentable and what is not patentable. The claims have to clearly define the patent-eligible innovation with the patent description clearly describing how to make and use the innovation.

For the near future, lawyers should familiarize themselves with the underlying concepts of AI, and conversely, IT professionals should familiarize themselves with the concepts of IP. For entrepreneurs who design or use AI systems, constant consideration of IP issues is essential to protect their achievements (Lavallée 2017).

In Europe, according to Article 52 of the 1973 *European Patent Convention*, computer programs are not patentable. Thus the underlying programming of an AI system would not be patentable under this legal system. Copyright is perhaps the most obvious form of IP for AI. Source codes have long been recognized as works within the meaning of the Canadian Copyright Act and in similar legislation in most other countries. Some jurisdictions have even enacted laws specifically aimed at software protection (Lavallée 2017). In addition to copyright, the protection afforded by trade secrets should not be underestimated. More specifically, in the field of computer science, it is rare for customers to have access to the full source code. Also, in AI, source codes are usually quite complex, and it is precisely such technological complexity that contributes to its protection (Keisner et al. 2015).

11.10   Knowledge acquisition

Attempting to answer the following questions involves acquisition of knowledge from this book and other books, documents, and the Internet.

- How did AI begin?
- What are the current trends in AI?
- What are the benefits of AI?
- What are the risks of AI?
- What does the future landscape of AI look like? What kind of concerns are there?
- How can AI both destroy and create jobs?
- How can AI threaten somebody's personal privacy?
- If you were to look five years ahead, how much more do you expect to use AI?
- Can AI be ethical?
- What is machine learning and how does it relate to AI?
- What is deep learning and how does it relate to AI?
- How do we design AI systems so that they function ethically?
- How is it possible to make a world with interconnected AI and autonomous devices safe and secure, and how can we gauge the risks?
- Does it make sense to speak about shared control and shared responsibility between humans and autonomous devices?
- How it is possible to ensure that designers, manufacturers, owners, and operators of AI are transparent, responsible, and accountable?
- How will AI change retail in the next few years?
- What competences might AI systems one day have, and what would be some possible social impacts?
- How it is possible to make a world with interconnected AI and autonomous devices safe and secure, and how do we gauge the risks?
- How it is possible to ensure safety for AI technology that is designed to learn how to modify its own behavior?
- Are machines the future of work?
- How should institutions and laws be redesigned to make autonomous cars serve the welfare of individuals and society and to make society safe for this technology?
- Should AI be allowed to get a patent?

11.11   Knowledge creation

Collaborate with peers on learning or work with others outside the class to narrow down the objectives of each activity. You may access online resources and analyze data and information to create new ideas and balanced solutions. High-level digital tools may be used to develop multimedia presentations, simulations or animations, videos and visual displays, digital portfolios, reflective practice (online publishing and blogging), or well-researched and up-to-date reports.

11.11.1   Autonomous weapons

While seamlessly autonomous weapons systems can be a source of alarm, a key challenge might well be their possible failure. Some claim that autonomous weapons can never be fully liable and dependable, and that a level of doubt will always remain. For this task, investigate the above subject by answering the following questions:

- What types of autonomous weapons might be developed within 10 years from now?
- What are the possible deployments of autonomous weapons?
- How likely is the development of relatively cheap autonomous weapons that are approachable and destructive in the hands of civilians?
- What sorts of regulatory actions might be required to head off this kind of possibility, and when would such actions be suitable?

11.11.2   Robots' rights

Once we consider robots as entities that can perceive, feel, and act, it is not a huge jump to consider their legal status. Should they be treated like humans? Or like animals of similar intelligence? Will we consider the suffering of feeling robots? Some ethical questions are about mitigating suffering, some about risking negative outcomes (Bossmann 2016). While considering these issues, investigate the subject in general, keeping in mind that, at the end, AI has vast potential to bring better lives for everyone, but its implementation is a responsibility.

11.11.3   AI security and safety

The more powerful a technology becomes, the more it can be used for nefarious reasons as well as good. This applies not only to robots produced to replace human soldiers or autonomous weapons, but to AI systems that can cause damage if used maliciously. Because these fights won't be fought on the battleground only, cybersecurity will become even more important. After all, we are dealing with a system that is faster and more capable than us by several orders of magnitude (Bossmann 2016). While considering this issue, investigate the topic and discuss the following:

- Is it possible that AI systems might prove valuable in refining defenses against hacking while at the same time being helpful for carrying out hacking?
- What are the dangers of AI-powered cyberattacks?
- What ethical issues arise from AI-powered cybersecurity?
- What are the ethics of counter-attacks?

11.11.4 The AI technology landscape

New possibilities for innovation based on AI technologies are emerging at a high rate. In every sector of industry, consider what possibilities might look like for AI as a driver of future change. For this task, develop a digital poster about AI technologies and related industrial examples. You may benefit from the following table while developing the poster.

Technology	Brief summary	Industrial example
Deep learning		
Machine learning		
NLP		
Chatbots		
Cognitive cyber security		
Neural networks		
Pattern recognition		
Others		

11.11.5 Unemployment

The hierarchy of labor is concerned primarily with automation. As we've invented ways to automate jobs, we could create room for people to assume more complex roles, moving from the physical work that dominated the pre-industrial globe to the cognitive labor that characterizes strategic and administrative work in our globalized society (Bossmann 2016). Look at trucking: it currently employs millions of individuals in the United States alone. What will happen to them if the self-driving trucks promised by Tesla's Elon Musk become widely available in the next decade? But on the other hand, if we consider the lower risk of accidents, self-driving trucks seem like an ethical choice. The same scenario could happen to office workers, as well as to the majority of the workforce in developed countries.

References

ACM. 2018. New conference: AAAI/ACM conference on AI, ethics, and society. https://sigai.acm.org/aimatters/blog/2017/09/20/new-conference-aaaiacm -conference-on-ai-ethics-and-society/.

Agrawal, A., J. S. Gans, and A. Goldfarb. 2017. What to expect from artificial intelligence. *MIT Sloan Management Review* 58(3): 23–26.

AI100. 2016. One hundred year study on artificial intelligence (AI100). Stanford University. https://ai100.stanford.edu.

Albert, P. H., and R. Block. 2018. How to make sure the owner of your intellectual property is you and not your AI. https://www.ailawadvisor.com/2018/0 3/how-to-make-sure-the-owner-of-your-intellectual-property-is-you-and-not-your-ai/.

Allianz. 2018. The rise of artificial intelligence: Future outlook and emerging risks. https://www.agcs.allianz.com/assets/Insights/Artificial%20Intelligence/ Artificial_Intelligence_Outlook_and_Risks.pdf.

Ashkenas, J., and A. Parlapiano. 2016. How the recession reshaped the economy, in 255 Charts. The New York Times. http://www.nytimes.com/.

Atikian, J. 2018. Robot, AI, and jobs: All three are coming. https://www.theglobe andmail.com/business/commentary/article-robots-ai-and-jobs-all-three-are-coming/.

Balfe, N., S. Sharples, and J. R. Wilson. 2015. Impact of automation: Measurement of performance, workload and behaviour in a complex control environment. *Applied Ergonomics* 47: 52–64.

Bench-Capon, T. J. M., and P. E. Dunne. 2007. Argumentation in artificial intelligence. *Artificial Intelligence* 171(10–15): 619–641.

Berman, F. 2008. Got data? A guide to data preservation in the information age. *Communication of the ACM* 51: 50–56.

Bossmann, J. 2016. Top 9 ethical issues in artificial intelligence. https://www.wef orum.org/agenda/2016/10/top-10-ethical-issues-in-artificial-intelligence/.

Bostrom, N., and E. Yudkowsky. 2011. The ethics of artificial intelligence. Cambridge Handbook of Artificial Intelligence. https://nickbostrom.com/ ethics/artificial-intelligence.pdf.

Bostrom, N., and E. Yudkowsky. 2014. The ethics of artificial intelligence. In Keith, F. and M. W. Ramsey. *The Cambridge Handbook of Artificial Intelligence.* Cambridge, UK: Cambridge University Press.

Brookfield. 2018. AI + public policy: Understanding the shift. Brookfield Institute for the Innovation and Entrepreneurship, Ontario. http://brookfieldins titute.ca/wp-content/uploads/2018/03/AI_BackgroundMaterials_ONLIN E-1.pdf.

Burton, E., J. Goldsmith, S. Koenig, B. Kuipers, N. Mattei, and T. Walsh. 2017. Ethical considerations in artificial intelligence courses. White Paper. https:// arxiv.org/pdf/1701.07769.pdf.

Bush, V. 1945. As we may think. *The Atlantic Monthly* 176(1): 101–108.

Campolo, A., M. Sanfilippo, M. Whittaker, K. Crawford. 2017. AI now. https://ai nowinstitute.org/AI_Now:2017_Report.pdf.

Cle, J. 2018. Thoughts on AI: How bias can shape data insights—and how to conquer it. https://medium.com/inside-machine-learning/thoughts-on-ai-how-bias-can-shape-data-insights-and-how-to-conquer-it-c00bf1f505f8.

Cockburn, I. M., R. Henderson, and S. Stern. 2017. The impact of artificial intelligence on innovation. NBER Conference on Research Issues in Artificial Intelligence, Toronto, September 2017. http://www.nber.org/chapters/c14006.pdf.

Davey, T. 2017. Towards a code of ethics in artificial intelligence with Paula Boddington. https://futureoflife.org/2017/07/31/towards-a-code-of-ethics-in-artificial-intelligence/.

Desai, N. 2018. The future is here: Artificial intelligence and robotics. http://www.nishithdesai.com/fileadmin/user_upload/pdfs/Research_Papers/Artificial_Intelligence_and_Robotics.pdf.

Dignum, V. 2017. Bringing accountability, responsibility, and transparency. https://aibusiness.com/bringing-responsibility-to-ai/.

Dignum, V. 2018. The ART of AI – Accountability, responsibility, transparency. https://medium.com/@virginiadignum/the-art-of-ai-accountability-responsibility-transparency-48666ec92ea5.

EC. 2018. Statement on artificial intelligence, robotics and autonomous systems. European Group on Ethics in Science and New Technologies. http://ec.europa.eu/research/ege/pdf/ege_ai_statement_2018.pdf.

EGE. 2018. Statement on artificial intelligence, robotics and 'autonomous' systems. European Group on Ethics in Science and New Technologies. http://ec.europa.eu/research/ege/pdf/ege_ai_statement_2018.pdf.

El-Attar, M.-S. T. 1997. Application of artificial intelligence in architectural design. PhD Thesis, Al-Azhar University, Cairo, Egypt.

EU. 2018. Statement on artificial intelligence, robotics and 'autonomous' systems. European Group on Ethics in Science and New Technologies, Brussels. http://ec.europa.eu/research/ege/pdf/ege_ai_statement_2018.pdf.

Evans, 2013. Artificial intelligence: Where we came from, where we are now, and where we are going. MSc Thesis, Department of Computer Science, University of Victoria. https://dspace.library.uvic.ca/bitstream/handle/1828/8314/Evans_Guy-Warwick_MSc_2017.pdf?sequence=1.

Faggella, D. 2017. Examples of artificial intelligence in education. https://www.techemergence.com/examples-of-artificial-intelligence-in-education/.

Felipe, J., C. Bayudan-Dacuycuy, and M. Lanzafame. 2016. The declining share of agricultural employment in China: How fast? *Structural Change and Economic Dynamics* 37: 127–137.

Foote, K. 2016. A brief history of artificial intelligence. http://www.dataversity.net/brief-history-artificial-intelligence/.

Hamid, S. 2017. The opportunities and risks of artificial intelligence in medicine and healthcare. http://www.cuspe.org/wp-content/uploads/2016/09/Hamid_2016.pdf.

Hammond, K. 2016. Ethics and artificial intelligence: The moral compass of a machine. https://www.recode.net/2016/4/13/11644890/ethics-and-artificial-intelligence-the-moral-compass-of-a-machine.

Hislop, D., C. Coombs, S. Taneva, and S. Barnard. 2017. Impact of artificial intelligence, robotics and automation technologies on work. Rapid evidence review. University of Loughborough. https://www.cipd.co.uk/Images/impact-of-artificial-intelligence-robotics-and-automation-technologies-on-work_2017-rapid-eveidence-review:tcm18-35319.pdf.

IEEE. 2018. Ethically aligned design. The IEEE Global Initiative on Ethics of Autonomous and Intelligent Systems. http://standards.ieee.org/develop/indconn/ec/ead_v2.pdf.

ITU. 2018. AI for good global summit. https://www.itu.int/en/ITU-T/AI/2018/Pages/default.aspx.

Kaplan, J. 2017. Artificial intelligence: Think again. *Communications of the ACM* 60: 36–38.

Karliuk, M. 2018. The ethical and legal issues of artificial intelligence. https://moderndiplomacy.eu/2018/04/24/the-ethical-and-legal-issues-of-artificial-intelligence/.

Keisner, A., J. Raffo, and S. Wunsch-Vincent. 2015. Breakthrough technologies – Robotics, innovation and intellectual property (No. 30). World Intellectual Property Organization – Economics and Statistics Division.

Kendall, A. 2018. Let's talk about ethics in artificial intelligence. https://alexgkendall.com/artificial_intelligence/lets_talk_about_ethics_in_artificial_intelligence/.

Keynes, J. M. 1937. The general theory of employment. *Quarterly Journal of Economics* 51(2): 209–223.

Kristin, L. 2017. Artificial intelligence, automation, and the economy. *Chinese American Forum* 32: 22–23.

Lavallée, E. 2017. Intellectual property and artificial intelligence. http://www.lavery.ca/en/publications/our-publications/3037-intellectual-property-and-artificial-intelligence.html.

Lund, S., and J. Manyika. 2017. Five lessons from history on AI. Automation, and employment. https://www.mckinsey.com/featured-insights/future-of-organizations-and-work/five-lessons-from-history-on-ai-automation-and-employment.

Luxton, D. D. 2014. Artificial intelligence in psychological practice: Current and future applications and implications. *Professional Psychology: Research and Practice* 45(5): 332.

MacCarthy, M. 2018. Tech policy perspectives. https://www.cio.com/article/3273324/artificial-intelligence/the-ethical-challenges-of-ai.html.

Marchant, G. E. 2018. Artificial intelligent and the future on legal practice. https://www.americanbar.org/content/dam/aba/administrative/litigation/materials/2017-2018/2018-sac/written-materials/artificial-intelligence-and-the-future.authcheckdam.pdf.

McCarthy, J. 1960. Recursive functions of symbolic expressions and their computation by machine (Part I). *Communications of the ACM* 3(4): 184–195.

McCarthy, J., M. L. Minsky, N. Rochester, and C. E. Shannon. 1955. A proposal for the Dartmouth summer research project on artificial intelligence. http://www-formal.stanford.edu/jmc/history/dartmouth/dartmouth.html.

McCorduck, P. 2004. *Machines Who Think: A Personal Inquiry into the History and Prospects of Artificial Intelligence*. Natick, MA: A K Peters, Ltd.

Medeiros, M., and J. Sanft. 2018. Artificial intelligence and intellectual property considerations. https://www.financierworldwide.com/artificial-intelligence-and-intellectual-property-considerations/.

Monthly, L. 2017. Robots and AI: Giving robots 'personhood' status. https://www.lawyer-monthly.com/2017/02/robots-and-ai-giving-robots-personhood-status/.

Nadimpalli, M. 2017. Artificial intelligence – consumers and industry impact. *International Journal of Economics and Management Sciences* 6(4): 1–3.

Nilsson, N. J. 2010. *The Quest for Artificial Intelligence: A History of Ideas and Achievements.* Cambridge, UK: Cambridge University Press.

Nissan, E. 2012. An overview of data mining for combating crime. *Applied Artificial Intelligence* 26: 760–786.

NSTC. 2016. Preparing for the future of artificial intelligence. National Science and Technology Council. https://obamawhitehouse.archives.gov/sites/de fault/files/whitehouse_files/microsites/ostp/NSTC/preparing_for_the_fu ture_of_ai.pdf.

OECD. 2015. *Data-Driven Innovation: Big Data for Growth and Well-Being.* Paris, France: OECD Publishing, Paris, http://dx.doi.org/10.1787/978926422 9358-en.

Petropoulos, G. 2018. The impact of artificial intelligent on employment. http:// bruegel.org/wp-content/uploads/2018/07/Impact-of-AI-Petroupoulos.pdf.

PWC. 2018. 2018 AI predictions 8 insights to shape business strategy. https:// www.pwc.es/es/publicaciones/tecnologia/assets/ai-predictions-2018.pdf.

Ramsey, J. 2017. Advances in artificial intelligence: A primer and its impact on business and the law. https://www.torys.com/insights/publications/2017/ 04/advances-in-artificial-intelligence-a-primer-and-its-impact-on-busin ess-and-the-law.

Russell, S., and P. Norvig. 2010. *Artificial Intelligence: A Modern Approach.* Third edition. Upper Saddle River, NJ: Prentice Hall.

Russell, S., and P. Norvig. 2016. *Artificial Intelligence: A Modern Approach.* Third edition. Essex, UK: Pearson Education Limited.

Russell, S., S. Hauert, R. Altman, and M. Veloso. 2015. Ethics of artificial intelligence. *Nature* 521(7553): 415–418.

Schultebraucks, L. 2017. A short history of artificial intelligence. https://dev.to/ lschultebraucks/a-short-history-of-artificial-intelligence-7hm.

Sobowale, J. 2016. Beyond imagination: How artificial intelligence is transforming the legal profession. http://www.abajournal.com/magazine/article/ how:artificial_intelligence_is_transforming_the_legal_profession.

Stanford. 2016. Artificial intelligence and life in 2030. https://ai100.stanford.edu/ sites/default/files/ai100report10032016fnl_singles.pdf.

Turing, A. 1950. Computing machinery and intelligence. http://www.abelard.o rg/turpap/turpap.htm.

Turing, A. M. 1937. On computable numbers, with an application to the Entscheidungsproblem. *Proceedings of the London Mathematical Society* 2(1): 230–265.

van Est, R., J. T. Gerritsen, and L. Kool. 2017. Human rights in the robot age: Challenges arising from the use of robotics, artificial intelligence, and virtual and augmented reality. Rathenau Instituut. https://www.rathenau.nl/ sites/default/files/2018-02/Human%20Rights%20in%20the%20Robot%20Ag e-Rathenau%20Instituut-2017.pdf.

Wallach, W., and C. Allen. 2009. *Moral Machines: Teaching Robots Right from Wrong.* New York, NY: Oxford University Press.

Witten, M. 2018. The techno-ethicist. https://www.queensu.ca/gazette/alum nireview/stories/techno-ethicist.

Woolf, B. P., H. C. Lane, and J. L. Kolonder. 2013. AI grand challenges for education. *AI Magazine* 34(4): 66–84.

Zicari, R. 2018. How to make artificial intelligence fair, transparent and accountable. http://www.odbms.org/2018/01/how-to-make-artificial-intelligence-fair-transparent-and-accountable/.

module twelve

Professional and career development

12.1 Knowledge and understanding

Having successfully completed this module, you should be able to demonstrate knowledge and understanding of:

- Professional and career development activities to develop an individual's skills, knowledge, and expertise
- Future work that is influenced by the continuing march of digital paradigm transformation, automation, and AI
- Types and categories of work and key approaches for work readiness
- The future shape of the workforce as a result of changing and competing forces
- The workplace that is constantly changing with new technologies, new generations of employees, and new approaches of emerging work
- Ethics, moral principles, and standards of behavior in the workplace
- Digital and physical platform economies and their abilities to support entrepreneurship
- Critical need for digital leaders with a combination of skills, attitudes, knowledge, and experience to drive digital change
- Skills and attributes to approach work readiness
- Basic attributes required by graduates before they join the workforce
- Key elements of professionalism in the workplace
- Keys for a successful career and competences for job satisfaction

12.2 The changing nature of work

> If opportunity doesn't knock, build a door.
>
> **Milton Berle**

Professional and career development as a lifelong activity, in the sense cited in the quotation above, is not only about how work is perceived as tasks or jobs separated from other activities, but a vision to developing an individual's door for essential knowledge, competencies. Today's doors to digital world are changing mindsets and transforming the way people live, learn, and work significantly (Figure 12.1).

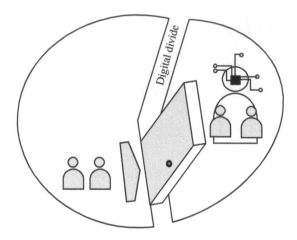

Figure 12.1 Digital divide and beyond.

In the early part of the twentieth century, career choice and progression were dictated by tradition, socio-economic status, family, and gender. For most men, career choice and status were determined by what their fathers and other male family members had accomplished before them. For women, the career choice options were even more limited by convention and social norms. After WWII, the corporate organization became the driving force. Both employers and employees operated under an implied contract. In the latter part of the twentieth century, however, this trajectory of a person's career at one employer became a thing of the past. From the late 1970s onward, the economy experienced several boom-and-bust cycles, causing many organizations to undergo massive layoffs and restructuring. The shift away from a manufacturing to a knowledge-based economy caused a further weakening of the once-implied contract of employee loyalty for lifetime employment (SHRM 2015).

The traditional career still exists today, but it operates in an environment where workers witness continuous and intense changes. The way work is organized and executed constantly evolves and changes. Jobs are divided into tasks, which are then outsourced. Work is redesigned to accommodate increased demands for flexibility, such as teleworking hubs, online connectivity with global colleagues, and virtual worlds. To examine this changing nature of work, it is valuable to look at some of the key trends that are impacting the above scenario. Several of those trends are listed in Figure 12.2.

There are many fascinating technology trends in automation and digitization that are dramatically starting to impact the way people work. Social media and the Internet are becoming widespread, making people and workers more collaborative. This trend is observed across all

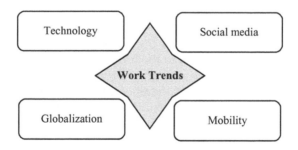

Figure 12.2 Key trends shaping the future of work.

demographics and geographies around the world (Morgan 2014). Today, with the advances in mobile technology, employees can work from anywhere, anytime, and on any device. The technological framework is there, but many are striving around the deliberate attitude to enable this change. Importantly, talents do not need to be local. Organizations can be comprised of international teams and can also operate in any part of the world without boundaries.

Technology is shifting how people think about the workforce. The increasingly sophisticated technologies have caused the nature of work to shift away from relatively routine work environments to ones filled with growing diversity and complexity (Moses and Garia 2017). Thus, the work will depend on how well organizations merge and expand the capacities of humans and technology by making them collaborative. However, humans and technology may be considered different in complementary, rather than conflicting, ways.

The evolving nature of work could create more good jobs, if organizational leaders are able to develop their jobs by crafting them to make the most out of their employees' inherent nature to be social creatures, lifelong learners, and creative problem-solvers. The anticipated AI technologies may allow more good jobs to be created as work begins to leverage the essentially human qualities of social and critical skills (Ramani and Garia 2017; Ton 2014).

12.3 Types and categories of work

> *Choose a job you love, and you will never have to work a day in your life.*

Unknown

There have been several ideas related to current work types and categories. This section will combine these ideas together, as well as serve as a place to discuss additional suggested categories or work types of the future.

12.3.1   What influences future work?

One of the key workplace trends of the future would be the downfall of the corporate ladder, dating back to the Industrial Revolution when thriving businesses were developed on a strict order (Fox and O'Conner 2016). Society today is experiencing a fundamental transformation in the way people work. Automation and thinking machines in the digital age are replacing human tasks and jobs and changing the skills that organizations are looking for in their employees. Automation will not only alter the type of jobs available and their supply, but also their perceived value. By replacing workers engaged in routine and methodical tasks, machines can amplify the comparative advantage of those workers with skills in problem-solving, leadership, EQ, empathy, and creativity (PWC 2018). Automation adoption will take decades, however, across a wide range of possible scenarios. Accordingly, only a small percentage of occupations can be fully automated by adopting current technologies, although work activities of almost all occupations could be automated (Manyika et al. 2017).

The future of work is fast approaching and requires consideration of the biggest questions of our age: What influence will the continuing march of digital transformation and AI in particular have on where people work and how they work? Will people need to work at all? What is the role of workers in an automated world? The real answer is far more complicated. This might be less about technological innovation and more about the manner in which humans decide to embrace, adopt, and manage those technological tools (PWC 2018).

AI will change the future of work through automation by the use of technology to complete tasks and augmentation by the use of technology to assist in completing tasks. These technologies bring a seismic shift in the work environment, making some roles outdated and improving other roles while creating new jobs and even reproducing new professions.

The work is also becoming increasingly improved by technology, which frees up greater capacity for higher-order cognitive tasks. For example, the advent of AI makes it possible and desirable to intellectualize work, not as a set of discrete tasks laid end-to-end in a predefined process, but as a collaborative problem-solving effort where humans define the problems, machines help find the solutions, and humans verify the acceptability of those solutions (Evans-Greenwood et al. 2017).

Large organizations are currently facing an enormous challenge in attracting the millennial generation to come and work for them. Those people expect much more entrepreneurial environments. One of the ways to do this is through a series of "intrapreneurship" programs, which encourage employees to think and act like entrepreneurs within the confines of their organizations (Fox and O'Conner 2016). This means individuals will have the freedom to take full ownership of particular domains or projects, with the least supervision or bureaucracy, and be able to pitch directly to high management without having to go through numerous layers of management.

12.3.2   Major types of work

As the world of work continues to evolve at a rapid pace, innovation continues to become both a top priority and a highest challenge. Types of work is a way to plan and develop future career objectives. Based on the nature of tasks, work may be classified into four major categories that map engineering and computing to a large extent: people, ideas, data, and information- building and producing, as shown in Figure 12.3.

The first type of work can be classified as people work, referring to a job that consists of working primarily with people and communities. Examples of people work include counseling, teaching, coaching, health, and charity. This type of work requires people skills, which refers to interpersonal skills, or the ability to work well with others. Examples of people skills might include listening and speaking effectively, resolving conflicts, and acting with authority. Most of engineering management careers highlight people skills.

"Ideas" is the second type of work, which involves the development of new ideas, strategies, and/or creative solutions to complex problems. Such workers are the thinkers, and their work involves designing new products and services, new business ideas, and ways of doing everyday activities.

The third type revolves around data and information, which requires working with numbers and data. Jobs that include solving math problems, gathering and managing information, and analyzing data, databases, and other sources of information would fall into this type of work, which largely suits the various disciplines of engineering and computing.

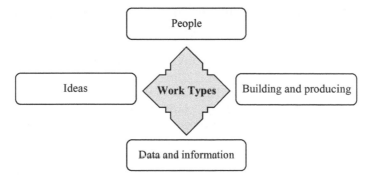

Figure 12.3 Major types of work.

The fourth type of work is classified under building and producing using machines and tools. These people take ideas and convert them into reality. Technical process skills combined with problem-solving proficiencies to implement effective solutions are needed for this type of work. Many disciplines of engineering prepare graduates in large numbers to work in manufacturing and production facilities.

Few of the above types of work are at the front end demand for engineering and computing professionals; some bulge in the middle; some are heavily weighted towards high demand. Most industries need engineers and computing professionals from a range of different disciplines for the numerous knowledge and skills that they bring.

12.3.3   Major categories of workers

The industrial world was about reducing choices; however, the pre-digital world is about expanding choices. Industrial firms have provided society with remarkable well-being over the last few centuries but are increasingly being evaluated as unsuitable for meeting the needs of today. These firms need to excel in innovation and to meet new demands for change and must embrace uncertainty.

The current innovative era with the entrepreneurial experience of work is very different from the industrial era. It is about acting on the unknown, not necessarily working towards a goal. It is about creating a future together through interaction, not about reductionist job roles and separations. It is more about improvising together rather than following scripts. It is more about emergence than causality. It is more about sciences of complexity than system-based thinking (Kilpi 2018).

To meet the above emerging needs and with regard to engineering and computing, candidate skills and competencies can be divided into several categories, each with certain attributes, interests, and strengths, as shown in Figure 12.4.

Technical skills are the abilities and knowledge needed to perform specific tasks. Technical candidates are practical and enjoy being the technical know-how. They relate to electrical, mechanical, civil, IT, mathematical, or scientific tasks. They can be involved with details, analysis, or in implementing technical processes.

Managerial skills often overlap with leadership skills, as both involve problem-solving, decision-making, planning, communicating, and time managing. Good managers are often good leaders, although the two roles are distinct. The managerial category includes people who can manage and organize teams with the goal of achieving results.

The entrepreneurial category is defined by a fast-paced and challenging environment. Among the significant qualities related with successful

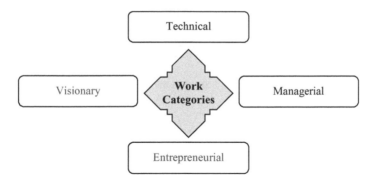

Figure 12.4 Major categories of work.

entrepreneurship is passion, creativity, self-confidence, self-reliance, willingness to take risks, and ability to finish tasks.

The visionary category consists of the creative or strategic thinkers in an organization for the development of new ideas and setting the direction for teams or organizations. Visionary leaders are charismatic leaders, excellent communicators, strategic-planners, and risk takers. They have a convincing vision for their tasks. They can see beyond the uncertainty and challenges to an inspiring picture of the future.

12.4   Future Workforce

> *To prepare for the workforce, you have to understand the world.*
>
> **Tae Yoo**
> *[from "5 Ways We Can Prepare the Next Generation of Workers for Tomorrow's Technology" (Huffpost 2017)]*

The workforce is about people. Because emerging digital communities are just starting to enter the workforce, and the role of technology is constantly shifting, it is important to understand the effects for how people approach work and how work could be reshaped in the future. In that future, do people need to work at all?

12.4.1   Future workforce skills

The digital workforce has developed many competencies in the course of their interactions with technology that may be leveraged at work. With the increasing prevalence of technology, new graduates may join the workforce with high levels of digital fluency. New technology platforms are

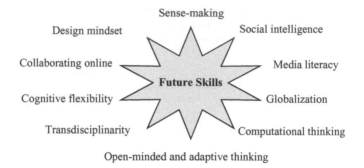

Figure 12.5 Future workforce skills.

driving an unprecedented reorganization of new skillsets for the future workforce, as outlined in Figure 12.5.

The future workforce requires improvements in education in order to use digital technology and AI tools efficiently. As AI begins to dominate industries, there will be an increasing demand for the kinds of skills that machines are not good at. These are higher-level thinking skills that cannot be codified, skills that help people create unique insights critical to decision-making. Socially intelligent employees are able to quickly assess the emotions of those around them and adapt their words, tone, and gestures accordingly. This has always been a key skill for workers who need to collaborate and build relationships of trust. Digital media literacy provides workers with a foundation of knowledge and skills to use technology in the workforce. This competency can be valuable to organizations in a number of different ways. However, the future workforce will require new competencies in addition to digital fluency to anticipate and respond to the powers of change.

12.4.2   Workforce skill

Many of today's worldwide problems are just too composite to be solved by one particular discipline. These multifaceted problems require transdisciplinary solutions, which refers to the ability to understand and adapt concepts across multiple disciplines to challenge primary skills. Contrary to current times, the future will see transdisciplinary approaches take the center stage. People who can connect knowledge from diverse sources and obtain substantial results will be valuable in the future workplace. This is because problems are multifaceted and too complex to be solved by a single discipline.

The "T-shaped person" is a concept popularized by Tim Brown, CEO of design firm IDEO, which refers to the transdisciplinary mindset. T-shaped individuals possess deep knowledge in a primary field but cultivate a broad curiosity about areas of expertise outside of that field. Brown cites empathy, enthusiasm, and a readiness to collaborate as hallmarks of the T-shaped person (Staff 2012). Figure 12.6 reflects the nature of knowledge and skills of the future workforce.

Educational institutions should ensure that breadth of learning, beyond the technical aspects of the specialist discipline, is a major drive in education. For graduates, this means not only possessing deep technical skills, but also having acquired broader attributes such as critical thinking skills and entrepreneurial mindset, compassion, written and verbal communication skills, team-building, client interaction skills, and the ability to collaborate.

Workers of the future will need to become adept at recognizing the kind of thinking that different tasks require and making adjustments to their work environments that enhance their ability to accomplish these tasks (Davies et al. 2011). Cognitive flexibility is an important skill needed by the future workforce so that workers are able to adjust the way they work when difficulties arise or a shift is needed. As leaders of virtual teams, individuals need to develop strategies for engaging and motivating a dispersed group.

Employees of the emerging and future workforce will be more independent and skilled than ever before. The employees will take control of their careers in ways former workers did not. They will be sought more on a project basis for their skills and competencies rather than as permanent workers. They will gain more skills and value to add to their ever-growing experience with the completion of each project.

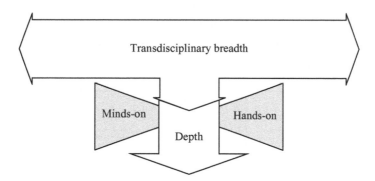

Figure 12.6 Transdisciplinary nature of knowledge and skills of future workforce.

12.5　*Future workplace*

> *What we know is the workplace is more demanding than ever before.*

Margaret Spellings

The workplace is the environment in which people work. It is constantly changing with new technologies, new generations of employees, and new emerging approaches of working. The above technologies will affect every aspect of the workplace and its workers. They will considerably change the type and number of jobs available.

12.5.1　*The evolving digital workplace*

The digital workplace is an environment where employees are able to quickly and easily share their knowledge and find what they need with consistent experiences across devices and locations. It can best be considered as the natural evolution of the workplace. Technically, the digital workplace consists of the holistic set of tools, platforms, work environment, and all the technologies people use to get work done in today's workplace. It ranges from core business applications to email, instant messaging, enterprise social media tools, and virtual meeting means (Deloitte 2018). In most organizations, the digital workplace paradigm (Figure 12.7) can be broadly defined in several categories to support the ways in which employees communicate, collaborate, connect, and deliver day-to-day services. The bulk of the digital workplace tools available today are either on data centers or on the cloud.

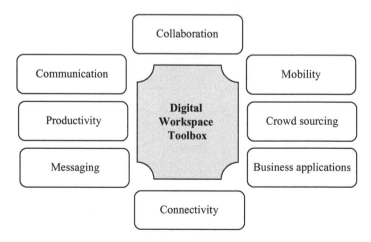

Figure 12.7 Digital workplace paradigm.

The evolving workplace will require several areas of expertise, including a deep knowledge of work; a facility with technology, ranging from email and office productivity software to imaging, database management, health informatics, coding, cybersecurity, systems engineering, or robotics; an ability to engage in critical thinking and problem-solving and work in interdisciplinary, cross-functional teams; and people skills, including interpersonal communication, flexibility, and EQ (Hrabowski 2015).

Collaboration represents methods and tools that enable people to connect in a network manner. It facilitates cooperation between employees and partners via team rooms, communities, and web conferencing. The digital workspace also promotes mobility, which enables employees to access tools away from the physical office or workplace by using PCs and laptops, smartphones, home offices, and remote scanners. It means that people connect with others and with data anywhere, anytime, and on any device. Organizations are becoming increasingly familiar with crowdsourcing practices and are achieving remarkable results in gathering ideas, input, and thoughts from employees, including ideation platforms, polls, surveys, and forums. Business applications are also useful features for organizations to provide access for employees to self-service applications including expense claims, HR systems, enterprise resource planning, and customer relationship management. Connectivity helps locate experts and colleagues across the organization by using employee directories, organization charts, and rich user profiles. Messaging provides a fast way to communicate with colleagues and others including email, instant messaging, micro blogging, and mobile messaging. Greater degrees of productivity are achieved with tools such as Word processors, spreadsheet software, and presentation software, enabling knowledge workers to complete tasks efficiently (Deloitte 2018). Communication addresses the degree to which robust communication capabilities exist that may reach all employees in a variety of formats. It supports information sharing and internal publishing, including portals/intranet, blogs, and personalized homepages.

An important dynamic to witness is related to the generational differences between educators and their students. During this key transitional period, many educators are "digital immigrants", while their students are "digital natives". While teachers can follow with some consistency the patterns and needs of today's education, students are much more complex, in large part due to the varying attitudes towards digital technology, based mostly on their age (Guest 2018).

12.5.2   Networking and social media

Networking is defined as the building of mutually beneficial relationships, which are developed by interaction, exchange of information, and developing contacts. It is one of the most essential career developments that is often overlooked by students and job seekers. Professional networking, in particular, is the process of developing relationships with people in occupations.

Professional meetings offer opportunities to find like-minded people, to expand networks, to become informed about research frontiers and new products and services, to share research results, to find employment, to gain speaking experience, and to reconnect with people from the past. Although the Internet or other virtual approaches can be beneficial, they should only be used as supplements for traditional networking approaches, such as face-to-face meetings, phone calls, and handwritten notes.

Social media has transformed social interactions and is beginning to transform workplace communication (Davison et al. 2017). The use of the internet and social media has grown substantially over the last decade and has become a great resource for building CoPs with common interests. The use of new web-based technologies for work-related activities has been a major part of that. While Internet usage has grown, the way people are using the Internet has also changed. Social networking sites (such as Facebook and Twitter), professional networking sites (such as LinkedIn), and other innovations which are part of greater interactivity and user-generated content that characterize the so-called Web 2.0, are becoming increasingly important job search and recruitment tools (Dutton et al. 2009). Table 12.1 outlines a few examples of Web 2.0 and social networking sites.

Table 12.1 Examples of Web 2.0 and social networking sites

Site	Summary
Facebook	A social networking service where users create personal profiles. Users may join common-interest user groups, organized by common workplaces.
Twitter	Tweets are text-based posts displayed on the user's profile page. Users may subscribe to other users' tweets.
LinkedIn	A business-related social networking site mainly used for professional networking.
Myspace	An online community of users' personal profiles, typically including photographs, information about personal interests, and blogs.
YouTube	A video-sharing website on which users can upload, share, and view videos.
Wikipedia	A collaborative web-based encyclopedia project written collaboratively by volunteers around the world; almost all articles are freely editable by any visitor.

Work in the future will be more interconnected and network-oriented in the workplace. Employees and employers will require the competencies to work across different disciplines, to collaborate virtually, and to demonstrate cultural sensitivity. More innovations are expected to take place at the borders of disciplines and sectors. The spread of disciplines and jobs across sectors will also stimulate the hybridization of skills, which will provide some individuals with a strong position to compete within an increasingly demanding workplace (Störmer et al. 2014).

Educational systems will also need to evolve for a changed workplace, with policymakers working with education providers to improve basic skills in the STEM fields and put a new emphasis on creativity as well as on critical and systems thinking. For everyone, developing agility, resilience, and flexibility will be important at a time when everybody's job is likely to change to some degree (Manyika et al. 2017).

The consensus among HR professionals and employment lawyers is that it is possible for employers to take action against employees who make comments using social media sites. This is particularly the case where employee comments can be clearly considered defamatory (Whincup 2011). Aside from the legal issues, some commentators have examined the ethicality of social media usage by employees and responses from employers (Valentine et al. 2010). The question is important for a number of reasons, not least because if a dismissal is seen as unfair, it has the potential to generate discontent within the workplace (Broughton et al. 2009).

12.5.3   Ethics in the workplace

Ethics form the heart of any workplace culture and are reflected through the values an organization demonstrates in its goals and policies. The quality of experience in an organization depends on the quality of its culture (SHRM 2013). Work ethics is a value based on hard work and diligence. It is also a belief in the moral benefit of work and its ability to enhance character. A work ethics of any kind not only includes how one feels about their place of employment or position, but also how they perform the duties of the job (MANAGE 2018).

Ethics in the workplace is the application of moral principles, standards of behavior, and a set of values regarding proper conduct in the workplace as individuals and in a group setting. Every workplace is different, but they all should take the following into consideration: trustworthiness, respect, responsibility, fairness, and caring. Ethics applies to any relationship, whether it is between management and supervisors, colleagues and employees, or customers (EPCC 2018).

Good workplace ethics includes a variety of attributes and qualities, including determination, productivity, respect for others, honesty and accountability for actions, initiative, the ability to think critically to solve problems, cooperation and promptness, professionalism, operating with integrity, and taking pride. Employees are expected to avoid conflicts of interest, which refer to situations in which financial or other personal interests may be in conflict with the interests of the workplace.

12.6 Digital platforms and entrepreneurship

To have a great idea, have a lot of them.

Thomas Edison

Digital platform business models are rapidly becoming the privileged notion of the digital revolution. A digital platform is a shared technology-enabled business model that creates value by enabling exchanges between two or more interdependent groups. It brings together end users and producers to exchange transactions.

12.6.1 Platform economy

Work is being disconnected from jobs, and jobs and work are being disconnected from organizations, which are increasingly becoming platforms (Moses and Garia 2017). Numerous terms are used to describe the new platform work relationships; one among those is the platform economy. Today, digital platform companies are disrupting markets and rank among the most influential enterprises in the world. Workers are attracted to the platform economy for a variety of reasons, including the ability to earn extra income and enjoy work flexibility.

The platform economy exists in various industries and includes work at all wage and skill levels. The advantage of platforms is their ability to allow organizations to broaden and share information, services, skills, and technologies across a wider ecosystem that connects new networks of partners, suppliers, and customers. And as the Internet of Things (IoT) and the wider digitalization of society continues, there will be further opportunities for companies that imagine and anticipate the potential they offer (Walker 2016).

In the platform economy, the value depends on the extensiveness and functioning of the network. Companies provide services for connecting actors around an activity or need, and they enable them to collaborate, allocate, and use resources more efficiently, and co-create value for each other (Dufva et al. 2017).

The platform economy has the potential to fill the gap for those who appreciate independence in their work but look for less risk than starting their own firm. Work in the platform economy can be full-time or

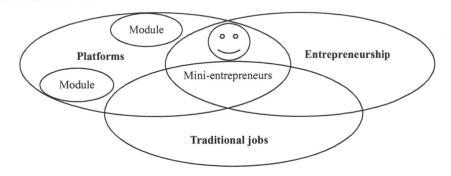

Figure 12.8 Today's typical overlapping types of work.

part-time, and may be the primary or supplemental source of income for workers. For example, a worker may engage in the platform economy for a temporary period of time to make enough money to help with start-up costs for a future business.

Figure 12.8 shows the existing three typical overlapping types of work. Modules are an add-on software subsystem that connects to the platform to add functionality to it.

12.6.2 Digital platforms

Today's platforms are empowered by new digital technologies. Their ecosystems encompass together customers, producers, and innovators. Companies such as Amazon, Etsy, Facebook, Google, Airbnb, and Uber are creating online structures that enable a wide range of activities. These digital platforms are diverse in their functions and structures. They offer broader opportunities for communication, collaboration, and computing skills to support innovation and entrepreneurship. Google and Facebook are digital platforms that offer search and social media, but they also provide an infrastructure on which other platforms are built. Amazon is a marketplace, as are Etsy and eBay. Amazon Web services provide infrastructure and tools with which others can build yet more platforms. Airbnb and Uber use the newly available cloud tools to force deep changes in a variety of incumbent businesses (Kenney and Zysman 2016). The above digital platforms have proliferated as engines of innovation for other firms to build complementary products and services in ecosystems as diverse as PCs, video games, and smartphones to newer Webs orchestrated by Facebook, YouTube, Twitter, and others (Srinivasan and Venkatraman 2017)

The emergence of software-based platforms is shifting competition towards platform-centric ecosystems. The algorithmic revolution and cloud computing are the foundations of the platform economy. Unlike traditional software development, they leverage the expertise of a diverse developer community with skills and an appreciation of user needs that platforms owners might not possess (Neittaanmäki et al. 2016).

While the industry as a whole engages in lively debate about the IoT, Industry 4.0, digitalization, predictive maintenance, and other assorted buzzwords, many smaller firms in this line in particular stay definitely critical and/or still see platforms as relatively irrelevant to their type of business.

12.6.3   Phygital platforms

Digital and physical worlds and their supporting industries differ widely. When it comes to production and transport, for instance, costs and speeds vary greatly. The digital sphere is immediately more scalable and offers greater potential for abstraction and simulation. With the evolution of machine-to-machine (M2M)/IoT advances, digital platforms can also enhance everyday lives and the ways people interact with physical objects. A multi-layer platform and approach can merge physical and digital into a "phygital" platform (Achillias 2015). Convergence happens when these two worlds come together harmoniously to enhance each other; physical things are enhanced by digital insights, and digital graphics are augmented on the physical world.

Digital platforms give plant and machinery manufacturers the opportunity to understand their customers on a deeper level. In the engineering sector, two categories of platforms are of general relevance: the digital marketplace for industrial goods and services, and industrial IoT platforms (Berger 2018). In conjunction with IoT technology, digital platforms make it possible to interconnect plant and machinery and harness scale effects in the use of digital services.

Physical goods from the manufacturing industry that are offered for sale and transactions are processed on digital marketplaces. Such marketplaces have been around since the earliest beginnings of the Internet economy. The best-known include Mercateo, SAP Ariba, Wucato, and Zamro. In conjunction with IoT technology, digital platforms make it possible to interconnect plant and machinery, and to harness scale effects in the use of digital services. The resultant platform landscape and the growing number of successful applications will give a powerful boost to the digitalization of mechanical and plant engineering (Berger 2018).

Lego and Philips are two product manufacturers that also created multi-layer platforms. They each took two simple physical elements (bricks and light bulbs) and made those objects the foundations of complex platforms that not only serve a need but are, in fact, ecosystems (Achillias 2015).

12.6.4   Entrepreneurship in digital platforms

An emerging area of entrepreneurship focuses on how new organizations born in the digital era can develop and adapt their strategies and business models when their products and services are to be organized within and across digital platforms. In digital entrepreneurship, an entrepreneurial venture uses ICT technology infrastructure to exist digitally instead of in more traditional structures. Digital enterprises can be region- or country-specific but can reach international markets. Furthermore, digital entrepreneurship creates opportunities to work remotely, in different time regions, at any place, or even on mobility. Over time, as entirely new platforms emerge or newer generations of current platforms evolve, entrepreneurs will succeed by capitalizing on opportunities to reuse their specialized knowledge to relaunch their existing businesses to newer business models.

Digital entrepreneurship ventures ranging from large firms that develop hardware, software, and networking technologies to small start-up firms have been developed over the last decade. Today, several digital disruptor supporting platforms such as Apple iOS, Alphabet/Google, Facebook, Twitter, Netflix, and Amazon, are supporting a variety of digital entrepreneurial ventures. While entrepreneurship is a valuable alternative for securing economic independence, the risk of failure is not something everyone can accept. Platforms are efficient in terms of their flexibility, transactional speed, and ability to support what is called "mini-entrepreneurs", which can provide goods and services, usually but not necessarily virtually, for platforms such as app stores, YouTube, or Amazon self-publishing (Srinivasan and Venkatraman 2017).

12.7   Digital leadership

> *IT leaders, CIOs specifically, need to stop being so passive. I view the role of IT, the role of the CIO as being frankly one of the most important, if not the most important role at the leadership table today. Because company CIOs that can't understand how to use technology to change their business models are going to find themselves somewhat out of jobs.*

> **Jeff Immelt**

Digital transformation requires digital leaders with different combinations of skills, attitudes, knowledge, and experience to drive digital change (Detecon 2016). Leadership is no different today than it was many years ago. However, if we are to accomplish the grand task of preparing future generations for a dynamic world that is more socially connected as a result of technology, the style and focus of leadership needs to change.

12.7.1   Doing digital to becoming digital

Digital leadership takes into account recent changes such as ubiquitous connectivity, open-source technology, mobile devices, and personalization. It represents a dramatic shift from how schools have been run and structured for over a century (Sheninger 2014). Digital leadership is also the strategic use of a company's digital resources to achieve business goals. Digital leaders recognize the impact of digital technologies on the expectations of customers and markets. Therefore, such leaders are critical actors for most organizations to develop digital capabilities.

Leadership is critical in making the transformation from an organization doing digital things to one that is becoming digital. For both the organization and its leaders, this involves three different types of transformations (Deloitte 2017):

- Cognitive transformation: Leaders need to think differently.
- Behavioral transformation: Leaders need to act differently.
- Emotional transformation: Leaders need to react differently.

Taken all together, these transformations show how radical the digital transformation will be. Accordingly, organizations should have certain core expectations from their digital leaders. They need to help their organizations imagine the digital nature; distort the internal and external boundaries in ways that assist the digital transformation; educate and train workers; enhance technical expertise; and use design thinking approaches to foster innovation.

12.7.2   High-performing digital leaders

Digital leadership is in high demand as business increasingly relies on digital technologies. It is not about attractive tools but a strategic mindset that leverages available resources to improve what is done while expecting the changes needed to cultivate a school culture focused on engagement and achievement. Digital leaders are technology and business savvy, data-driven, and are able to inspire teams to engage in fast investigation that drives transformation and firm outcomes. Figure 12.9 outlines the characteristics of high-performing digital leaders.

Digital leaders tackle problems in novel ways, are willing to take risks, are capable of considering changes of approaches, are comfortable with uncertainty, and influence positive outcomes. They create ways for cultivating innovation, operate effectively, look ahead to future possibilities, engage and inspire in organizations, and achieve results even under difficult circumstances. Digital leaders prefer entrepreneurial approaches, unstructured work environments, and are encountered by challenges

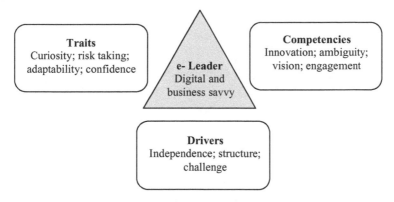

Figure 12.9 The characteristics of high-performing digital leaders.

(Korn Ferry 2018). They should be able to influence, educate, and collaborate with other key leaders across the organization.

12.8   Work readiness

> *Sometimes, we don't know that we are ready until someone tells us we are.*

Srividya Srinivasan

Work readiness is an ongoing process, beginning when students first arrive on campus and continuing through college or university and beyond. It never truly comes to an end during an individual's career.

12.8.1   Model of long-term career readiness

While moving quickly into the digital future, reviewing the prevailing definitions of work and career readiness underscores the uncertainty that any one set of skills and abilities can predict success for graduating students as entry-level employees (JA 2013). Students in colleges and universities are immersed in a variety of learning experiences, from navigating a new town or city to being a part of a club; from living in a student residence to participating in a seminar where views and opinions are challenged. University life provides students with an opportunity to lead teams and projects and enhance their communication skills through co-curricular activities, such as clubs and events. In addition to the skills in critical thinking and problem-solving that are derived from their studies, the university experience is rich with opportunities for personal development. Figure 12.10 shows the framework toward future career readiness.

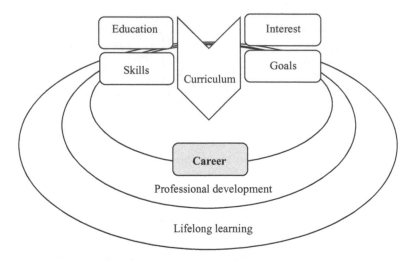

Figure 12.10 Typical model for career readiness.

The education process or learning experience of students varies from one discipline to another, but the objective is broadly to prepare them for their chosen career. When graduates enter the workforce, they must make a transition from an academic to a professional responsibility. Educational institutions should be helping students to understand what professional roles mean and what is encompassed by them. While academic curricula ensure that graduates possess sufficient qualifications to start a professional career, the outcome of these curricula in terms of how graduates interpret themselves as professionals is not well established.

In its original meaning, being a professional meant putting doing good work, attitude, and the quality of the work ahead of economic gain and the economic efficiency of work (Balthazard 2015). Perhaps the most important aspects of professional attitude are composure, EQ, motivation, and career orientation. As young people proceed into more independent experiences and begin to value skill-building, they need to learn to listen to and accept both positive and constructive feedback. Ultimately, students should be proactive about asking for feedback while building relationships with supervisors and adult coworkers who can serve as mentors. While some employers identify leadership as an important concept on its own, many people mention traits that could also be considered as communication skills, professional attitude, or teamwork skills (Klein 2018).

12.8.2 *Graduate attributes and new tools*

There is an indisputable consensus among researchers, service providers, and employers that soft skills are far more important for success in a first job or internship than any particular technical skill, regardless of the job (Klein 2018). In addition, Lave and Wenger (1991) highlighted the importance of social interaction as a critical component of learning, and social practice by itself is a learning process. Therefore, education programs have a responsibility to prepare students to create meaningful careers with confidence and enthusiasm. What tools or skills can the education system provide them? What education or training is appropriate? The consensus is to introduce educators, employers, and emerging workers to a system of training that should be delivered concurrently. The system will identify and develop a recognized set of foundation skills; teach students to learn for themselves; and adopt a hierarchical model of work-readiness preparation that is both practical and measurable. Such framework should be used to prepare the emerging generations for global, futuristic readiness.

Once they have graduated from university or college, graduates start their career to be practitioners of the subject. They work in teams to develop and test new products, to find solutions for problems, and to work on new inventions. Figure 12.11 outlines the basic graduate attributes required before joining the workforce. In addition to technical competence in terms of applying math and a range of engineering sciences to the solution of technology problems, students need to set goals and enhance their interests in the discipline. Such attributes are rooted in a

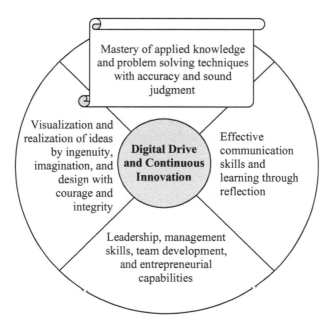

Figure 12.11 Basic graduate attributes.

soft context: the need for graduates to realize the essence of the practice and have the necessary skills and interest, especially in creating technological solutions that are aligned to society's needs.

12.8.3   Foundational milestones

The transition from study to the workplace can be challenging for recent graduates. Therefore, major approaches are necessary to produce skilled graduates that future employers seek. Employers and educational institutions need to collaborate to provide the desired competencies. Figure 12.12 outlines three key milestones for work readiness. The foundational milestone involves key knowledge and skills acquired through typical educational circles including digital literacy, communication comprehension, collaboration, listening, motivation to learn, self-control and self-efficacy,

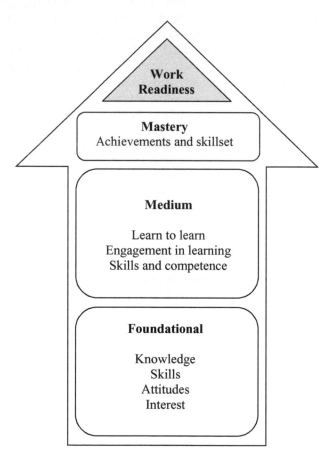

Figure 12.12 Key approaches for work readiness.

creativity, empathy, and use of professional tools and programs. The medium milestone comes through autonomous learning engagements during and after graduation, and it is understood to encompass the self-motivated, voluntary, and ongoing pursuit of knowledge, organization, time management, prioritization, sequencing, understanding of professional tools and programs' functionality, active listening, judgment, and social intelligence. The mastery milestone is a lifelong journey for one's own achievement by intentionally participating in analysis and synthesis, critical and design thinking, leadership, business conduct and protocol, resilience, the entrepreneurial mindset, and job searching (for example, resume writing and interviewing skills).

A career-ready person is proficient in the core academic subjects as well as in technical topics. It also includes a level of technical-skill proficiency aligned to a chosen career field and pathway, as well as the ability to apply both academic and technical learning in the context of a career. Many careers also require deeper learning and mastery in specific academic or technical subjects.

Technical skills like design, coding, statistics, and applied math remain important, but softer skills like adaptability, critical thinking, problem-solving, and creativity are critical. Remember, university education is far from being the single most important skill-building resource; it does not even crack the top two milestones of Figure 12.12. This implies that the best way to shape the future workforce is to concentrate on important knowledges and get more AI-focused training, not advanced degrees only (Genpact 2017).

12.9   The career path

> *Choose to live life. Choose your own career paths. Choose your own destiny.*
>
> **Lailah Gifty Akita**
> *[from Think Great: Be Great! (2014)]*

Choosing a career is probably one of the most important decisions most graduates will ever make. For former generations, it was a clear-cut choice. Today's generation is predicted to have more complex career paths, making it harder still to know what skills they will need to acquire because the nature of work itself is evolving.

12.9.1   The perfect candidate

A career can be developed in various ways, ranging from the formal to the informal. It can be made formal within schools where development is provided through coaching, teaching, and the sharing of good practices.

And it can be informal in the form of projects and competitions, workshops and conferences, individual or collaborative research, observational visits to other learning networks, and engaging in informal discussion with peers.

Digital technology and the anticipated applications of automation and AI are changing the face of work at an increasingly rapid rate. Some jobs are completely disappearing, while new ones are being created. Considering the above challenge, one must consider the all-time question: What makes a great candidate for future work? Sure, academic achievement in university or college is a great asset, but that is not everything. To succeed in the business world, skills not taught in school are necessary. Key skills needed in this regard are shown in Figure 12.13.

The most popular word given to make a successful graduate is creativity. This is because many of the problems society faces cannot be solved using outdated approaches. Knowledge and principles learned in school should be applied, through research or on the job, and should be used to create a unique solution. The biggest challenge the candidate should be prepared for is to know and understand the anticipated career and keep pace with changes and competencies including technological ones in the related industry.

Three words can be considered to be good descriptions of successful competencies: "determined", "diligent", and "dedicated". A certain stick-to-it characteristic is needed to solve the very complex and time-consuming problems career candidates face today (Engineering 360 2018).

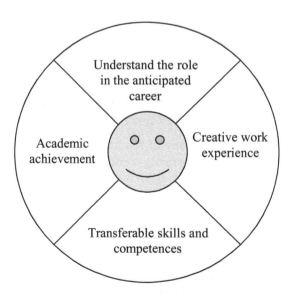

Figure 12.13 Key characteristics of an ideal job candidate.

12.9.2 Possible employers

The rapid developments in engineering and digital transformation have presented the added need to seriously consider how to prepare graduates to be economically active in a society built on emerging computing technologies rather than on industrial settings only.

Possible employers for today's graduates are industry, government, academia, or ventures. Some may become entrepreneurs either in product or service sectors. Many engineering and computing graduates are employed into non-engineering fields like banking, entertainment, medicine, law, and others. In industry, an engineer may work as a technical specialist leading and contributing to critical technical capabilities; as a project or program manager leading technical and business efforts to meet customer needs; or as an organizational manager leading engineering organizations, major business units, or corporations. Figure 12.14 lists the profession progress in the industry.

12.9.3 Career path planning

Career path is a traditional method by which an employee can develop and progress within an organization. It encompasses varied forms of career progression, including the traditional vertical career ladders and career progression outside the organization. Career ladders are the progression of jobs in an organization's specific occupational fields ranked from bottom to uppermost based on level of duty, responsibility, and pay.

Career path planning is an effective tool for producing an employee's development strategy; however, it requires time, patience, and persistence. Whether aspiring for a better position in existing organization, looking for a specific career somewhere else, or being interested in future graduate studies, career path planning is a proven way by which successful transitions in the workplace can occur.

Key elements of a successful career path plan offer two major benefits that are essential for employee retention: direction and motivation.

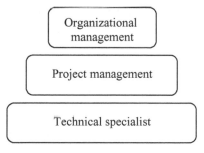

Figure 12.14 Profession progress in industry.

Planning is almost always a challenge, and although getting help from trusted sources can make it easier, it is undoubtedly a journey of challenges along the way. However, a well-designed plan should include a list of short- and long-term career prioritized goals with vision, taking into consideration interests, destination, benefits, challenges, outcomes, and barriers. The goals should be explicit, measurable, achievable, and appropriate.

Thinking and planning one's career is an ongoing effort that is helped along by building a positive mindset that is open to opportunities. Expanding one's knowledge network is always a good idea, although it is a demanding task. The ability to convey the developed process and how it will benefit an organization is critical to convincing the organization that one will add more value in a new and different position. Usually such value is reflected in the curriculum vitae and job interviews.

12.9.4   Skills gap analysis

A skills gap is the difference between skills that employers want or need and skills their workforce offers. Conducting a skills gap analysis helps workers identify skills they need to meet organization or business goals. It can also inform employee development and hiring programs (Bika 2018). A gap analysis also involves comparing the skills and competencies needed in one position with the skills and competencies needed in another position. In a company-driven career path approach, the gap analysis is a simple mathematical equation:

$$A - B = C$$

Where A is the skills and competencies needed in the future position, B is the skills and competencies needed in the current position, and C is the gap or the skills and competencies to be obtained to prepare for the future position. After completing this step, the career path designer will have a listing of the skills and competencies needed to move along each identified path.

There are three ways to fill skills gaps: education, training, and hiring. For workers to meet the requirements of employers, education and training are significant. However, for employers, hiring introduces new skills to the organization, while training and developing staff helps fill existing skill gaps.

12.10   Keys for a successful career

Successful and unsuccessful people do not vary greatly in their abilities. They vary in their desires to reach their potential.

John Maxwell

Goals are the vehicle that transform a career path vision into reality. For goals to be effective they must be specific, considerable, achievable, realistic, and time-bound. Every career path has a range of critical success goals and factors. Identifying these factors is crucial to achieving success in building career paths (Akporado 2015).

Career goals are a subjective indicator of career success primarily because it reflects an individual's attitude towards career based on a personal appraisal. Education in its broadest sense is an orderly accumulation of factual knowledge and progressive ability to interpret and apply that knowledge to human needs.

To make a move from the life of a college or university student into professional life is like emerging from the relative warmth and security of a well-defined area into an area where one once again must be established. What competences lie ahead of that? Tomorrow's workplace demands increasing levels of skill among its employees, and the skill-sets in demand will be different from those required today. As skills needs and career paths change, development is a continuing process in every workplace, with culture and management playing a crucial role. Figure 12.15 outlines the few key competences that are required for a successful career.

- **Practice. Practice. Practice.**
- Have a flexible work environment, anytime and anywhere.
- Shape and define own career.
- Exhibit confidence and be a reliably high-level performer.
- Embrace change and learn new things.
- Build relationships and work well with others to achieve goals.
- Expect changes, challenges, and constraints.
- Have the opportunity to become a leader.
- Know own strengths and weaknesses.
- Learn from past, live in present, prepare for future.
- Be transparent and efficient with communication.
- Shift from being knowledge worker to learning worker.
- Build strength and limit impact of weakness.
- Do not try to solve one big problem, instead, break it into sub-problems, which are much easier to solve.
- Improve competences of digital fluency, knowledge of design thinking, media literacy, computational thinking, and virtual collaboration.
- Stay current with skills and strive to upskill and reskill throughout career.

Figure 12.15 Traits of good graduates transitioning into the workforce.

Education makes all the knowledge available for students to learn and help them to progress and develop further. The challenge for educators is not to dismiss or keep up with students' latest technological know-how, but to create meaningful learning experiences in which students are taught how to apply their knowledge to solve real-world problems. Teachers more than ever have a vital role to play in helping students realize their futures by providing them with instruction that gives direction and allows them to hone their new cognitive and technological skills (Daggett 2010).

12.11   Knowledge acquisition

Attempting to answer the following questions involves the acquisition of knowledge from this book and other books, documents, and the Internet.

- How have changes in the nature of work practices impacted career development over the past few years?
- What is the future of work? What are the changing patterns of the workforce and their impact on the workplace?
- When should a student make a decision about his/her future career?
- What does the changing nature of work mean for entrepreneurship?
- Is there an identifiable set of core knowledge, skills, and attitudes that will ensure our students are prepared to face the unfamiliar challenges of the workplace?
- What is the digital workplace?
- What are work ethics?
- Is an employees' personal use of social networking sites such as Facebook, LinkedIn, and Twitter an issue for an organization?
- Are there currently any general restrictions on employees accessing the Internet/specific websites on working time?
- Which professional networking tools are most effective and why?
- What influence will the continuing march of digital transformation and AI in particular have on where people work and how they work?
- What are the central determinants of success in digital entrepreneurship?
- What is work readiness?
- What does it mean for a new engineering graduate to be ready for the workplace?
- Why do employers demand professionalism?
- What does professionalism entail?
- What is networking?
- Why is networking important when planning a career?
- What do great digital leaders look like?

12.12   Knowledge creation

Collaborate with peers on learning or work with others outside the class to narrow down the objectives of each activity. You may access online resources and analyze data and information to create new ideas and balanced solutions. High-level digital tools may be used to develop multimedia presentations, simulations or animations, videos and visual displays, digital portfolios, reflective practice (online publishing and blogging), or well-researched and up-to-date reports.

12.12.1   What does the workforce look like after 10 or 15 years?

What are the major factors that will shape the future of work, and how are those factors likely to evolve over the next 10 to 15 years? What are the consequences of these future trends on the future workforce and workplace, including size, composition, and skills; the nature of work and workplace arrangements; and worker compensation? Investigate the above issues to answer the given questions in a class presentation.

12.12.2   Undergraduate experience for the future workplace

Describe the most useful learning experience in your years of study at the university or college (it could be a lecture, a project, a whole subject, etc.). How did it help to prepare you for work in your field? If you are turning that experience into a learning task like a lecture or workshop, what sort of content, learning activities, and/or assessment would you include to help students prepare for the workplace?

12.12.3   Future digital workplace toolbox

A digital toolbox is comprised of the tools and technologies employees of an organization need to do their jobs. All organizations have a digital toolbox, but their tools vary depending on the industry, business strategy, and job functions. For this task, identify a workplace of your choice and create a digital toolbox in an e-Poster that meets the needs of the organization.

12.12.4   Social networking and employment law

Employer responses to the use of social media usage by employees receive a high level of attention, particularly through the press and high-profile individual disputes between individuals and their employers. Much of the attention in this area is focused on the so-called work bloggers and employees' references to their work on social networking sites such as

Twitter and Facebook. While a large amount of activity on social media is either entirely harmless or non-work-related, employers have in some circumstances taken exception to online postings made by employees and have taken disciplinary action (Broughton et al. 2009). For this task, prepare a five-page report to investigate the legal and ethical aspects of social networking in the workplace and their mutual impact on employment law. If you are asked to formulate a policy, what sort of areas would you want to cover?

12.12.5   Workplace ethics

Ethics allow us to distinguish the difference between right and wrong. For this task, develop a piece of art or an e-Poster that reflects the above and answer the following two questions:

- What are some examples of correct ethics in the workplace?
- What are some examples of weak ethics in the workplace?

References

Achillias, G. 2015. Phygital platforms: Merging physical and digital. https://wi prodigital.com/2015/09/15/phygital-platforms-merging-physical-and-digital/.

Akporado, A. 2015. 7 Keys to building a successful career path. https://www.lin kedin.com/pulse/7-keys-building-successful-career-path-aghogho-akporid o-mba--1.

Balthazard, C. 2015. What does it mean to be a professional? https://www.hrp a.ca/Documents/Designations/Job-Ready-Program/What-it-means-to-be-a-professional.pdf.

Berger, R. 2018. Platform economics in mechanical engineering. file:///C:/Users/ Dr%20Habash/Downloads/roland_berger_plattformoekonomie_en.pdf.

Bika, N. 2018. How to conduct a skills gap analysis. https://resources.workable. com/tutorial/skills-gap-analysis.

Broughton, A., T. Higgins, B. Hicks, and A. Cox. 2009. Workplaces and social net-working: The implications for employment relations. http://www.acas.org. uk/media/pdf/d/6/1111_Workplaces_and_Social_Networking.pdf.

COU. 2015. My career: How Ontario university career services prepare students for the future. Council of Ontario Universities. http://cou.on.ca/wp-conte nt/uploads/2015/05/MyCareer-Report-on-Ontario-university-career-servic es.pdf.

Daggett, W. R. 2010. Preparing students for their technological future. http:// www.leadered.com/pdf/Preparing%20Students%20for%20Tech%20Future %20white%20paper.pdf.

Davies, A., D. Fidler, and M. Gorbis. 2011. Future work skills 2020. Institute for the Future for University of Phoenix Research Institute. http://www.iftf.org/ uploads/media/SR-1382A_UPRI_future_work_skills_sm.pdf.

Davison, R. M., X. J. Carol, M. G. Martinsons, A. Y. Zhao, and R. Du. 2017. The communicative ecology of Web 2.0 at work: Social networking in the workspace. Wiley Online Library. https://doi.org/10.1002/asi.23112.

Deloitte. 2017. Rewriting the rules for the digital age. Deloitte University Press. https://www2.deloitte.com/content/dam/Deloitte/global/Documents/About-Deloitte/central-europe/ce-global-human-capital-trends.pdf.

Deloitte. 2018. The digital workplace: Think, share, do: Transform your employee experience. https://www2.deloitte.com/content/dam/Deloitte/mx/Documents/human-capital/The_digital_workplace.pdf.

Detecon. 2016. Are you a digital leader? Detecon Consulting. https://www.detecon.com/sites/default/files/20160331_digital_leadership_v1.4.pdf.

Dufva, M., R. Koivisto, L. Ilmola-Sheppard, and S. Junno. 2017. Anticipating alternative futures for the platform economy. Technology Innovation Management Review. https://timreview.ca/article/1102.

Dutton, W., E. Helsper, and M. Gerber. 2009. The Internet in Britain. Oxford Institute for the Internet, University of Oxford. http://oxis.oii.ox.ac.uk/wp-content/uploads/sites/43/2014/11/oxis2009-report.pdf.

Engineering 360. 2018. What makes a successful engineer? 5 Career Skills Employers Value. file:///C:/Users/Dr%20Habash/Downloads/Engineering_Career_Skills.pdf.

EPCC. 2018. Ethics in the workplace. http://www.epcc.edu/CareerServices/Presentations/Ethics%20in%20the%20Workplace.pdf.

Evans-Greenwood, P., H. Lewis, and J. Guszcza. 2017. Reconstructing work automation, artificial intelligence, and the essential role of humans. file:///C:/Users/Dr%20Habash/Downloads/DUP_Reconstructing-work-reprint.pdf.

Fox, K., and J. O'Conner. 2016. Five ways work will change in the future. https://www.theguardian.com/society/2015/nov/29/five-ways-work-will-change-future-of-workplace-ai-cloud-retirement-remote.

Genpact. 2017. The workforce: Staying ahead of artificial intelligence. http://www.genpact.com/downloadable-content/the-workforce-staying-ahead-of-artificial-intelligence.pdf.

Guest. 2018. Preparing students for the reality of the modern workplace. http://www.technologyrecord.com/Article/preparing-students-for-the-reality-of-the-modern-workplace-62851.

Hrabowski, F. A. 2015. The future of work: Preparing students for a changing world of work. https://psmag.com/education/the-future-of-work-preparing-students-for-a-changing-world-of-work.

JA. 2013. Are students prepared for the workplace? New Tools for a New Generation. https://www.juniorachievement.org/documents/20009/20652/Are+Students+Prepared+for+the+Workplace.pdf/c1b75524-016d-4bd1-b8aa-74395f51021a.

Kenney, M., and J. Zysman. 2016. The rise of the platform economy. http://issues.org/32-3/the-rise-of-the-platform-economy/.

Kilpi, E. (ed.). 2018. Perspectives on new work: Exploring emerging conceptualizations. https://media.sitra.fi/2017/02/28142631/Selvityksia114.pdf.

Klein, R. 2018. Job readiness skills for youth. http://www.seattle.gov/Documents/Departments/economicDevelopment/workforce/JRT-Report-and-Continuum-R4-Web.pdf.

Korn Ferry. 2018. Digital leadership in Singapore. Korn Ferry Institute. https://focus.kornferry.com/wp-content/uploads/2015/02/Korn-Ferry-Digital-leadership-in-Singapore.pdf.

Lave, J., and E. Wenger. 1991. *Situated Learning: Legitimate Peripheral Participation*. Cambridge, UK: Cambridge University Press.

MANAGE. 2018. Work ethics for development professionals. National Institute of Agricultural Extension Management. http://www.manage.gov.in/study material/workethics.pdf.

Manyika, J., M. Chui, M. Miremadi, J. Bughin, K. George, P. Willmott, and M. Dewhurst. 2017. A future that works: Automation, employment, and productivity. https://www.mckinsey.com/~/media/mckinsey/featured%20insight s/Digital%20Disruption/Harnessing%20automation%20for%20a%20future %20that%20works/MGI-A-future-that-works-Executive-summary.ashx.

Morgan, J. 2014. The future of work. http://otgo.tehran.ir/Portals/0/pdf/The% 20Future%20of%20Work.pdf.

Moses, R., and K. Garia. 2017. Forces of change: The future of work. Deloitte Insights. https://www2.deloitte.com/content/dam/insights/us/articles/4 322_Forces-of-change_FoW/DI_Forces-of-change_FoW.pdf.

Neittaanmäki, P., E. Galeieva, and A. Ogbechie. 2016. Platform economy and digital platforms. https://www.jyu.fi/it/fi/tutkimus/julkaisut/it-julkaisut/pla tform-economy-verk.pdf.

PWC. 2018. 2018 AI predictions 8 insights to shape business strategy. https://www. pwc.es/es/publicaciones/tecnologia/assets/ai-predictions-2018.pdf.

PWC. 2018. Workforce of the future: The competing forces shaping 2030. https://www.pwc.com/gx/en/services/people-organisation/workforce-of-the-fut ure/workforce-of-the-future-the-competing-forces-shaping-2030-pwc.pdf.

Ramani, M., and N. Garia. 2017. Forces of change: The future of work. https://ww w2.deloitte.com/content/dam/insights/us/articles/4322_Forces-of-change _FoW/DI_Forces-of-change_FoW.pdf.

Sheninger, E. 2014. Pillars of digital leadership. Leadership in Education. http://www.leadered.com/pdf/LeadingintheDigitalAge_11.14.pdf.

SHRM. 2013. Shaping an ethical workplace culture. Society for Human Resources Management. https://www.shrm.org/hr-today/trends-and-forecasting/special-reports-and-expert-views/Documents/Ethical-Workplace-Culture. pdf.

SHRM. 2015. Developing employee career paths and ladder. https://www.shr m.org/resourcesandtools/tools-and-samples/toolkits/pages/developi ngemployeecareerpathsandladders.aspx.

Srinivasan, A., and N. Venkatraman. 2017. Entrepreneurship in digital platforms: A network-centric view. https://onlinelibrary.wiley.com/doi/full/10.1002/ sej.1272.

Staff. 2012. Transdisciplinarity: A future work skill. https://talentmgt.com/201 2/10/18/transdisciplinarity-a-future-workforce-skill__trashed/.

Störmer, E., C. Patscha, J. Prendergast, C. Daheim, P. Glover, and H. Beck. 2014. The future of work: Jobs and skills in 2030. Evidence Report 84, UK Commission for Employment and Skills, Wath-upon-Dearne.

Ton, T. 2014. *The Good Jobs Strategy: How the Smartest Companies Invest in Employees to Lower Costs and Boost Profits*. Boston, MA: Houghton Mifflin Harcourt.

Valentine, S. G. Fleischmann, R. Sprague, and L. Godkin. 2010. Exploring the ethicality of firing employees who blog. *Human Resource Management* 49(1): 87–108.

Walker, S. 2016. The platform economy: What it is and why it matters. https://www.digitalistmag.com/iot/2016/10/14/what-is-platform-economy-and-why-it-matters-04582851.

Whincup, D. 2011. Weekly dilemma: Tweeting employees. Personnel Today. http://www.personneltoday.com/hr/weekly-dilemma-tweeting-employees.

Index

Milton Keynes UK
Ingram Content Group UK Ltd.
UKHW031139141024
449569UK00024B/1226